The European Discovery of American Surgery

Volume I
Land of Unlimited Possibilities

Perspectives in Health Humanities

UC Health Humanities Press publishes scholarship produced or reviewed under the auspices of the University of California Health Humanities Consortium, a multi-campus collaborative of faculty, students, and trainees in the humanities, medicine, and health sciences. Our series invites scholars from the humanities and healthcare professions to share narratives and analysis on health, healing, and the contexts of our beliefs and practices that impact biomedical inquiry.

General Editor

Brian Dolan, PhD, Professor, Department of Humanities and Social Sciences, University of California, San Francisco (UCSF)

Other Titles in this Series

Heart Murmurs: What Patients Teach Their Doctors
Edited by Sharon Dobie, MD (2014)

Humanitas: Readings in the Development of the Medical Humanities
Edited by Brian Dolan (2015)

Follow the Money: Funding Research in a Large Academic Health Center
Henry R. Bourne and Eric B. Vermillion (2016)

Soul Stories: Voices from the Margins
Josephine Ensign (2018)

Fixing Women: The Birth of Obstetrics and Gynecology in Britain and America
Marcia D. Nichols (2021)

Autobiography of a Sea Creature: Healing the Trauma of Infant Surgery
Wendy P. Williams (2023)

Medical Humanities, Cultural Humility, and Social Justice
Edited by Dalia Magaña, Christina Lux, and Ignacio López-Calvo (2023)

www.UCHealthHumanitiesPress.com

This series is made possible by the generous support of the Dean of the School of Medicine at UCSF, the UCSF Library, and a Multicampus Research Program Grant from the University of California Office of the President. Grant ID MR-15-328363 and Grant ID M23PR5992.

The European Discovery of American Surgery

Volume I
Land of Unlimited Possibilities

Edited by David Eugene Clark, MD

© 2024 University of California Health Humanities Press

University of California
Center for Health Humanities
Department of Humanities and Social Sciences
UCSF (Box 0850)
490 Illinois Street, Floor 7
San Francisco, CA 94143-0850

Cover Art: Professor Vincenz Czerny of Heidelberg, Germany (standing in gown at center) preparing to perform a gastroenterostomy at the Cooper Medical College in San Francisco, October 1901 (see Chapter 4). Standing next to him (in street clothes) is Levi Cooper Lane, the surgeon who founded the Cooper Medical College, which would become the Stanford University School of Medicine in 1908. Photograph courtesy of Stanford Medical History Center.

Book design by Virtuoso Press

Library of Congress Control Number (LCCN): 2024943168
ISBN for Volume 1 (Hardback): 979-8-9899229-8-7

Printed in USA

Table of Contents

VOLUME 1: Land of Unlimited Possibilities

Background

1. **Introduction**   1
   A time of rapid growth and transition – European surgical leadership in the 19th Century – The Columbian Exposition, Chicago 1893 – The origin and plan for this study and this volume

2. **European Immigration and Immigrant Surgeons**   15
   European immigration to America in the late 19th Century – Immigrant surgeons and their contributions

3. **"American Highlights"**   23
   Carl Beck (1856-1911) of New York, a German immigrant surgeon – His articles about America for German medical readers, 1901-1906

Reports from European surgical visitors, 1901-1907

4. **Vincenz Czerny (1901), Heidelberg, Germany**   36
   Visits Buffalo World's Fair (and Niagara Falls) just after McKinley's assassination – Travels on to California via Chicago and Colorado – Finds wonderful scenery, energetic people, ugly cities (except Washington), uncomfortable railroads, and poor food – Briefly visits Johns Hopkins Hospital in Baltimore, but unimpressed

5. **Justus Barth (1902), Kristiania, Sweden-Norway**   67
   Enjoys a longer and more rewarding visit to Johns Hopkins and elsewhere – Describes the extraordinary hospitality of Howard Kelly, including a memorable canoe trip – Visits Minnesota but only finds homesick Norwegians

6. **Francis Munch (1902-1903), Paris, France**   81
   Delivers periodic reports for a year from all over the USA – Many surgical topics, plus radiation therapy, infectious diseases, therapeutic whiskey, alcoholism, climate, and racial differences – Describes medical education, practice, associations, and meetings – Finds everything "business-like" in America, including the surgical practice of two brothers he does not name in rural Minnesota.

7. **Roman Barącz (1902-1904), Lemberg, Austria-Hungary**   196
   Gives detailed descriptions of surgical practice in New York and Chicago, including aseptic methods, anesthesia, suture materials, and radiation therapy – Praises American hospital construction and well-trained nurses

8. **Jean-Louis Faure (1904), Paris, France**   223
   Briefly describes his grand tour of America, including the Northeast, Florida, New Orleans, California, Grand Canyon, Mexico, Canada, and Minnesota (where the Mayo brothers are doing good work) – Considers France still the leader

9. **Albert Hoffa (1904), Berlin, Germany**   233
   Writes home from the "Land of Unlimited Possibilities" – Admires the work of orthopedic colleagues in New York, Philadelphia, and Chicago – Visits the AMA Meeting in Atlantic City and the St. Louis World's Fair – Notes the popularity of sports in America

10. **Julius Hirschberg (1905), Berlin, Germany**   245
    Journeys first-class to the AMA Meeting in Portland, Oregon, displaying his classical education, professional connections, and travel experience – Returns via San Francisco, Los Angeles, Salt Lake City, Denver, Chicago, and Boston – Sees energy and progress in America – Considers Germany still the leader

11. **Gunnar Nyström (1905), Uppsala, Sweden**   299
    Describes American medical schools, a few of them outstanding and many others poorly equipped or unscientific – Finds American hospitals generally quite good, with excellent nurses – Reports nothing of interest from Minnesota, having met one poorly educated Swedish-American doctor there

12. **Edvin Helling (1906-1907), Gothenburg, Sweden**   336
Visits the Mayo brothers in Minnesota, as well as prominent surgeons in the Northeast and Chicago – Notes the strong influence of German surgery – Describes intracranial, abdominal, and thyroid surgery in some detail

[Editorial Note: A full Index for Volumes 1 and 2 appears at the end of Volume 2]

1
Introduction

These two volumes trace how the attitudes of European surgeons toward American surgery developed around the beginning of the twentieth century, based upon contemporary articles written by some of those surgeons. Although they focus on surgery, they reflect more generally upon the differences and changes in European-American science and society.

Volume 1 starts with some background on the transatlantic surgical relationships that existed at the end of the nineteenth century, during which time a massive wave of immigration from Europe to America was also in progress. The historical figure of Christopher Columbus is invoked intentionally to symbolize the first few surgeons who bravely explored the New World without knowing exactly what they would find. The subtitle for this volume is taken from a book published in 1903 entitled *Das Land der unbegrenzten Möglichkeiten* [*The Land of Unlimited Possibilities*],[1] which will be mentioned by two of the authors.

At the end of the nineteenth century, American surgeons could point to some notable achievements, including the first successful abdominal operation (Ephraim McDowell's 1809 "ovariotomy" in rural Kentucky), the introduction of ether anesthesia in 1846, and an extensive experience with battlefield wounds during the Civil War. However, nearly every leading surgeon had felt it necessary to complete his education with several months or years of study at a European university hospital.

In the early part of the century, most of these American postgraduate students had gone to Great Britain or France,[2] but a growing number were now attracted to the research in anatomic pathology and innovative operative methods that had been developed at the German universities.[3] A central figure in the rise of German surgery was Bernhard von Langenbeck, Professor of Surgery in Berlin from 1848-1882.[4] Langenbeck was the principal founder of the *Archiv für klinische Chirurgie* in 1861 (a journal known today as *Langenbeck's Archives of Surgery*)[5] and the *Deutsche Gesellschaft für Chirurgie* (DGCh, German Surgical Society) in 1872.

By the 1870's, several surgeons who had worked with Langenbeck were themselves professors of surgery elsewhere in central Europe, including

Friedrich von Esmarch in Kiel, Richard von Volkmann in Halle, Johann von Nussbaum in Munich, and especially Theodor Billroth in Vienna. Billroth's former assistant Vincenz Czerny had become professor first in Freiburg and then in Heidelberg, and many other European leaders would follow from this "Vienna School."

The eminent Samuel D. Gross of Philadelphia (age 63) and the young J. Collins Warren of Boston (age 26) separately visited Berlin in 1868, and each remarked on Langenbeck's courtesy, his skill, his fluent English, and his teaching sessions that started at 6 A.M.[6, 7] Warren, whose grandfather had introduced ether anesthesia in Boston, was impressed that Langenbeck "split the soft palate in order to remove a large tumor from the posterior wall of the pharynx. After removal of the tumor he applied actual cautery to the wound – all without chloroform."[7] William W. Keen, later Gross's successor in Philadelphia, was also studying in Berlin around this time and agreed that Langenbeck was "an excellent clinical teacher."[8]

These current or future American surgical icons also visited Theodor Billroth at the *Allgemeines Krankenhaus* [General Hospital] in Vienna. While acknowledging Billroth's educational contributions, Gross reported:

> As an operator he is fearless and bold almost to the verge of rashness. The principal operation which I saw him perform was excision of a carcinomatous rectum – a tedious procedure, attended with great loss of blood, the patient, an elderly man, being under the influence of chloroform. Upon asking him the following morning how his patient was, he replied, with a significant shrug of the shoulder, "He is moribund," and passed on.[6]

Keen was also struck by the disregard for patient suffering and even dignity throughout the European centers, writing after a visit to Vienna:

> I thought that in Paris the patients were made subservient enough to the instruction & Enlightenment of the Students but here they are nothing but animals trotted out for the gaping crowds … but it's certainly jolly for the Students. It's a magnificent place to learn & in many respects is far superior to Paris.[2]

Warren praised Billroth as a teacher and observed him performing a thyroidectomy "with great fearlessness and rapidity, but I fear the mortality was high … it was well known that his wards contained their quota of pyemia and erysipelas in undiminished frequency."[7]

It was at this moment in history that Joseph Lister of Glasgow published his initial reports of surgical antisepsis using a spray whose active ingredient was carbolic acid (a chemical now called phenol).[9-11] Lister noted that "continental surgeons visiting our Infirmary [were] already familiar with the use of carbolic acid as an ordinary antiseptic dressing," and were therefore quick to adopt the concept. After a favorable clinical experience with Lister's method during the Franco-Prussian War of 1870, German surgeons led by Volkmann became its most prominent supporters.[12-14] However, they soon realized that phenol was not really a very good disinfectant and that in fact an antiseptic aerosol was unnecessary if bacterial contamination could be avoided in the first place (asepsis).[15]

Lister visited America 1876, encountering enthusiasm among the younger generation but skepticism from Samuel Gross and other established surgeons.[16] However, by 1882, even Gross acknowledged Lister's contributions to surgical progress: "If only one tithe be true of what his admirers claim for him, enough remains to entitle him to the credit of being one of the world's eminent benefactors."[17] After Gross's death in 1884, the American Surgical Association (which he had founded) elected Lister an Honorary Fellow (*in absentia*), along with three other British surgeons, two Frenchmen, and all the Germans mentioned above.[18]

German surgeons and physiologists now applied their microscopic expertise to the expanding field of bacteriology,[15] their pioneering operations could be performed with less risk to the patients, and their well-organized university clinics, scientific lectures, and operative cadaver labs became even more attractive to Americans who lacked these things in their own country.[3] The young William S. Halsted spent the years 1878-1880 at several of the German centers, and would uphold their educational ideals for the rest of his career.[19] John Benjamin (J. B.) Murphy of Chicago visited Billroth in 1882, by which time the professor had developed a "reputation for being a careful and meticulous surgeon";[20] when Murphy was later a famous teacher he acknowledged that his lectures were modeled after those of Billroth.[21]

Thomas Bonner, the leading historian of this era of European-American medical relationships, has estimated that 15,000 American doctors visited the German-speaking universities of Europe for educational purposes, and that two-thirds of them went to Vienna.[3] The enthusiasm began to fade during the 1890s, but prospective academic surgeons still dutifully made the journey, generally returning with admiration for the scientific work but abhorrence of the disrespect with which patients were treated.[22-25]

Roswell Park had been to Europe in the 1880's after graduating from Northwestern Medical School in Chicago, but by the time he was teaching his own students in Buffalo in the 1890s he wrote:

> ... thanks to the influence of the foreign schools and the receptivity and natural quickness of the American mind, we have reached a point in this country when it is no longer necessary for American students to visit the foreign centres ... Americans are in all respects as good practitioners as – and in most respects better than — their foreign colleagues.
> They evince more of humanity, more of real interest and care in their patients, and more consideration for their comfort and welfare ...[26]

In any case, since most American medical graduates who wanted to specialize in surgery or other areas could not afford to spend months or years traveling around Europe, facilities for postgraduate study had begun to appear closer to home. The most famous of these were the Polyclinic and the Post-Graduate Medical School in New York City, both founded in 1882.[27-29] Not long thereafter, Chicago had its own "Policlinic" (started in 1886) and Post-Graduate Medical School (started in 1888 by Franklin H. Martin, among others).[30-31] Similar but generally less successful schools were also established in other cities across America, and collectively these schools provided an opportunity for thousands of American medical school graduates (including the Mayo brothers) to remedy their often deficient education.

The model that would eventually dominate American surgical training was the residency system at Johns Hopkins University, established during the early 1890s under Halsted's direction.[19] He later acknowledged, "It was our intention originally to adopt as closely as feasible the German plan, which, in the main, is the same for all the principal clinics of the German universities."[32] Although European approaches had to be modified to meet American conditions and sensibilities,[33] the emphases on scientific knowledge and graduated clinical responsibility in surgical education persist to this day.

However, in 1894, when Harvey Cushing wrote to Halsted asking for a position in his residency, the professor initially turned him away, responding "I think it would be well for you to go to Europe as soon as you can, and to remain as long as possible before coming to us. ... You probably know that there is little if any scientific work done in this country in medicine, and that most of it is done in Germany."[34]

Indeed, these American efforts were barely getting started as the nineteenth century entered its last decade, which may be considered a turning point in the history of surgical science. The flood of medical visitors from

America to Europe was slowing down, while a small countercurrent of visits in the opposite direction was slowly starting to grow.

The Columbian Exposition of 1893

Christopher Columbus is dismissed by popular historians today as a greedy, cruel, and culturally-insensitive adventurer unworthy of special recognition. However, on the 400th anniversary of his accidental 1492 discovery, the rapidly growing nation that now dominated the American continent was eager to use the occasion for a celebratory event. The story of how the 1893 World Columbian Exposition came to be in Chicago, and its struggles with the many challenges (including an undetected serial killer), has been recently presented in an enlightening and entertaining fashion.[35]

In the *Official Guide* to the Exposition,[36] between descriptions of the exhibits from alms-houses and prisons, is a brief mention of exhibits from American medical and surgical hospitals, especially "models of modern war hospitals." In addition, American pharmaceutical and medical device companies were expected to showcase their products.

Adam Politzer was officially designated as the medical delegate of the Austrian Empire to the Columbian Exposition. Politzer had studied medicine and surgery at the University of Vienna, and now specialized in surgery of the ear, nose, and throat. He extended his assignment to look at some of the other medical facilities in the northeastern United States and Canada, and his report spread out over several issues of the *Wiener Medizinische Wochenschrift* in 1894.[37] Regarding the fair itself, he concluded that "the main credit for the great success of the medical-hygienic exhibition undoubtedly belongs to Germany, whose contributions exceeded those of all other nations put together." He noticed that many of the American drug companies, instrument makers, and other medical industries from the East were not participating and attributed this to the rivalry between eastern and western companies. He commented on various technical innovations, most of them from Europe, but including the ten cases reported by J. B. Murphy in which intestinal anastomosis had been performed using his invention of a metal "button" (the forerunner of today's stapling methods).

During his travels, Politzer was impressed with the Army Medical Museum in Washington and the Mütter Museum in Philadelphia but found that medical schools did not have enough cadavers for proper anatomic study and research. He did observe that most surgeons used good aseptic technique, and especially admired the new hospitals being built in New York, entirely with private support:

> In the United States, the federal government does nothing at all for public welfare and the states do very little. Not only the humanitarian institutions but even the universities and other educational facilities are built and maintained by private contributions and gifts. In view of this, we have to express our unbounded admiration for the generosity and charitable spirit of the American people. We must acknowledge without envy that America has overtaken Europe in its idealistic efforts to achieve the greatest benefits of science and education, while also addressing the pain and suffering of the poor.[37]

Franz von Winckel, Professor of Gynecologic Surgery in Munich, also attended the fair, first visiting a friend who had emigrated to St. Louis, and concluding with an extensive tour of North America. Reporting in the *Münchener Medicinische Wochenschrift*,[38] Winckel had little to say about the commercial exhibits but was disappointed in the presentations by German universities. In particular, he thought the northern (Prussian) schools were greatly overrepresented compared to the south German schools.

Winckel looked at several American educational institutions in some detail, including the ten ("yes, I said *ten*") medical schools in St. Louis and the Universities of Southern Illinois, Wisconsin, Washington, Berkeley, Stanford, Johns Hopkins, and Harvard. He recognized that most of the medical schools were primarily business ventures but acknowledged that competitive pressures might produce good teachers and that the European system of state-appointed tenured professors also had its drawbacks. He predicted that "the public spirit, the energy, the endurance, and the intelligence of the American people promises their universities, now still young but designed on a large scale, a future that will be envied by their European sisters."[38]

Samuel Pozzi of Paris, also an academic gynecologist, was an official representative of France at the fair. He too was impressed by the superior construction and management of hospitals in Chicago, staffed by well-educated nurses in addition to the religious sisters customary in Europe.[39] The final committee report to the French government took note of the excellent hospitals and nurses and acknowledged that "there are undoubtedly physicians and especially surgeons of the highest quality in the United States," but was highly critical that the medical meetings at the fair "did not energetically demand what the best American practitioners have been demanding for a long time: The reform of medical education in the United States."[40]

The recognition of some strengths and optimistic predictions about the future did not alter the general perception that "Europe is vastly ahead."[41]

Vincenz Czerny turned down a personal invitation from the president of the American Surgical Association to attend one of the medical meetings associated with the Columbian Exposition, taking offense that presentations had to be made in one of the official languages of North or South America. "I do not think that the physicians of Germany can take part in the proceedings of the Pan-American Medical Congress, if they are not permitted to read their papers in German," he responded in an open letter that was reprinted (with an equally polite but pointed reply) in the *Journal of the American Medical Association*.[42-43]

The Berlin ophthalmologist Julius Hirschberg also travelled across North America on his way around the world in 1892-1893, but skipped the Columbian Exposition, apparently more interested in seeing the Canadian Rocky Mountains. During a previous tour of the natural wonders of the United States in 1888, he had already made a brief inspection of Chicago's seven medical schools, concluding that "in Germany the smallest university has far better facilities than all these put together."[44]

Graduates of the Chicago medical schools by that time included J. B. Murphy, Roswell Park, Franklin H. Martin, Nicholas Senn, Albert J. Ochsner, Arthur Dean Bevan, and Charles H. Mayo (his brother William J. Mayo had graduated from the equally undistinguished University of Michigan). Along with their colleagues from the somewhat more established eastern schools, these surgeons would attract an increasing number of European visitors in the coming years, whose voyages of discovery in the early twentieth century constitute the main body of this study.

Editorial Background

I was initially attracted to this period in surgical history as an officer of the New England Surgical Society, which was celebrating its centennial in 2016. This interest was enhanced during my time as Archives Fellow for the American College of Surgeons during 2018-2019. The more I learned about the early years of the twentieth century, the more interested I became in this time when America was confident and optimistic, investing generously in public institutions, and harnessing the energy of its many immigrants. (Could we not recapture this spirit today?) A few explorers from the Old World were beginning to appreciate the scientific progress in the New World, and looking forward to a time of mutual growth, but this era ended abruptly in a catastrophic World War. (Will we ever truly recover, and did things really have to happen this way?)

In the course of my reading, I encountered the figure of Paul Clairmont, whose interesting life story and connections to American surgery I have described elsewhere.[45] As an appendix to that article, I included my translation of his report about visiting surgical centers in the United States during 1908. I was fascinated to read his impressions from that time not only about surgery, but also the observable and implicit differences between the European and American societies. It struck me that other Americans might be interested in reading objective first-hand reports about their country from similarly intelligent and relatively open-minded observers, translated into English and placed in context.

It made sense for me to focus on surgery, since I have spent a career immersed in this subject and can understand most of the specific topics discussed by the European visitors. I have since retired, and the year when I started medical school (1971) is now almost halfway back to the time period being described; consequently, I have personally experienced or at least have heard discussed many of the ideas and practices that may now be forgotten. My retirement from clinical practice also afforded me the time to sort through all this material and to organize it for others who might take an interest.

Previous historians have discussed European medical visitors, and have provided brief quotations from some of their reports.[3,46-49] Readers looking for summary descriptions of this period could consult these authors, especially Thomas Bonner's many publications about German-American medical relationships.[3,31,46,50] However, I believe that the complete and authentic voices of the original authors are intrinsically interesting. The historical overviews by previous authors did provide a starting point for identifying others, which I have pursued using index and internet searches and the systematic review of selected publications.

I limited my sample to European surgeons who returned home and published a report soon thereafter addressed to colleagues in their own countries. Surgery was a very broad field in those days, and although some authors had specialized in gynecology, orthopedics, or some other field, they all had general surgical training and were active in other areas as well. Indeed, Charles Mayo continued to perform eye surgery until 1908,[51] so I felt justified in considering ophthalmology as part of surgery, which allowed me to include Julius Hirschberg's erudite report of his third visit to America.

Historical research of this era is greatly simplified by the expiration of copyrights and the consequent scanning and freely accessible electronic publication of books and journals by the Hathi Trust, Internet Archive, and others. Of course, there is still no substitute for good libraries, and I am fortunate to live not far from Harvard University. Additional materials have been obtained for me by librarians and archivists at Tufts University, the University of Maine, the New York Public Library, the New York Academy of Medicine, and the W. Bruce Fye Center for Medical History at the Mayo Clinic. The University of California Health Humanities Press has turned my draft manuscript into a beautiful publication. I am grateful for this assistance, without which this book would not have been possible.

Although I have formally or informally studied the major European languages, translation is greatly simplified today by the computer-based dictionaries, spell-checkers, and other available methods. Of course, the process still requires a lot of sentence-by-sentence and word-by-word interpretation, especially when orthography or usage has changed over the past century, but I believe I have understood the general sense of each author. More challenging (and more fun!) has been the investigation of various persons, places, and things referred to by the different authors, presumably familiar to most of their intended readers but not necessarily to a twenty-first-century American, which I have annotated at the end of each report and incorporated into the index.

I expect that most readers of these volumes will themselves have some medical background, although there may be others with a more general interest in American scientific history or European-American academic relationships prior to the First World War. Only a few of the authors spend much time on technical descriptions of surgical procedures, so these sections can be skimmed over by those with less interest in such details. I have used anatomic, chemical, and surgical terminology as it would appear in an English language publication today and have assumed that the reader will be familiar with these words or can easily look them up. I have retained Latin or Greek terms that are still in common use and translated others where appropriate.

When the authors quote American publications, I have consulted the books and articles written by those who are cited to ensure that the back translation into English restores the original meaning, and in most cases the original words. My translations have not otherwise attempted to mimic the style or vocabulary of an American or British author writing at the beginning of the twentieth century, but I have tried to avoid any anachronisms that would have been incomprehensible to an English-speaking person at the time. I have corrected the many misspelled names, sometimes with a note but always with an independently verified entry in the index, which also supplies first names or at least initials.

Most of the authors whose reports are included exhibited some national pride and assumed superiority, which were covered by the veneer of a common European civilization but would soon lead to disaster. I have not attempted to review the voluminous literature about the causes of the First World War, but the anxieties and resentments of the German and French surgeons are especially apparent. Frank Trommler has provided interesting background on the deterioration of German-American academic relationships during this time,[52] although the authors included in this study were *ipso facto* among those who were trying to maintain and improve them.

Some of the authors (and the Americans they cite) also had obvious prejudices about the characteristics of different "races," which I have not hidden. None of them used crudely insulting words, and in translation I have used the terms "Colored," "Negro," "Asian," or "Indian," which were standard and not considered derogatory at the time (e.g., the National Association for the Advancement of Colored People, the United Negro College Fund, the Indian Health Service).

Long-distance travel in those days was principally by the relatively recent innovations of steamship and railroad, and indeed the descriptions of first-class or even second-class travel sound much more pleasant than modern airlines and highways. Most of the reports predate the *Titanic* disaster of 1912, and there is only a tangential reference to it afterwards by one of the authors (Robert Proust). Unless an automobile or motor car is specifically indicated, I have assumed that local vehicles were drawn by horses, whose maintenance and inconveniences are also barely mentioned.

Stefan Zweig has provided a memorable description of the apparent security, immutability, and dominance of imperial Europe at the beginning of the twentieth century.[53] This "World of Yesterday," also taken for granted by the authors in this study, was destroyed by the First World War, although some of its characteristics certainly persist. By contrast, an American can recognize many of our own current attitudes in the descriptions that follow, and an American surgeon can recognize many practices that have persisted for more than a century. American popular culture and scientific approaches (including the English language) are now dominant, and students from all over the world come to our universities and laboratories. In what other places should we now be looking for new ideas?

Notes

1) Goldberger LM, *Das Land der unbegrenzten Möglichkeiten: Beobachtungen über das Wirtschaftsleben der Vereinigten Staaten von Amerika*, Berlin: F. Fontane, 1903.

2) Warner JH, *Against the Spirit of System: The French Impulse in Nineteenth-Century American Medicine*, Princeton NJ: Princeton University Press, 2014.
3) Bonner TN, *American Doctors and German Universities*, Lincoln NB: University of Nebraska Press, 1963.
4) Luther B, "Zur Geschichte der Chirurgie an der Berliner Universität," *Zentralblatt für Chirurgie* 1985; 110:778-785.
5) Beger HG, "From *Archiv für klinische Chirurgie* to *Langenbeck's Archives of Surgery*: 1860-2010," *Langenbeck's Archives of Surgery* 2010; 395(Suppl 1):S3-S12.
6) Gross SD, *Autobiography of Samuel D. Gross, M.D,* Philadelphia: George Barrie, 1887.
7) Churchill ED, editor, *To Work in the Vineyard of Surgery: The Reminiscences of J. Collins Warren*, Cambridge MA: Harvard University Press, 1958.
8) James WWK, editor, *Keen of Philadelphia: The Collected Memoirs of William Williams Keen Jr.,* Dublin NH: William L. Bauhan, 2002.
9) Lister J, "On the antiseptic principle in the practice of surgery," *Lancet* 1867; 90:353-356.
10) Lister J, "An address on the antiseptic system of treatment in surgery," *British Medical Journal* 1868; 2:53-56.
11) Lister J, "Remarks on some points in the history of antiseptic surgery," *Lancet* 1908; 171:1815-1816.
12) Willy C, Schneider P, Engelhardt M, Hargens AR, Mubarak S, "Richard von Volkmann: Surgeon and renaissance man," *Clinical Orthopedics and Related Research* 2008; 466:500-506.
13) Godlee RJ, *Lord Lister*, London: MacMillan and Co., 1918.
14) Upmalis IH, "The introduction of Lister's treatment in Germany," *Bulletin of the History of Medicine* 1968; 42:221-40.
15) Schlich T, "Asepsis and bacteriology: A realignment of surgery and laboratory science," *Medical History* 2012: 56:308-334.
16) Rutkow I, "Joseph Lister and his 1876 tour of America," *Annals of Surgery* 2013; 257:1181-1187.
17) Gross SD, "Preface," In: Gross SD, *A System of Surgery*, Sixth Edition, Philadelphia: Henry C. Lea's Son & Co., 1882.
18) Sparkman RS, Shires GT, editors, *Minutes of the American Surgical Association*, Dallas TX: Taylor Publishing Co., 1972.
19) MacCallum WG, *William Stewart Halsted: Surgeon*, Baltimore: Johns Hopkins Press, 1930.
20) Davis L, *J. B. Murphy: Stormy Petrel of Surgery*, New York: G. P.

Putnam's Sons, 1938.
21) "Editor's preface," *Clinics of John B. Murphy* 1916; 5:985-987.
22) Finney JMT, *A Surgeon's Life*, New York: G. P. Putnam's Sons, 1940.
23) Crile G, *George Crile: An Autobiography*, Philadelphia: J. B. Lippincott, 1947.
24) Bruce HA, *Varied Operations*, Toronto: Longmans, Green and Co., 1958.
25) Bliss M, *Harvey Cushing: A Life in Surgery*, New York: Oxford University Press, 2005.
26) Park R, *An Epitome of the History of Medicine*, Philadelphia: F. A. Davis, 1897.
27) Beck C, "Die Medizinische Fortbildungsschule in New-York," *Münchener Medizinische Wochenschrift* 1903; 50:515-517.
28) Peitzman SJ, "'Thoroughly practical': America's polyclinic medical schools," *Bulletin of the History of Medicine* 1980; 54:166-187.
29) Rutkow I, "The education, training, and specialization of surgeons: Turn-of-the-century America and its postgraduate medical schools," *Annals of Surgery* 2013; 258:1130-1136.
30) *History of Medicine and Surgery and Physicians and Surgeons of Chicago*, Chicago: Biographical Publishing Corporation, 1922.
31) Martin FH, *Fifty Years of Medicine and Surgery*, Chicago: Surgical Publishing Company, 1934.
32) Halsted WS, "The training of the surgeon," *Bulletin of the Johns Hopkins Hospital* 1904; 15:267-275.
33) Bonner TN, "The German model of training physicians in the United States, 1870-1914: How closely was it followed?," *Bulletin of the History of Medicine* 1990; 64:18-34.
34) Fulton JF, *Harvey Cushing: A Biography*. Springfield IL: Charles C. Thomas, 1946.
35) Larson E, *The Devil in the White City*, New York: Crown Publishers, 2003.
36) *Handbook of the World's Columbian Exposition*, Chicago: Rand, McNally, 1893.
37) Politzer A, "Bericht über die medizinisch-hygienische Abtheilung der Weltausstellung in Chicago 1893," *Wiener Medizinische Wochenschrift* 1894; 44:1323-1325,1359-1362,1403-1406,1435-1438,1477-1480,1509-1512,1613-1614,1643-1645,1732-1735. Note that this Austrian journal already used the spelling "Medizin" in the nineteenth century, while other German publications wrote

"Medicin" until 1901.

38) Winckel Fv, "Ein Studienreise in der neuen Welt," *Münchener Medicinische Wochenschrift* 1894; 41: 7-10, 31-33, 53-55, 71-73, 92-94.

39) Vanderpooten C, *Samuel Pozzi: Chirurgien et Ami des Femmes*, Ozoir-la-Ferrière : V&O Éditions, 1992.

40) de Chasseloup-Laubat L, "Congrès de Chicago: 3. Congrès de la Médecine," *Exposition Internationale de Chicago en 1893: Rapports publiés sous la direction de M. Camille Krantz*, Paris: Imprimerie Nationale, 1894, pp. 25-28.

41) Baudouin M, quoted in "The surgical exhibits at the World's Fair," *Medical Record* 1893; 44:398-399.

42) Czerny [V], "Offenes Schreiben an Herrn Claudius H. Mastin, M.D., LL.D., in Mobile Ala., 1890 Präsident der American Surgical Association, betreffend den panamerikanischen medicinischen Congress," *Deutsche Medicinische Wochenschrift* 1893; 19:47.

43) Czerny [V], Reed CAL, "Germany and the Pan-American Medical Congress," *Journal of the American Medical Association* 1893; 20:222-223.

44) Hirschberg J, *Von New York nach San Francisco*, Leipzig: von Veit, 1888.

45) Clark DE, "Paul Clairmont and his connections to American surgery," *Langenbeck's Archives of Surgery* 2023; 408:94.

46) Bonner TN, "German doctors in America – 1887-1914," *Journal of the History of Medicine and Allied Sciences* 1959; 14:1-17.

47) Lesky E, "American medicine as viewed by Viennese physicians," *Bulletin of the History of Medicine* 1982; 56:368-376.

48) Schlich T, "'One and the same the world over': The international culture of surgical exchange in an age of globalization, 1870-1914," *Journal of the History of Medicine and Allied Sciences* 2016; 247-270.

49) Neid T, *Ärzte und Naturwissenschaftler auf Reisen. Reiseberichte aus der Deutschen Medizinischen und der Münchener Medizinischen Wochenschriften 1890-1930*, Dissertation, Martin-Luther-Universität Halle-Wittenberg, 2012.

50) Bonner TN, "Friedrich von Müller of Munich and the growth of clinical science in America, 1902-1914," *Journal of the History of Medicine and Allied Sciences* 1990; 45:556-569.

51) Henderson JW, "Ophthalmic practice of Charles H. Mayo, M.D.," *Mayo Clinic Proceedings* 1994; 69:1011-1014.

52) Trommler F, "Inventing the enemy: German-American cultural relations, 1900-1917," In: Schröder H-J, editor, *Confrontation and Cooperation: Germany and the United States in the Era of World War I, 1900-1924,* Providence: Berg, 1993.

53) Zweig S, *The World of Yesterday*, New York: Viking, 1943.

2
European Immigration and Immigrant Surgeons

The ships that transported European surgeons comfortably to and from America for their study tours had many other passengers below decks on the outward journey who had decided to leave Europe forever, and this massive emigration was surely on the mind of any temporary visitor from the Old World.

The population shifts that occurred in North America during the decades after the Civil War were the largest in human history. These included the forcible confinement of native tribes to reservations, the internal migration of emancipated African-Americans from southern plantations to northern cities, and Asian immigration to the Pacific coast. However, even these fundamental changes in American society were vastly overshadowed by the massive influx of European immigrants to North America, which is an important consideration in this study both as a background to the events that will be described and because it included a significant number of European-educated physicians and surgeons.

Of course, North America had been receiving European immigrants since the time of Columbus, with Spanish settlements in Florida and Mexico followed by British, French, and other colonies further north. However, at the beginning of the nineteenth century, the territory of the United States was confined to the Atlantic coast. Outside of the native tribes and the mostly enslaved Africans, its three million inhabitants were almost entirely of English origin, with a few Scottish and Irish. In a study based on family names of citizens in the US Census,[1] the only exceptions were the well-assimilated descendants of the original Dutch colonists in New York (16% in that state) and the "Pennsylvania Dutch." The latter were actually Germans, many of whom still spoke their own language (*Deutsch*); they constituted 26% of the population in Pennsylvania itself, and also 2-6% in Maryland, Virginia, and the Carolinas. No other country of origin accounted for more than 1% in any state.

In contrast, the 1900 US Census recorded 10.3 million foreign-born inhabitants, the vast majority from Europe, out of a total population (including free African-Americans) of 76.0 million (13.6%); another

15.7 million Americans (20.6%) had at least one foreign-born parent.[2] In Massachusetts, Rhode Island, Connecticut, New York, New Jersey, Michigan, Illinois, Wisconsin, Minnesota, the Dakotas, Montana, Utah, Nevada, and California more than half of the people were either immigrants or children of immigrants.

About 33.1% of these first- and second-generation Americans at the beginning of the twentieth Century were from the German-speaking countries of central Europe, and another 15.8% were from Scandinavia or eastern Europe, where the educational systems were modeled on the German example.[2] The exceptions to this pattern were the New England states (where Irish and French-Canadian immigrants predominated), Utah (whose immigrants were mostly British), and the Southeast (which attracted very few immigrants).

In the middle of the nineteenth century, the immigrants included a number of well-educated liberals and socialists who had abandoned their hope of reforming the monarchies of central Europe, including some who had participated in the unsuccessful revolutions of 1848. These "Forty-Eighters" fleeing their homelands to avoid prosecution spread the German language and culture across the United States, especially in the Middle Atlantic, Midwest, and California. During this time, the number of German immigrants was exceeded only by those from Ireland.[3]

New York was the port of entry for most immigrants, and those with a medical education often stayed in that city. William Detmold graduated from Göttingen and served as an army surgeon until emigrating in 1837 and establishing a surgical practice in New York.[4] Detmold and a few colleagues started a New York German medical society, which published a journal called the *New Yorker Medicinische Monatsschrift*.[5] This organization failed after a few years, but was soon revived by the influx of "Forty-Eighters," who also founded the German Dispensary (later called the German Hospital) in 1857. The initial hospital staff included the surgeon Ernst Krackowizer, a graduate of Vienna,[6] and the gynecologist Emil Noeggerath, a graduate of Bonn.[7] The German Hospital (today called the Lenox Hill Hospital) would become one of the leading hospitals of New York City by the end of the century, and is frequently mentioned in the reports that follow. The Irishman John Byrne, a graduate of Edinburgh, also emigrated in 1848 and would become a prominent gynecologist in Brooklyn.[8]

After the Civil War, during which many recent immigrants served in the Union Army, immigration accelerated, especially from Germany. In addition to economic and social restrictions, the political and religious intolerance of European monarchies continued to be important factors. Now, immigrants with medical training brought with them the bacteriologic discoveries of Pasteur and Lister, which were being most enthusiastically pursued by German surgeons.

New York remained the largest community of immigrants with a European medical education, and its German-speaking contingent became particularly active. The "German Medical Society of the City of New York" had more than 300 members at the beginning of the twentieth century, and had re-established a regular journal, again eventually entitled the *New-Yorker Medizinische Monatsschrift*.[5]

The most prominent immigrant surgeon in New York at the end of the nineteenth century was Arpad Gerster, who had been born in Hungary (then part of the Austrian Empire), received his doctorate in Vienna, and studied Lister's methods with Richard von Volkmann in Halle.[9] He had come to New York in 1874, practiced surgery using the new aseptic principles, wrote an influential textbook, and taught popular courses at the "Polyclinic Medical School" that had been started in 1882.[10] He was later a professor at the College of Physicians and Surgeons at Columbia University. Although Gerster himself was Catholic, he was a leading member of the surgical staff at the predominantly Jewish Mount Sinai Hospital,[11] an institution that will be mentioned frequently in the reports that follow.

Willy Meyer came to New York in 1884 after having been an assistant to Friedrich Trendelenburg in Bonn.[12] Otto Kiliani came to New York in 1891, having been like Gerster an assistant to Volkmann.[5,13] Another prominent immigrant surgeon was Carl Beck,[14] who was on the faculty of the New York Post-Graduate Medical School, a friendly rival of the Polyclinic Medical School where Gerster taught.[10] The following chapter will examine Carl Beck's many publications about American medicine, including one summarizing the medical contributions of German immigrants.[15]

Chicago was the second-largest city in the United States by 1900 and had the second-largest collection of immigrant surgeons. Wilhelm Wagner, another "Forty-Eighter," started a German Medical Society here in 1857. Although the society fell apart later after an argument about aseptic technique, it was reinstated in 1897 and had grown to 43 members by 1899.[16]

The leading academic surgeon in Chicago by the end of the century was Christian Fenger.[17-19] Fenger was originally from Denmark, graduated from the University of Copenhagen, received further training in Vienna, and joined his brother's practice in Egypt, where an American Army officer persuaded him to emigrate to America in 1877. He settled in Chicago, joined the German Medical Society, and soon became a leading surgical pathologist and eventually a surgeon known for meticulous operations that applied his profound knowledge of pathology. In addition to teaching at the Policlinic, he was Professor of Surgery at Northwestern University and later at the Rush Medical College.

Another influential immigrant surgeon in Chicago was Carl Beck from Bohemia in the Austrian Empire.[20-21] Beck had received his medical degree from the University of Prague, and studied pathology and surgery in Leipzig, Berlin, and Vienna. Having possibly contracted tuberculosis, he took a position as a ship's surgeon in 1890, where an American doctor recruited him for the faculty of the Chicago Post-Graduate Medical School. He obviously shared a name with Carl Beck of New York, but Carl Beck of Chicago had an eventful career well past the time considered in this study and is much better known today than his New York namesake.

By the end of the nineteenth century there was a "German Hospital" not only in New York but also in Chicago, Philadelphia, Cleveland, San Francisco, and other cities with large German minorities. German medical associations in Chicago, Cleveland, and San Francisco were associated with the *New Yorker Medizinische Monatsschrift*, and others existed in Philadelphia, Buffalo, and St. Louis.[5] A "French Hospital" could be found in New York, San Francisco, Los Angeles, and New Orleans.

Although the southeast had few immigrants, New Orleans was somewhat of an anomaly, with 10.6% of its 1900 population foreign-born, mostly from Germany, Italy, or Ireland.[2] Rudolph Matas, himself the son of Spanish immigrants, maintained that the "pioneer of antiseptic surgery in America" was Moritz Schuppert, a German who had come to that city after being educated at the University of Marburg.[22-24] However, the earlier French influence in medicine and surgery also remained strong in Louisiana for most of the nineteenth century.[24-25]

Texas likewise attracted some notable surgical immigrants.[26] Ferdinand Herff, a graduate of the University of Giessen in Germany, led a group of "Forty-Eighters" to Texas and established a surgical practice in San Antonio,[27] which was already home to George Cupples, a surgeon who had graduated from the University of Edinburgh. Berthold Hadra, trained in Berlin, emigrated to Texas and became chief of surgery in Galveston.[26] Later, James Edwin Thompson, a graduate of the University of London, became an outstanding teacher and practitioner of surgery in that city.[28]

Other immigrants with European surgical training were scattered across the country: Albert Walker, a graduate of Königsberg, emigrated to Pittsburgh, and performed one of the first recorded laparotomies for trauma in 1859.[4] Martin Stamm, a graduate of Bern, settled in northwestern Ohio, where he published a method of gastrostomy still used today.[29] John Fairbairn Binnie was a Scot who had graduated from Aberdeen, studied further in Germany, and then moved to Kansas City, where he became a surgeon with a national reputation.[30] Robert Gilmore was an Irishman trained in Edinburgh, who settled in Omaha and became its leading surgeon.[31] Morris Herzstein trained in Berlin, emigrated and practiced surgery in San Francisco,[31] and later endowed a professorship at Stanford University. Friedrich Fehleisen graduated from Würzburg and did important research with Robert Koch,[32] but eventually became the principal surgeon at the German Hospital in San Francisco.[33] Carl Beck (of New York) named several others, and he was only referring to the Germans.[15]

In addition to those who immigrated with a European medical education, some children of immigrants born or raised in America also retained the necessary language skills to obtain a medical degree from a European university before returning home to a surgical practice. These included Frederic Kammerer in New York, August Bernays in St. Louis, and Nicholas Senn in Chicago (who already had a degree from the Chicago Medical School).[34-36] As described in the previous chapter, thousands of other American-born medical graduates also traveled to Europe for postgraduate study.

Two other immigrants with surgical training at European universities will be mentioned frequently in the following pages, although they were distinguished much more by their research than by their surgical practice. One was Samuel Meltzer, who was born in Russia, graduated from the University of Berlin, and came to New York City in 1883, initially supporting his active research career from his own practice income.[37-38] The other was Alexis Carrel, who trained in Lyon, France, and met Carl Beck (of Chicago) at a meeting in Montreal;[21,39] Beck convinced him to continue his research in Chicago, where he worked with Charles Guthrie to improve methods of vascular suture.[40] Meltzer and Carrel would both join the Rockefeller Institute for Medical Research in New York, where their investigations would have a profound effect on European visitors and modern surgery.

William W. Mayo was also an immigrant from England, although he did not attend university there; nevertheless he deserves some credit for the outstanding achievements of his two sons, who also freely acknowledged their debt to Gerster, Fenger, and several European-educated surgeons in Minnesota.[41-43] The Mayo brothers are the prime example of how American surgeons were able to measure themselves against an international standard represented by European-educated immigrants, and to use that base in the pursuit of their own initiatives. The following chapters will explore how well they did so.

Notes

1) *A Century of Population Growth: From the First Census of the United States to the Twelfth 1790-1900*, Washington: Government Printing Office, 1909.
2) *Abstract of the Twelfth Census of the United States 1900*, Washington: Government Printing Office, 1902.
3) *Profile of the Foreign-Born Population in the United States*, Current Population Reports, Series P23-206, Washington: Government Printing Office, 2000.
4) Kelly HA, Burrage WL, *American Medical Biographies*, Baltimore: Norman, Remington, 1920.
5) Hoffmann KF, "The history of the Rudolf Virchow Medical Society in the city of New York," In: Berberich J, Lax H, Stern R, editors, *Rudolf Virchow Medical Society 100th Anniversary Jubilee Volume*, Basel and New York: S. Karger, 1960, Pages 12-47.
6) Boas EP, "A refugee doctor of 1850," *Journal of the History of Medicine* 1948; 3:65-94.
7) Reichle HS, "Emil Noeggerath (1827-1895)," *Annals of Medical History* 1928; 10:77-79.
8) *The National Cyclopaedia of American Biography*, Volume IX, New York: James T. White, 1899.
9) Halajian EB, Wheat TA, Bloom DA, "Arpad G Gerster, MD, and the first photographic surgical textbook," *Journal of the American College of Surgeons* 2006; 203:116-23.
10) Rutkow I, "The education, training, and specialization of surgeons: Turn-of-the-century America and its postgraduate medical schools," *Annals of Surgery* 2013; 258:1130-1136.
11) Aufses AH, Niss BJ, *This House of Noble Deeds: The Mount Sinai Hospital, 1852-2002*, New York: New York University Press, 2002.
12) M[eyer] HW, "Dr. Willy Meyer," *American Journal of Surgery* 1932; 17:287-92.
13) "Dr. Otto G. T. Kiliani," *New York Times*, 13 June 1928, Page 27.
14) *The National Cyclopaedia of American Biography*, Volume X, New York: James T. White, 1900.
15) Beck C, "Der Einfluss deutschen Aerztetums in Amerika," *Münchener Medizinische Wochenschrift* 1904; 51:1792-3.
16) Lutterbeck EF, Widenhorn HL, "The German Medical Society of Chicago: 1897 to the present," *Illinois Medical Journal* 1962; 122:269-272,374-379.

17) Senn N, "Life and work of the late Professor Christian Fenger," *Journal of the American Medical Association* 1902; 39: 4-8.
18) Billings F, "Christian Fenger," *Surgery, Gynecology & Obstetrics* 1922; 35:365-369.
19) Rosen G, "Christian Fenger, medical immigrant," *Bulletin of the History of Medicine* 1974; 48:129-145.
20) Blair SJ, *The Doctors Beck of Chicago: Men of Integrity*, Chicago: Chauncey Park Press, 2013.
21) Baader W, Nyhus LM, "The life of Carl Beck and an important interval with Alexis Carrel," *Surgery, Gynecology & Obstetrics*. 1986; 163:85-88.
22) Matas R, "Surgical operations fifty years ago," *American Journal of Surgery* 1941;51:40-53.
23) Cohn I, Deutsch HB, *Rudolph Matas: A Biography of one of the Great Pioneers of Surgery*, Garden City: Doubleday, 1960.
24) Duffy J, editor, *The Rudolph Matas History of Medicine in Louisiana*, Volume II, Baton Rouge: Louisiana State University Press, 1962.
25) Duffy J, "French influence on the development of medicine in Louisiana," *Biomedicine & Pharmacotherapy* 1990; 44:147-152.
26) Singleton AO, "The surgeon in the romantic story of Texas," *Annals of Surgery* 1940; 111:673-687.
27) Lekisch K, "Dr Ferdinand von Herff, idealistic pioneer and distinguished Texas physician," *Texas Medicine* 1986; 82:48-52.
28) Burns OR, Campbell HG, "The extraordinary influences of two British physicians on medical education and practice in Texas at the turn of the Twentieth Century," *Vesalius* 1999; 2:79-84.
29) Jacobsen JH, "Martin Stamm, MD, FACS," *Transactions of the American Association of Obstetricians and Gynecologists* 1918; 31:352-358.
30) Rixford E, "John Fairbairn Binnie 1863-1936," *Annals of Surgery* 1937; 106:157-160.
31) *The National Cyclopaedia of American Biography, Volume XII*, New York: James T. White, 1904.
32) Schlich T, "Asepsis and bacteriology: A realignment of surgery and laboratory science," *Medical History* 2012: 56:308-334.
33) *Official Register and Directory of Physicians and Surgeons in the State of California*, Twelfth Edition, San Francisco: California Medical Society Board of Examiners, 1900.
34) Stetten D, "Frederic Kammerer," *Annals of Surgery* 1929; 89:315-318.

35) Bernays T, *Augustus Charles Bernays: A Memoir*, St. Louis: Mosby, 1912.
36) Beck C, "Nicholas Senn," *Surgery, Gynecology & Obstetrics* 1923; 37:398-400.
37) Harvey AM, "Samuel J. Meltzer: Pioneer catalyst in the evolution of clinical science in America," *Perspectives in Biology and Medicine* 1978; 21:431-440.
38) Meltzer A, "Samuel James Meltzer, M.D.," *Experimental Biology and Medicine* 2000; 223:114-117.
39) Hamilton D, *The First Transplant Surgeon: The Flawed Genius of Nobel Prize Winner, Alexis Carrel*, London: World Scientific, 2017.
40) Skladman R, Hanto DW, Sacks JM, "The story of Charles Guthrie and Alexis Carrel," *Journal of the American College of Surgeons* 2022; 235:559-565.
41) Clapesattle H, *The Doctors Mayo*, Garden City NY: Garden City Publishing Co., 1943.
42) Nelson CW, "Dr. Arpad Gerster and the Mayo Brothers," *Mayo Clinic Proceedings* 1992; 67:620.
43) Mayo WJ, "An appreciation of Dr. Arnold Schwyzer," *Minnesota Medicine* 1934; 17:151-2.

3

"American Highlights"

Carl Beck (1856-1911) was born in Neckargemünd, near Heidelberg, Germany. After attending local schools, he studied medicine at the Universities of Heidelberg, Berlin, and Jena, receiving his medical degree in 1879. He married Hedwig Loeser in 1881 and emigrated to New York the following year. He established a surgical practice there, working mostly at St. Mark's Hospital (which closed in 1930), and taught at the New York Post-Graduate Medical School.[1]

This Carl Beck must be distinguished from Carl Beck of Chicago (1864-1952), another German-speaking immigrant surgeon mentioned in the previous chapter.[2-3] The activities of both are prominently described in the *New Yorker Medizinische Monatsschrift* during 1904-1908, sometimes in the same issue, and they must have been aware of each other. Carl Beck of Chicago outlived his namesake by more than forty years, and is much better known today; unfortunately, library and archival catalogues often confuse the two.

Carl Beck of New York (the subject of this chapter) wrote extensively in German and English about the surgical issues of the day, including aseptic technique, fractures, and thoracic surgery (especially drainage of empyema).[4-6] Following the discovery of X-rays in 1895 he was quick to explore their use in both diagnosis and therapy, including the prevention of radiation burns.[7-8]

Beck was elected President of the German Medical Society of New York and was also President of the Union of Old German Students of America.[9] He wrote fondly of his boyhood and student years, especially in Heidelberg,[10] and sought to promote the continuation of German culture in the United States. Based on his background and literary abilities, Carl Beck was well-situated to explain the New World to the Old World, and for several years in the early twentieth century he regularly contributed articles, mostly to the *Münchener Medizinische Wochenschrift* (Munich Medical Weekly). Like many of the articles in the following chapters, these were partly for the benefit of the many German ecotourists and partly to describe the status of American medicine and surgery, of which he was increasingly proud.

In order to focus on the impressions of the surgeons who were still practicing in Europe, this study will not translate Carl Beck's articles in full, but summaries are provided below. These articles contributed to the concepts that the medical community in Europe was forming about American surgery during these years. Of course, the author knows that his German-speaking audience will welcome any compliments, but he does not hide his own admiration of German science and culture, and he regrettably reveals some of the prevailing prejudices about people from other backgrounds, cultures, or political opinions.

Letter from New York: At the medical congress in St. Paul and on to Wonderland (1901)[11]

The article starts with a description of the special train carrying New York City delegates, accompanied by their wives, to the 1901 Annual Meeting of the American Medical Association (AMA) in St. Paul MN. They pass through the "famous beer city" of Rochester NY, which is so thoroughly German that some shop windows have signs reading "English spoken here." They stop for several hours at Niagara Falls, endure an alcohol-free Sunday dinner in St. Thomas ON, and are amazed at the ferryboat that takes their entire train across from Windsor to Detroit. They pass quickly through Chicago and Wisconsin, admire the majestic and romantic Mississippi, and arrive in St. Paul.

"Sixty years ago, an enterprising Frenchman had the courage to settle here next to the wigwams," and now the city is the capital of Minnesota, with 650 factories, 20 hospitals, hotels in the best European style, and beautiful parks. It coexists in a friendly way with the larger city of Minneapolis on the other side of the Mississippi.

The opening address of the AMA President, Dr. Reed of Cincinnati, announces Rockefeller's gift of $200,000 to start an experimental laboratory in New York. In the surgical section, appendicitis is a controversial subject as always. Deaver advocates early operation, while Senn is more conservative.

The author describes in rather sarcastic terms the "Women Suffragists" convention that is also taking place in St. Paul. This group opposes the sale of alcoholic beverages in the "canteens" on Army bases, has convinced the US government to pass a law to this effect, and has formally requested the support of the AMA. A sizeable number of women doctors present this issue to the AMA general session, but an army doctor argues that the soldiers will just leave the base and drink cheap and possibly tainted alcohol elsewhere. The women's request is refused.

The author is more pleased with the dinners and receptions, where there is "not the slightest sign of abstinence" and which include the more proper ladies of St. Paul "as opposed to the ascetic zealots I have described." The AMA women's group makes an enjoyable excursion to Minnehaha Falls, and the four days of the meeting otherwise pass quickly leaving only pleasant memories.

A special train has been arranged to take 158 doctors, 3 chemists, and their families on an excursion from St. Paul to Yellowstone Park. Dr. Keen and his two daughters are part of the group, and occupy the compartments next to the author. Most of the other passengers are from the Midwest. Everyone is under the benign but strict authority of the Colored Pullman porters, who treat all the passengers with democratic equality (perhaps modified slightly by a generous tip), regulate the ventilation, and quietly patrol the corridors through the night.

During the long stretches across the prairie, the author recalls the German-American Heinrich Villard who created the Northern Pacific Railway, sees a few cowboys and Indians, and notes the widely separated farms. They cross the muddy Missouri, and he sends a postcard home from Bismarck ND. They pass near the site of Custer's last stand, see some prairie dogs, and on the next morning have a wonderful view of the Rocky Mountains. At Livingston MT they switch to a branch line, at the end of which 30 six-horse carriages are waiting to take the party to Yellowstone.

The National Park is like a wonderland, a fairy tale, or a Wagner opera setting. They visit the geysers, admire the animals and birds, and stay at a comfortable hotel. The author, two German chemists, and their wives tour the park together. They arrive at their next hotel and learn that a German tourist is there who had been burnt a week before by getting too close to Old Faithful. This turns out to be another German doctor whom the author knew during his time in Berlin. There are areas of necrotic skin on one lower leg, which the nearsighted patient did not realize, and the author excises them using the portable surgical kit he always carries. By the time of this report three months later, the patient has healed and is heading home.

The return trip is uneventful, but after 7 nights on the train the author is grateful to sleep in a real bed when they get to Chicago. He tours the Presbyterian Hospital there with Dr. Senn, and he also has the chance to talk with some army doctors who are meeting in Chicago. Then back to New York, where the Mohawk Valley reminds him of the Neckar Valley (although of course nothing in the world can really be as nice as his boyhood home.)

Medical Highlights from America: A vacation trip from the medical congress in Saratoga across the Adirondacks to Canada, the White Mountains, and Boston (1902)[12]

The author attended the 1902 Annual Meeting of the AMA in Saratoga NY. Arriving visitors were greeted by a band playing *Die Wacht am Rhein*, probably because of the recent visit of the German Prince; usually they play the *Marseillaise*. He reflects that some Americans seem to think of Germans only as tavernkeepers, barbers, musicians, or servants, which is resented by German visitors and immigrants.

The hotel has outstanding facilities, and its garden recalls the Heidelberg Castle; doctors greet each other that evening, and even many home-grown Yankees say "*Guten Abend, Herr Kollege.*" After an opening address by New York surgeon John Allan Wyeth, the sectional meetings begin, with the surgical section led by DeForest Willard of Philadelphia. Topics discussed include tuberculous peritonitis (Murphy, Richardson, Ransohoff), gunshot wounds (Rodman, LaGarde), gallstones (Tinker, Mayo), appendicitis (Deaver, Weir, Abbe), fractures (Matas, Roberts), and experimental cardiac wounds (Ricketts). In the ophthalmologic section, extraction of foreign bodies is discussed by Haab, Knapp, and others. The pediatric section discusses tonsillitis and milk intolerance. The neurologic section discusses peripheral neuropathy as a complication of whooping cough. The hygiene section discusses regulations regarding tuberculosis. Kelly describes methods and indications for ureteral catheterization.

Saratoga is a resort famous for its mineral waters, which remind the author of European spas and customs. The surroundings are very beautiful, and remind the author of their original inhabitants, the stories of Cooper, and the Battle of Saratoga. He visits Lake George, where many New York City doctors and their patients have summer homes, as does the "freedom fighter" Karl Schurz. The New York medical license is still valid here, whereas practicing at the resorts of New Jersey would require an additional difficult state examination thus creating a "Chinese wall."

Traveling further north, the author praises the beauty of Lake Champlain and the mountains, lakes, and woods of the Adirondacks, which have an aroma of balsam firs. The healthy air makes it ideal for patients with respiratory diseases, and many sanatoriums have been built here. He enters Canada, crosses the St. Lawrence River, and arrives in Montreal, where he perceives the separateness of the English and French citizens, and briefly discusses the historical background. Montreal has 18 hospitals, of which the "pearl" is the Royal Victoria, only 8 years old. He travels on to Quebec, where the Hôtel Dieu is the leading hospital, and then back onto "republican soil" in New

Hampshire.

The White Mountains of northern New Hampshire remind the author of the Harz Mountains in Germany, whereas the Adirondacks were more like the Black Forest. He is impressed by the famous "profile" at Cannon Mountain, the "flume," and the colorful rock formations contrasted with the green of the virgin forest. The mountain roads are steep, so the traveler needs a four-horse carriage like an aristocrat. The author mentions, but apparently does not ride, the cog railway up to the highest peak, Mount Washington. The Mount Washington Hotel has an orchestra composed of selected members of the Boston Symphony, of whom the principal violinist and cellist are "of course, good Germans."

From this point, the geography becomes confused, as the author says the train took four hours "through the wooded foothills of the White Mountains" to reach Plymouth, "the landing place of the Pilgrims," and then another two hours "along the coast of Maine and Massachusetts" to reach Boston. He likes this city because of its rather European appearance and emphasizes the German connections of Harvard University. Its medical school is still on Boylston Street, but Rockefeller has donated a million dollars for new facilities. On the way back to New York, the train stops briefly in New Haven, where Yale has just celebrated its bicentennial.

The Post-Graduate Medical School in New York (1903)[13]

The article begins by acknowledging the historically poor quality of medical education in America compared to Europe, but "to the credit of our American colleagues," this deficit is being rapidly diminished. An important part of this progress has been provided by postgraduate schools modeled after the "vacation courses" at German universities. The New York Post-Graduate Medical School was founded in 1882 under the leadership of Dr. Daniel Roosa, an eye-ear-nose-throat surgeon. In the next few years, it moved to a new building, added a hospital and nursing school, and became affiliated with the New York State University.

Now in 1903 the school has 51 full professors, 25 adjunct professors, and 74 instructors, all serving without pay. The students are all medical school graduates. Clinical instruction is at the attached hospital, although initially the faculty taught students at the other hospitals where they practiced. Surgical procedures are demonstrated on cadavers every day. Many of the surgical faculty have European training, but there is also Dr. Powell, "the eminent practical full-blooded American, from whom particularly the overeducated Germans could learn a great deal," and Dr. Morris, "the prototype of a true American gentleman."

Most students remain for a semester, some for a full year. There are also short courses lasting 6 weeks. Last year there were about 800 students in all. Instruction starts at 8 A.M. and continues until 9 P.M., with only a brief pause at lunchtime. The school issues a monthly journal, which has gone from being purely an institutional newsletter to a more general circulation.

Following the example of New York, most of the major cities in America now have a Post-Graduate Medical School. Furthermore, the better universities are steadily increasing their standards and quality. Ewald has written in the *Berliner Klinische Wochenschrift* that the rapid progress in America, unencumbered by tradition, will soon bring it to a comparable level with Europe. "The dawn of this new era is already shining auspiciously on the American horizon."

From the Fifth Congress of American Physicians and Surgeons in Washington (1903)[14]

The author attended what was actually the Sixth Congress of this organization that generally met every three years and included the American Surgical Association. A special train has been arranged for the New York and New England doctors traveling to Washington, and the author brings along his wife and child. In Jersey City they see an ocean liner arriving from Germany and he feels a bit homesick. They pass through Princeton, which he thinks is like a small German university town: The students are just as smart, exercise and compete through sports rather than dueling with swords, but of course they lack the romanticism of a German. Philadelphia reminds him of the tolerance of William Penn, the diligence of the "Pennsylvaniadeutsch" farmers, and the excellence of the University of Pennsylvania. Baltimore will always have a place of honor in American medical history.

The Hotel Raleigh in Washington is excellent, and after one generous dinner they are invited to another. Dr. Keen gives the opening address the following morning, but everyone is especially looking forward to the presentations of the invited guests Drs. Mikulicz, Tillmanns, Ewald, and Kehr. The first afternoon is free and devoted to seeing the city, whose layout reminds the author of Mannheim. He describes the principal buildings, praises President Roosevelt and the German ambassador (whose wife is American), and speculates about the skulls exhibited at the Smithsonian Institute, especially those of African-Americans. "Whether in the course of centuries the Negro will really achieve *Egalité* and *Fraternité*, as it says so nicely on paper? Who knows?" He asserts the "blood-brotherhood between Germany and America" which cannot be altered by "the cry of the yellow journalist vultures." After the conference, the author returns home via Pittsburg (spelled without an "h"), "the American Chemnitz," where thousands of factories pour smoke into the air.

The author says very little about the meeting itself, including the talks by the German professors, since these have already been published in German journals. These visitors will travel to Baltimore, Philadelphia, Boston, and Chicago, will receive many honors, and will speak at the New York County Medical Society and German Medical Society. Professor Tillmanns is especially celebrated because of his new textbook that is obligatory at every American university.

The worthy goals of the German Medical Society of New York City (1904)[15]

In the past, it was thought that the principal mission of the German Medical Society was to mentor German doctors who had recently immigrated and often did not speak English. Today, however, the author thinks its role is expanding. Society members are contributing to the rising educational standards in America, and we should be proud that American students often finish their education at the German universities.

We physicians especially remember the names of the famous German scientists. Even our greatest poets – Schiller and Goethe – were once medical students. The wonderful achievements of industry are in no small part due to German chemistry and physics. What would medicine be without Müller, Graefe, Virchow, and Koch, or surgery without Dieffenbach, Langenbeck, Billroth, Volkmann, Virchow, Esmarch, Bergmann, Czerny, and König? Without denying the immortal contributions of Pasteur and Lister, the scientific renaissance of medicine, including asepsis and radiology, is largely a German creation.

One of the main goals of our society should be to make our fellow Americans aware of these accomplishments. It is more difficult for those who do not speak German, but perhaps we could sometimes allow our native colleagues to speak in English, and those who have studied at a German university may appreciate the opportunity to continue with our language.

Educated Americans appreciate the German characteristics of modesty and thoroughness. These are valuable counterweights to the typical American optimism and practicality, which run the risk of superficiality and fanaticism. We should not forget that Germans can also be pedantic and obstinate, but fortunately Americans are very tolerant and ready to compromise.

In medicine, the era of one-sided German contributions is past, and we should acknowledge the importance of McDowell, Mott, Morton, Warren, Sims, and Parker. Our knowledge of appendicitis comes from America, as do Senn's bowel suture, methodical thoracentesis, operations for club foot, the Murphy button, and the Pravaz syringe. Asepsis is better developed in the United States than anywhere else. Our second great mission is to introduce American science to our colleagues in Germany. Long live the German Medical Society of New York City!

The influence of German doctors in America (1904)[16]

This article describes how, even in the early years of the United States, Americans made many innovations in surgical practice, and here and there some German immigrants were influential. In 1846, they founded the organization that became the German Medical Society of New York City. However, the first great influx of German doctors came to the New World following the Freedom Movement of 1848. The most important were Krackowitzer, Noeggerath, Jacobi, and Roth in New York, who founded the German Hospital, and the excellent surgeon Hammer in St. Louis. Others included Herff in Texas, Zipperlen in Cincinnati, Kiefer in Detroit, and Emmerling in Pittsburg. Hermann Knapp gave up his professorship in Heidelberg to become the Father of American ophthalmology. Schilling, Althof, Kammerer, Schnetter, and Schwedler also contributed to the development of the German Hospital in New York.

Heitzmann helped develop histology, and Lange transplanted the aseptic method to America. Only a few have been named, but there are hundreds more. Every year more Germans arrive, no longer as pioneers, but as worthy colleagues, in many cases with a reputation already established. The German Hospitals of Brooklyn and Philadelphia have developed into exemplary institutions in addition to the German Hospital of New York already mentioned. The success of German-Americans is an honorable contribution to the land that welcomed them.

From the International Congress in St. Louis (1905)[17]

The author attended the International Congress of Arts and Science at the St. Louis World's Fair. He thinks it demonstrated that in science, one can still say "Deutschland über alles." The Americans did a good job in organizing the Congress, whose overall chairman was the astronomer Newcomb, but the plans were actually made by Hugo Münsterberg, formerly professor at Freiburg and now at Harvard. Germany, France, England, Italy, and Japan all sent illustrious scientists.

Dr. Jordan, President of Stanford University, led off the medical section with a talk on immunology, which was largely based on German discoveries. Some of the subsequent addresses have already been published in the

Münchener Medizinische Wochenschrift. The author himself was chairman of the surgical subsection, where Waldeyer, Orth, and Escherich were featured along with the well-known American surgeons Dennis, Murphy, Bernays, Tuholske, and Binnie. He acknowledges that in technical areas the Americans lead the way, while in the basic sciences they still have much to learn from Germany. Those who talk about an "American danger" should be ashamed; there is actually a brotherhood between America and Germany, which was apparent in the surgical subsection.

The Congress of Arts and Science was only a relatively small part of this great World's Fair, where the German industrial, scientific, educational, and hygienic exhibits were also excellent. The French artistic presentations were almost as good as those from Germany, but even some of the French art had German themes like Siegfried or Faust. Art depicting the Franco-Prussian War is generally not exhibited in America, as if to deny the German victory.

America has the best hospitals. German architects should not be permitted to build a new hospital unless they have studied the construction of American hospitals. It must be admitted that American hospitals, like American hotels and boarding houses, are even cleaner than those in Germany. The outpatient clinics especially pay attention to cleaning up recent immigrants from Poland and Italy, about whom the author makes some rather disparaging comments.

There were a lot of Japanese at the fair, and many of them spoke good German. There was an excellent reproduction of Dr. Kitasato's laboratory.

On the first evening, the Ladies' Committee gave a reception, where the German professors mixed easily with the rest of the crowd, the "Wacht am Rhein" was played along with the Marseillaise, and everyone got along fine. On the second evening, a reception had been planned at the elegant French Pavilion, but it was postponed and then cancelled. The reception at the German Pavilion was the social highlight of the week; German immigrants like the author tried to express their loyalty to the culture of the old country while fulfilling their duty to their adopted land. On the following evening, there was a reception for all the foreign scholars, which the author skipped in order to attend a meeting of the Old German Students in America. On the final evening, there was a reception at the "Tyrolean Alps" pavilion, where a giant beer hall had been prepared, but the French band assigned to play at the reception at first did not appear and then only did so unwillingly; they played the national anthems of each speaker, but refused to play "Die Wacht am Rhein."

The author has traveled the world but has never seen anything as enchanting as the Cascade Garden. From a semicircular façade, three fountains 24 feet high produced cascades down the marble steps into a basin 600 feet wide, flowing into a large canal that flowed by the "Tyrolean Alps" pavilion. At night it was lit by electric lamps and looked like something from a fairy tale. We knew that the Yankees could make amazing buildings and machines, but did not expect anything with such artistic taste. It made the author proud to be an American.

St. Louis played a decisive role in the Civil War, and specifically through its German citizens, who were the only ones who opposed the rebellion. They seized Camp Jackson, which General Grant said was "one of the best things in the whole war." Many of the street names, and the name of the city itself, are reminders that it was founded by the French; Napoleon sold it to the young republic in 1803. Now it is one of the greatest commercial cities of the world, with the largest tobacco and shoe factories and the largest brewery in the world, whose owner Busch has made major contributions to the arts and sciences.

Most of the delegates to the Congress had to return to Europe at the end of the sessions, but some went on to visit other American cities. For the hundreds of people who attended, the Congress will be an unforgettable memory, and a new pillar of the wonderful bridge that is being built from the Old World to the New.

A vacation trip across the Atlantic Ocean (1905)[18]

The author traveled from New York to Bremen on the *Großer Kurfürst* [Great Elector], a North German Lloyd ocean liner. The passengers watch New Jersey and Long Island disappear behind them, many at first feel seasick, and they run into fog at the Grand Banks. Then things improve, the young people flirt, the musicians play, and the food and drink are excellent. They encounter the liner *Deutschland* and then an American naval squadron that is headed for Cherbourg to obtain the body of John Paul Jones, which will be reinterred with honor on American soil.

The ship reaches Plymouth, lets off some passengers, and continues. Then they hear "Man overboard!" The ship stops, a boat is lowered, and the crew rescues a 26-year-old Hungarian, who is cold and exhausted but survives. The author goes to the lower deck to offer his medical services and is appalled by the crowded and unhealthy conditions. Various national groups tend to cluster together, with some brave working-class families among the crowds of rougher elements.

The author praises the captain, officers, and crew of North German Lloyd. He recalls a previous voyage when they managed to deal with a fire on board (probably from a short circuit), and another when they ran aground leaving New York Harbor (the fault of the harbor pilot, not the captain). He recommends that the management provide them with better medical facilities, instead of spending so much on luxuries for the passengers.

The *Großer Kurfürst* arrives safely in Bremerhaven late in the evening. The shadows of the houses are barely visible, but the feeling of home glows in the author's heart.

To Florida at Christmas time (1906)[19]

The author traveled with his family to Florida for Christmas. From Richmond, where they notice the separate "White" and "Colored" waiting rooms, they intentionally take a local train in order to see more of the South. They observe more and more Blacks, whose appearance the author considers repulsive, but he is careful not to speak aloud any racial epithet that might be highly offensive and even cause a violent reaction. They perceive that the great majority of southern Whites hate and fear the Blacks, they pass some battlefields of the Civil War, and they wonder how this racial animosity will ever be resolved.

They are happy to see so many Christmas decorations. 30-40 years before, only the German-Americans had a Christmas tree, and it was not generally considered a holiday. Now Americans from Alaska to Mexico, Whites and Blacks, all observe this solstice celebration of the heathen Germanic tribes. By evening, they are in Charleston, and the author recalls the beginnings of the Civil War, observing that this harbor is now the most important naval base on the Atlantic Coast.

The train continues through Savannah, Jacksonville, and Saint Augustine, and the author reviews the history of this oldest American city, the Spanish and British empires, the Seminoles, and the Spanish-American War. They travel on past orange and pineapple plantations, palm trees, and numerous beach towns, finally arriving at the "queen" of winter resorts, Palm Beach. "How can I find the words to describe this Paradise on Earth?" The author extensively praises the resort, the climate, the natural vegetation, and the cultivated plants. He visits the farm of "Alligator Joe," who collects the reptiles for which he is named and is happy to show them off. The author has his picture taken with a Seminole (who charges 50 cents, after some bargaining), but he declines the opportunity to be photographed with a live alligator. From the pier by the hotel, fish of many shapes and colors are being caught, including a shark 17½ feet long.

After a week, the vacation is over. The final point of interest is Miami, where the author marvels over the active commerce with the Caribbean region, one more evidence of the increasing power of the United States.

Carl Beck republished most of these articles from the *Münchener Medizinische Wochenschrift*, along with some others primarily dealing with German-American organizations, in a book entitled *Amerikanische Streiflichter* [American Highlights].[20] In a forward, he expresses his goal to share his honest opinions about America with his fellow Germans, since they are too often presented with superficial or even distorted caricatures. He feels that his twenty-five years in New York, in contact with all kinds of Americans through his medical practice and academic positions, has given him a meaningful perspective, and that his writings have been a modest contribution toward brotherhood between Germany and America.

After a period of declining health, Carl Beck died of pneumonia in 1911, at the age of 55, and so he did not have to witness the end of the peace and the devastating effect of the First World War on German-American relationships. A century later, it is easier to distinguish the admirable aspects of the European science and culture he celebrated from other attitudes that were ultimately rejected.

Notes

1) *The National Cyclopaedia of American Biography, Volume X*, New York: James T. White, 1900.
2) Blair SJ, *The Doctors Beck of Chicago: Men of Integrity*, Chicago: Chauncey Park Press, 2013.
3) Baader W, Nyhus LM, "The life of Carl Beck and an important interval with Alexis Carrel," *Surgery, Gynecology & Obstetrics*. 1986; 163:85-88.
4) Beck C, *A Manual of the Modern Theory and Technique of Surgical Asepsis*, Philadelphia: W. B. Saunders, 1895.
5) Beck C, *Fractures*, Philadelphia: W. B. Saunders, 1900.
6) Beck C, *Surgical Diseases of the Chest*, London: Rebman, 1907.
7) Beck C, *Die Röntgenstrahlen im Dienste der Chirurgie*, München: Seitz & Schauer, 1902.
8) Beck C, *Röntgen Ray Diagnosis and Therapy*, New York: D. Appleton, 1908.
9) "Obituary: Carl Beck, M.D," *Boston Medical and Surgical Journal* 1911; 164:869.
10) Beck C, *Feuchtfröhliches und Feuchtunfröhliches*, Berlin: Leonhard Simion, 1906.
11) Beck C, "New-Yorker Brief: Zum St. Pauler Aerztecongress und

nach Wunderland," *Münchener Medizinische Wochenschrift* 1901; 48:1367-1368,1397-1401,1430-1432,1637-1639,1685-1687,1729-1732.

12) Beck C, "Medizinische Streiflichter aus Amerika: Eine Ferienrundfahrt vom Aerztekongress in Saratoga über die Adirondacks nach Canada, den weissen Bergen und Boston," *Münchener Medizinische Wochenschrift* 1902; 49:1934-1936,2023-2026.

13) Beck C, "Die medizinische Fortbildungsschule in New-York," *Münchener Medizinische Wochenschrift* 1903; 50:515-517.

14) Beck C, "Vom 5. Kongress der amerikanischen Aerzte und Wundärzte in Washington," *Münchener Medizinische Wochenschrift* 1903; 50:1898-1901,1936-1938.

15) Beck C, "Ueber erstrebenswerte Ziele der Deutschen Medizinischen Gesellschaft der Stadt Newyork," *Münchener Medizinische Wochenschrift* 1904; 51:395-396.

16) Beck C, "Der Einfluss deutschen Aerztetums in Amerika," *Münchener Medizinische Wochenschrift* 1904; 51:1792-1793.

17) Beck C, "Vom internationalen Kongress in St. Louis," *Münchener Medizinische Wochenschrift* 1905; 52:285-289,333-336,374-377.

18) Beck C, "Eine Ferienreise über den atlantischen Ozean," *Münchener Medizinische Wochenschrift* 1905; 52:1735-1737.

19) Beck C, "Um die Weihnachtszeit nach Florida," *Münchener Medizinische Wochenschrift* 1906; 53:915-918,978-981,1025-1027.

20) Beck C, *Amerikanische Streiflichter*, Berlin: Leonhard Simion, 1905.

4
Vincenz Czerny (1901)

Vincenz Czerny was born in 1842 in Trautenau (at that time part of the Austro-Hungarian Empire, today Trutnov, Czech Republic). He studied at the University of Vienna, receiving his Doctorate in Medicine with highest honors in 1866. He was primarily interested in laboratory research, but caught the attention of Theodor Billroth, who brought him into clinical surgery and advanced his career. Czerny became Professor of Surgery in Freiburg in 1871 (age 29) and in Heidelberg in 1877. He developed a special interest in cancer. He spoke several languages, traveled extensively to visit surgical centers in Europe, and was one of twelve European surgeons elected *in absentia* as Honorary Fellows of the American Surgical Association in 1885.

In 1901, at the age of 60, he traveled to the United States with his wife, primarily as a tourist. A report of his visit is given in the following pages.

In 1906, Czerny established a Cancer Research Center in Heidelberg which became a model for Europe. He formally retired as Professor but remained active in international cancer organizations and the Société Internationale de Chirurgie, whose Second Congress he chaired in 1908. He died in Heidelberg in 1915.

Ein Ferien-Ausflug nach San Francisco
Frankfurter Zeitung 1902; 46:
33 (*2. Februar 3. Morgenblatt*) 1-2,
36 (*5. Februar 3. Morgenblatt*) 1-2,
40 (*9. Februar 3. Morgenblatt*) 1-2,
43 (*12. Februar 3. Morgenblatt*) 1-2,
47 (*16. Februar 3. Morgenblatt*) 1

A holiday excursion to San Francisco
by Dr. Vincenz Czerny (Heidelberg) [1]

Almost at the same hour when our *Columbia* left the harbor in Cherbourg, the assassin's bullet struck McKinley.[1] Just before that, in a long speech, the President had expressed the justifiable pride felt by him and the entire American public in the unprecedented progress that this great country has made in recent years. At the same time, he warned of the need to avoid the thoughtless egoism that would threaten to put many companies in the Old World out of business by a vexatious tariff, since there is nothing to be gained by depleting a business partner to the point where it has no purchasing power. "Live and let live" was the basic theme of his speech, which seemed well designed to bring peace to an anxious world.

We first got news of the assassination from the customs officials. When we landed on September 13th, we learned that the President's condition was hopeless. He died the following night.

Our arrival in the splendid harbor of New York was unfortunately spoiled by the annoying customs procedures. After a long wait, you are allowed to declare under oath that you are not carrying anything subject to customs duties. False testimony is punishable by five years in prison and thousands of dollars in fines. Then follows a cumbersome search of boxes and trunks in the giant customs hall in Hoboken. My experience with customs procedures in Russia, Spain, and Turkey was never so aggravating. Already you get the feeling that the free country of America will unscrupulously alter its principles when it can get a temporary advantage. After all, it fought for its independence from England because the British Parliament wanted to put a small tax on coffee and tea.

We had just reached the Statue of Liberty when I was able to go back on deck. She may have the most wonderful location that could be found for a statue in the middle of New York Harbor, but despite her dimensions she seemed insufficient for the size of the space.

Gradually we began to see the great buildings of New York which cover the southern end of Manhattan Island: Planted irregularly among them appeared the towering four-sided "skyscrapers," which increasingly dominate the business district with their unappealing shapes and are turning Broadway into a canyon. From the depths rise some church steeples, which once were landmarks that mariners could see from afar but now look like stalagmites in a cavern, barely reaching to the rim of the canyon. We too had to rest from our tiring sea journey in a twenty-story hotel. These fantastic creations of the American architects now reach up to Central Park and include the paragons of the American hotel industry, whose greatest example is the Waldorf-Astoria.

It is amazing to me how human caprice has managed to create an elegant and apparently comfortable habitation for thousands of people on such a narrow, incredibly expensive piece of land, but from the standpoint of public health it would be better to prohibit building above a certain height depending on the width of the streets, as was done in time for Berlin. I have to admire how the engineers have provided plumbing and drainage for the baths and toilets in every apartment, keeping the pipes out of sight and in working order, but in some circumstances the ventilation is insufficient. If your bedroom is not on the street side, so that you can sleep with the window open, the interior of the building develops a definite air of anxiety. Beyond this, the American custom is to heat the lower rooms that are used for dining and conversation in the evening, even if it has been unbearably hot all day. This custom has to be suffered even more on the railroads, where one is at the mercy of the Negroes in the Pullman cars, who have inherited the need for warmth from their ancestors in Guinea and now force the whites to sweat with them.

When you see how the Americans eat, you can easily understand why they so often have to deal with stomach problems. Breakfast starts with melon or other fruit, then ice water, warm bread, mush, pork chop, fish, or bacon with eggs, and coffee or tea. Most foods are robbed of their natural flavors by the addition of herbs. In the best hotels in the East, you can dine as well as in Europe, but after working through the complicated menu you find that it is best to keep having one of the same two or three simple dinners every day.

The service in the restaurants is good, but they also expect a good tip. In other situations, service is quite poor, whether you tip or not. It is well known that getting clothing or boots cleaned in an American hotel is difficult. Ladies have to brush their own boots. Gentlemen go to the bootblack who works in the servants' washroom or on the street.

It is even more difficult to get something to drink than something to eat while traveling. As mentioned, they usually drink only ice water with meals. Cocktails or whiskey are consumed in a private room before or afterwards. The heavy California wines are poor due to the dry, stimulating air in the mountains and California. The American beers can seldom compare to our local brews. If I had stayed longer in the West, I might have gone back to being an abstainer, since they do have excellent milk and coffee, although unfortunately poor tea in general.

New York is still in the summer doldrums in September. The nearby seaside resorts are already closed, since it is not worth keeping the large hotels open, but all the good company is either headed back to Europe or is still living in the mountains to avoid the heat, or is hunting or fishing in Canada. Our Sunday excursion in the beautiful Central Park was gilded with the colorful display of early autumn but not very enjoyable due to the sultry heat. We saw only a few occurrences of the lively traffic of cars and carriages that we had enjoyed the week before in the *Bois de Boulogne*.[2]

We did enjoy a quick visit to the Museum of Arts. This contains a small but interesting collection of mostly French masters. Here and in the other cities I was sorry not to see a larger collection of American artists. Some might say that it is too soon, that American art has not yet reached this point, but I disagree. In the Art Section of the Exhibition in Buffalo, a large number of quite good paintings and sculptures had been assembled, so that you start to wonder how it might be possible to follow the historical development of American art from its roots in England and France.

Among the American Maecenates,[3] who donate millions for libraries, universities, hospitals, etc. and buy famous paintings for gigantic sums, there is no Tretiakov,[4] who pursued Russian talent with his sense of good taste over decades and created a National Museum in Moscow that could be envied by Kensington, the Luxembourg, and the Berlin National Gallery. It would be timely for the federal government in Washington, like its sister republic in France, to support domestic artists systematically by purchasing their works, in order to create national art collections in the great human conglomerations that are called American cities.[5] Understanding and appreciation of this is beginning to grow in America, as shown by the enthusiastic visitors at all the museums that I saw. The artistic sense has made real progress, which one can see best by comparing the interior decoration of the Capitol in Washington, which incidentally is undergoing a thorough renovation, to the decoration in the new Library of Congress there. The latter may be a bit too colorful and ostentatious for its serious purpose but is as beautiful and poetic as I have seen anywhere.

After a three-day stay, we escaped the heat of New York to rest at Niagara Falls and from there to visit Buffalo and its Exposition. The location is made to order for a vacation. The first rain of autumn spoiled our trip along the Hudson somewhat but brought with it a welcome cooling. In the changing sunlight, a walk through Goat and Three Sisters Islands afforded wonderful views of the rapids and roaring waters of Niagara. Even more wonderful is the view from the Canadian side of the Horseshoe Falls, which receives most of the flow of the Niagara River. Staying in the rapidly growing Niagara Falls City on the United States side is more interesting and inviting for fascinating walks. The Americans have used their portion of the Niagara Falls much more for power generation than the Canadians. Fortunately, both sides have recognized the falls as a national treasure and protected them from further depredations and displacements by modern industrial enterprises. Anyway, one would notice the low water level if the concessionaires took the entire 3 million horsepower from the stream. So far, they have only used about half of this.

On September 19, the Exposition in Buffalo was closed for McKinley's funeral. We made use of the day for an excursion with the electric train along the Niagara, to see the famous rapids and the whirlpool, where the river makes a right-angled turn and the roiling waters circle in a giant pool, slowly exiting into a peaceful channel toward Lake Ontario. Unfortunately, the holiday applied not only to Buffalo but also to the entire region. Endless excursion trains brought several thousands of people to the banks of the Niagara. Although we had reserved tickets, it was hard to find space on the overfilled cars. We had to deal with the Sunday public, who attempted to replace their delayed dinner hour with chewing tobacco among the men and chewing gum among the ladies. With admirable patience, the men stood on the steps and running boards in order to make the trip. This detracted from our enjoyment of the beautiful landscape. The ascent of the train from the gorge to the top of the cliff (Great Gorge Route) is very steep and in places somewhat worrisome. The slopes of the gorge, at the bottom of which the Niagara roars, are partly geologic rifts in the terrain and partly embankments covered with the original vegetation. The American arbor vitae and the Virginia juniper form stands of trees with the fine-needled white pine, mingled with oaks, lindens, and hazelnuts. Yellow and red creepers adorned the bushes, while the slopes were covered with pink and white branches and yellow panicles of goldenrod. Large brown-red butterflies with black wingtips, whose exotic character reminded us that we were at the 42nd latitude, floated in the light of the autumn sun. From the edges of the gorge, we enjoyed beautiful distant vistas of Queenstown on Lake Ontario and the wooded hills of Canada.

Even if the funeral of the President did not produce much evidence of national mourning on the faces of the passengers enjoying the holiday, I have to say that the rather demonstrative outpouring of sadness in the country did make a strong and correct impression. From the great office buildings adorned from roof to ground with flags and funeral decorations to the little wooden shack with an old sackcloth star banner at half-mast on a willow pole, every house had at least a picture of the President. Print shops, leaflets, and newspapers did their business with the unfortunate event. Not only were the final hours depicted repeatedly in the minutest detail, but phonographs endlessly repeated the President's last speech and words. Cinematographs attempted to depict how the wounds were inflicted. The newspapers did not speak very highly of the doctors, since they at first gave the false hope that the President would recover by operative closure of the stomach wounds. The immediate tachycardia should have made them more cautious. At laparotomy they found an injury of the pancreas, which resulted in retroperitoneal sepsis gradually leading to heart failure and death. Gunshot wounds of the pancreas are always serious injuries.

In the main streets of Buffalo, a coffin store stimulated our curiosity by the splendor of its satin-lined coffins and its expensive very modern mourning clothes of heavy colorful silk brocade. As we entered, the owner immediately turned on all the electric lights for the showroom and showed us a facsimile of McKinley's coffin, which was of relatively simple construction using black wood. We were also shown the little gray villa (Milburn House) on Delaware Avenue, where McKinley stayed during his final days. It was guarded by two policemen. As you know, the democratic custom that the President must shake hands in public with anyone who wishes to approach him enabled the murderer to strike his fatal blow. I fear that this assassination will not suffice for long to protect the endangered person of the President, although for now the new President will be diligently watched over in the White House. For the greatest tyranny in America is established custom, and is only surpassed by the power of money, whose pursuit is here an end in itself. There are different reasons why this tyranny is so little appreciated. For one thing, the American has an unbelievable tolerance for anything that is frequently repeated. Then he tells himself, if we are poorly governed, it is our own fault. Since he can do little by himself, he joins some organization, whose insignia he wears even more than the French wear their red ribbons.[6] He hopes then he can exert some influence in the direction he thinks best at the next election and acquiesces in the winning majority. Finally, the great fortunes are divided in the second or at most the third generation and since it is easy to partake in the increasing wealth of the land, everyone hopes it will be his turn at some point. That will last as long as there are still unsurveyed districts of land, new mineral deposits can be extracted from the extensive mountain lands, and new industries find inexhaustible areas of application. If these circumstances ever change, which will still take some time, then the plutocracy will soon be overthrown.

In addition to the general mourning, I was impressed by the peacefulness with which this immense country underwent the change in its Presidents. The new 43-year-old President has the reputation of an honest, independent man. Of old Dutch ancestry, he is nevertheless American from head to toe. In his address on the "History of the City of New York" he stated that an American citizen, no matter what language he speaks, can only have one point of view, which is as an American. At Yale University,[7] which just celebrated its 200th year, he was educated so well in body and mind that he was able to pursue his independence as a cowboy in the West and publish historical and biographical studies. He left a high administrative position to lead the Rough Riders in the Spanish War in Cuba, and returned as Governor of New York State, supported by the American ladies. It is an open secret that the Republican Party feared his independence and strength of will and therefore wanted to sideline him as Vice-President. Now the hand of a murderer has raised him to the top position. As is well-known, the Democrats more than the Republicans are fearful of imperialism, which has appealed to Americans since their easy victory over the Spanish. I saw captured Spanish cannons at several railroad stations, set up in pretty gardens and widely admired. In the museum in Washington various trophies of this war are the central and chief attractions. Great mausoleums for generals are being built on the Hudson.[8] The patriotism of the Americans, their pride on the progress they have made during the last decade, could be easily escalated by external conditions into a fever pitch, as indeed the explosion of the battleship "Maine" led to the outbreak of the Spanish War.

The newspapers and brochures of the great railways always deal in superlatives like "the most beautiful, the greatest, the biggest" etc. "in the world." So, it is no surprise that those Americans who have never been abroad think that their own circumstances are unsurpassed, and suffer from excessive self-importance. Every state, every county, indeed every town of 20,000 inhabitants wants its Capitol to be like the one in Washington even if it costs a terrific amount of money that would be better spent on streets and drinking water. Even Washington itself has no purification system for drinking water and suffers from malaria due to inadequate regulation of the river. I was often ashamed to recall how our German Reichstag, with a false sense of economy, cut the proud cupola off the top of its own assembly hall and thus did away with the splendid façade of Master Wallot,[9] which otherwise would have surpassed the Capitol of Washington.

[February 5]
The Pan-American Exposition of Buffalo was put on as a patriotic initiative by the citizens of this city, supported by the State of New York and the federal government. It closed with a deficit of 1 million dollars and suffered from the competition of its predecessors in Chicago and Paris. Americans did not find it worthwhile to travel to Buffalo since Chicago was "the most beautiful in the world," and for Europeans it was certainly too long and uncomfortable a journey.

Nevertheless, the fair deserved more visitors than it received. Even if the Spanish-Moorish central building did not have the grace of the *Giralda* in Seville, it alone still made the visit worthwhile, lit by thousands of electric lights powered by Niagara Falls and surrounded by broad canals and beautiful gardens. The wonderful rotunda of pillars behind it, with copies of the best statues from all the museums, the huge stadium used for numerous athletic competitions, and the baroque Midway Fair on the other side were remarkable arrangements. The whole area was framed by the great water surfaces of an old park containing the music pavilion and the exhibition hall with proper sections for industry, electricity, and art. With characteristic buildings, the different American states had tried to emulate the *Rue des Nations* in Paris. Although this was bound to fail, since the individual states of North America are not really so different, it can still be said that the overall impression of the fair in Buffalo was only surpassed by that in Paris because of the enchanting views from the Pont Alexandre and the Trocadero, while the buildings were not as crowded together and therefore detracted less from each other than was frequently the case in Paris.

There is not much to say about the city of Buffalo,[10] except that it is a relatively attractive city with a proud City Hall and government buildings in Gothic style and is an active harbor. With 10 million tons it is said to be the sixth largest harbor, which I can believe because on the American Great Lakes alone the tonnage is apparently larger than the combined total for all German railroads. Buffalo is wrapped in a gray cloud of smoke, since the generators of Niagara do not come close to providing sufficient power for its industries. Natural gas is brought by a hundred-mile-long pipeline from the Pennsylvania oilfields and is four times cheaper for heating and motors than the usual coal gas. However, it does not burn brightly enough for illumination.

On September 21, we traveled with the Michigan Central Railroad through Detroit to Chicago, where we arrived an hour late. In the Annex of the Auditorium Hotel[11] we stayed in Room 1962. The high number is explained by the fact that the main building and the annex each have 10 stories, and that in each story the room numbers start with 1. Thus, we were in Room 62 of the 19th floor, that is the 9th floor of the Annex. In such a large hotel one might be treated simply as a number, but if the hotel is famous throughout America, it should be a good room. Unfortunately, this was not true. There was no view, and despite repeated efforts by the bellman the lock did not work, and no other room was available, so we had to keep the door closed as well as possible with our suitcase straps.

Chicago is the most unpleasant city that I have ever seen. The streets, darkened by the 10- to 20-story buildings, with their streetcars and elevated trains making a hellish cacophony of rumbling, honking, and noise could provide a modern Dante with useful materials for depiction. The streets are dirty, poorly paved, and end in village-like rows of wooden houses. A new post-office building with a giant pillared hall is the only break in the gray monotony of skyscrapers. The library, museum, and park grounds on the lake are points of light in the otherwise unbearable city appearance.

We sped through Denver to Colorado Springs, where we checked into a nice hotel called "The Antlers." The journey there through the broad valleys of the Missouri and Mississippi was monotonous. It was mostly huge cornfields being harvested, separated by small woods which showed their golden-brown colors in the autumn sunshine. One does not see much of the towns other than a few saloons and cafés near the train stations. At Denver, nicely situated on the high plain with a wonderful view of the mountains, I saw low cacti and yucca bushes with their black fruits next to the train, the northern outliers of the remarkable cactus and agave flora characteristic of the hot and dry areas of New Mexico and Arizona.

Soon after my arrival in Colorado Springs I was interviewed by the editor of the local newspaper. After she had thoroughly obtained my views about America, about the death of the President, etc., I asked about her background and was not a little surprised to learn that she had immigrated from Karlsruhe[12] fourteen years before. I was even more surprised that my attempt to converse with her in German failed completely. I was involuntarily reminded of the physiologic weakness of women emphasized by Möbius,[13] who feels that they forget their old languages and customs as quickly as they learn new ones. The lady is from Germany and certainly must have attended the excellent school in Karlsruhe! She explained that she had no opportunity to speak German in Colorado Springs, and that it is not necessary for an American editor to read German newspapers or books. (*We think that the author has too easily accepted the superficial theories of Möbius based on this single case, which seems to us rather doubtful in itself. Probably the lady was not really from Germany and had her own reasons not to let herself be interrogated by a German scientist. The Editor [of the Frankfurter Zeitung].*) It was truly reassuring soon thereafter to meet a common old laborer who could not believe that just a month before I had been in his old Württemberg hometown Freudenstadt, which he had left as a boy; he not only retained his language but also his fondness for his old home.

Why do Germans in America so quickly lose their language and their sense of national identity? Observation and exchange of views with experienced men have led me to the following conclusions:

The English language is necessary for success in any business. It is a comfortable instrument, especially the slang common in America, which can be hard even for the British to understand. For most businesses only a small vocabulary is needed. Above all, it is the American school that serves to amalgamate the different kinds of people. The public schools are of course run for American purposes. It is not the job of the state or the communities that maintain the schools to do anything to preserve the German heritage. On the contrary, it is in the interest of the state to Americanize foreign people as quickly as possible. They do not want to conjure up a "German issue" along with the Negro, Chinese, and Mormon issues. We should be grateful that they do not interfere with the establishment of an occasional private German School. However, since the Germans find that they do better if their children are Americanized, they seldom feel the need to replace the free American education with an expensive German School. One does meet German families in America with excellent German education and orientation, who have kept their national identity into the third generation. However, these families have made the sacrifice of sending their children to Germany at a young age to be educated. A further reason why the descendants want to become full-blooded Americans as soon as possible is that if a German tends to mix up English and American words he makes himself an object of ridicule, like the old German caricature of an Englishman.

In spite of this rapid Americanization, the Germans in America constitute an important constituency by their wealth and customs, so that their votes in every election must be considered. They could have much more influence if they had not brought from the old Fatherland the habit of breaking into factions and having petty arguments.

Colorado Springs consists of two parts, a business and residential area, where neither saloons nor factories are allowed, and – just a quarter hour away – a working area with mills and industrial establishments. Because of its proximity to Cripple Creek with its numerous gold, silver, lead, and copper mines there is an active market in mining shares, which attracts a crowd of businessmen and speculators. Its location at over 6000 feet in a shallow depression on the eastern side of the Rocky Mountains has given Colorado Springs the reputation of an American St. Moritz. It has a bracing dry climate, with no rain from September to April, but is visited by dry southwest winds starting at 10:00 A.M., which sometimes develop into gales and stir up an unbelievable amount of fine sandy dust. Despite this, it is thought to allow about 25 days in the month in the open air for patients staying there. In sheltered locations one sees the camps that are common in America: Tents or shacks where entire families live almost in the open air. Since the days are very warm and it seldom snows, it is possible to live this way even in the spring or fall. It is very easy by electric train to make nice excursions to Manitou Springs at the foot of Pikes Peak and the interesting granite and porphyritic gorges of Cheyenne Canyon. In order to reach the picturesque crags of colorful sandstone and red slate called the "Garden of the Gods" and the idyllic property of General Palmer[14] it is necessary to travel over dusty roads by carriage. The return trip across the mesa, upon which are growing resinous smelling thyme and sage, offers beautiful views of the grand shapes of the Rocky Mountains and elegant sunset coloration.

On September 24 after luncheon, we made the journey with the cog railway up the 14,170-foot-high Pikes Peak. The train travels steeply upwards in a wooded gully along a rushing mountain stream that also provides drinking water for Colorado Springs. Everywhere you can see evidence of old forest fires. Charred trunks cover the floor of the new growth, which at lower elevations include stately silver firs and blue spruces, nicely adorned with the red leaves of barberry and sumac. White pines alternate with gold-leafed aspen and cottonwood trees. Halfway up there is a picturesque lodge, from which attractive trails lead into the valley of the wild brook. Higher up you can look across the mountain range, partly visible through the trees, which is covered with broad meadows at the base of which lie two small black alpine lakes in the ancient glacial valleys. In protected locations up to an altitude of 11,000 feet there are still some evergreen trees. The final peak is bare and covered with stone rubble and rises above the surrounding range rather like the Schneekoppe[15] towers over the crest of the Riesengebirge, only enlarged to giant size.

Despite the advanced season of the year, all the mountaintops were still free of snow. The panorama was wonderful, but monotonous across endless brown mountain ranges and forested valleys. The plains were covered with a veil of fog like an endless sea. My wife had symptoms of altitude sickness and urgently needed a cardiotonic, which was available in the signal house ("the highest telegraph station in the world"). I too found the rapid ascent in 2½ hours approximately from the altitude of Zermatt to that of Monte Rosa unpleasant due to increased pulse rate and lightheadedness. This is a good place to study altitude sickness since it is not confounded by any effects of physical exertion during the ascent.

Three railroad routes lead from Colorado Springs over passes of 9-10,000 feet traversing the eastern edge of the American highlands, in the center of which lie the Great Salt Lake and Salt Lake City. Since we had already had poor experiences with the punctuality of American railroads, we chose the main route of the Denver-Rio Grande line through the valley of the Arkansas, which now in the low water of September was about the size of the Nahe at Münster am Stein,[16] through the Royal Gorge, a picturesque rock valley, over the Tennessee Pass (10,440 feet), past Glenwood Springs and Leadville into the once desolate, now sacred land of the Mormons.

The mountains are bare, on the slopes extend small groups of scrubby firs, making a picturesque contrast with the golden colored alder bushes in some of the valleys. On the brown valley floor a few herds of cattle were grazing. As we descended into Utah, we saw the grey wormwood bushes, which are so characteristic of the rocky high plains, especially in Nevada. The broad plain of the Salt Lake was also once covered with the same thin brushwood and was given the name of Deseret (desert)[17] by Brigham Young, when in 1847 he led his Mormons here through wild Indian tribes and over the rocky mountain passes 2000 miles from the bank of the Mississippi.

As we arrived in Salt Lake City at noon on September 27, one hour behind schedule, an autumn rain the day before had cleared the air. The sun shone gently on the happy valley, which has been transformed into a flourishing garden and grain land from an old lake bottom by excellent irrigation systems that draw their water from the Jordan River and Utah Lake (which abounds in fish and reminded Young of the Sea of Galilee). Cows and horses grazed on the stubble fields and beautiful fruit and vegetable gardens surrounded the friendly dwellings. The picturesque mountains surrounding the plain, which were distinctly visible in the clear air, reminded me of the setting of the *campagna romana*,[18] except that the altitude of the Salt Lake at 4,300 feet is much higher and the mountains rise up another 5-6,000 feet. The flat Salt Lake is several kilometers distant from the city, but easy to reach by train and is used extensively for bathing in the summer. It is larger than all the Swiss lakes together, but is gradually shrinking through evaporation, probably because the forests have been cut down. The dry surfaces are gradually becoming desalinated through irrigation and rainfall, are first used for grazing of horses and sheep, and then are cultivated. A sulfur spring in the city center has been used for a large bath house with swimming pools. The surrounding mountains have been increasingly exploited for mining and have delivered a growing yield of precious metals. The ground is fruitful and produces all the crops of southern Germany in excellent quality. The air is stimulating and the winter almost cloudless, with only a few days of snowfall. The people look fresh and healthy. I consider Salt Lake City a much better location for a cure than Colorado Springs, since it has less wind and dust and is not at such a high elevation.

I will only briefly comment on the section of the city that is sacred to the Mormons, about which so much has been written. The Temple, a proud building with six towers of white marble, is difficult to classify architecturally. With its numerous, somewhat round windows it is a mixture of Romanesque design and Israelite temple. The interior is not accessible for non-believers. The Tabernacle, which can be viewed, resembles a giant elliptical circus. The Assembly Hall from the outside gives the impression of an elegant apartment building. The city continues to grow within the large boundaries that B. Young gave it. The broad, well-maintained streets are crossed by electric trains, and mostly planted with pretty trees. The houses were decorated in white and pink from top to bottom. Since McKinley's picture was displayed in all the windows, I thought at first that white and pink might be the Mormon mourning colors. Soon I was instructed that the "Elks," the largest club in the city, was celebrating a week-long festival with exhibits, concerts, parades, and presentations of every kind and that this was the reason why the city was decorated with their colors. At the fairgrounds there was a crowd of people every evening admiring a mighty elk, the symbol of this club, which had been borrowed from some zoo. The main attractions were a dozen well-managed cattle and 20 Indians of the Utah tribe, who risked consumption by dancing in the rather cool evening. The next morning, we saw the Indians sitting self-consciously in the rocking chairs of a Mr. Mehesy from Siebenbürgen,[19] where they were inspecting a large selection of grizzly bear pelts and Indian curiosities for sale by this old Forty-Eighter who had almost lost his life at Waghäusel.[20]

Just an hour by train from Salt Lake City, at the important junction of Ogden, one can connect with the express train that runs from Chicago to San Francisco. 26 hours before departure of the train, I wanted to reserve a drawing room at the Pullman office. I was put off until the following morning and discovered that I could not make a reservation because the connecting train of the Denver-Rio Grande line was several hours late. My request was reported to Ogden by telegraph, and I could see if I could obtain a place there. In fact, both competing lines (Colorado-Midland and Denver-Rio Grande) have extra trains for 150 passengers at the correct hour (1:00 P.M.).

[February 9]

When we went to the Pullman office, the agent said that the express train was also two hours late. He did not know if there would be any places available on it. When the train finally arrived, there was not a single vacant place. The entire company was now deferred to the delayed train of the Denver-Rio Grande line. Nobody knew whether it would be continuing on that day. When this train arrived at 5:00 P.M., we were told it would be held there until 4:00 A.M., when it would be attached to the scheduled passenger train. However, we could obtain places in the sleeping cars, which we were glad to do considering the limited hotel facilities in the little town of Ogden and the early hour of the planned departure. However, it was no great pleasure to spend the night at the station, where the freight trains were very noisy.

The 18-hour involuntary stay in Ogden, which punctual and effective communications could have allowed us to spend more enjoyably in Salt Lake City, gave us the opportunity to study a "rising city" in America: Two perpendicular streets with tall office buildings and electric trains in both directions, which ran for a half hour by small villas and country homes surrounded by gardens. The most handsome houses were the Catholic dormitories for boys and girls. The setting sun imparted a violet color to the nearby mountain ranges, whose peaks were covered with fresh snow, and gilded the Great Salt Lake shining in the distance. Thus, the day squandered by the inept American railroad system ended in a glorious harmony of colors.

Finally, around 8:00 the train headed slowly west, with 200 passengers and no dining car. A crowded train with no dining car in America means a prison with bread and water. The Negro in charge of the so-called buffet was indescribably arrogant in the awareness of his indispensability and was unwilling to make any extra effort even for a generous tip. The occasional railroad station restaurants were dismal cafés, with seating for at most 40-50 people. Those who had no place to sit could not get one of the expensive meals, which consisted of peppered soup, tomatoes, and incredibly tough mutton or roast, followed by pear cake. We were often glad just to get a glass of milk, a cup of coffee, and some bread. I was constantly amazed at the patience with which the Americans tolerate their mistreatment by the great railway companies, and always accept the excuse that 30 years earlier travel in the west was only possible with an oxcart or on horseback. For these pioneers, riding in a Pullman car may represent a great luxury, but for an experienced European who has always heard advertisements and glowing reviews about the unsurpassable American railroads, travel in the American West is a bitter disappointment. One begins to understand why if you ask 100 inhabitants of New York, at least half have been to Europe several times, but hardly one has been to California. Trains in the East leave on time, but always arrive several hours late. Since the different railroad companies generally pay no attention to each other, one can hardly count on an undisturbed continuation with connecting trains, even allowing for the usual delays. It is risky to make side trips, since one may have to wait a day to get back on the main line. The delays result from insufficient supervision at the stations, from the grade crossings, and from the general lack of a second track. Continuing tickets only allow changing trains if one reports to the ticket window on arrival and departure and confirms by signature that he is the same person. Usually, the conductor attaches a printed personal description. The supposed democratic arrangement that all trains have only one class is nothing but a monstrous license for the railroad company to rob the public. The usual sitting cars, which cost more than our Second Class, have very narrow seats with such low backs that you cannot rest your head. If you pay extra for a Pullman car, corresponding to our First Class, you are more comfortable than in our Second Class. But for a long trip, which is the rule in America, the added cost may not be affordable, and if you want a Drawing Room, which corresponds to our Double Coupé sleeping car, you have to pay for three beds. The Americans could learn something from the Russians about how to travel well and inexpensively on the train and be well taken care of.

The American train cars are long and heavy, with six axles, and are generally quieter than ours. The narrow doors at both ends, of which the Negro only opens one, make it difficult to load and unload the car. In a collision like that in Offenbach[21] all the passengers would die as if in a mousetrap. The beds are lengthwise on both sides of the car, and are somewhat wider than our sleeping car beds, but are uncomfortable for dressing and undressing and have no place for handbags. The noise and dust are at least as great as with us, but you notice them less because of the low double windows, which the Negro seldom opens. The abundant water for washing, soap and hand towels, the containers with ice-cold drinking water and a glass in each car, and the restriction of smokers to small smoking areas are some arrangements of the American railroads that are worth emulating. The arrival and departure arrangements for some companies, like the Pennsylvania Railroad in New York, are intelligently organized, but unashamedly expensive like all taxi rides in America; for example, a two-horse carriage from the steamer in Hoboken to the hotel in New York was five dollars. Also, the famous luggage transfer with check-system is complicated and expensive, if one is not traveling with very large trunks. Generally, you must drop off your trunks two hours before departure and only receive them much later at the hotel, which is very disruptive for a short stay. Once we had to wait an entire day for our luggage, and one time a missing piece only appeared two days later.

Once you have left behind the shimmering blue surface of the Great Salt Lake, the train enters the pitiless American desert of Nevada: Arid grey plains with dried-up saltbeds, marl, and gravel, here and there covered with gray sage, wormwood, and yellow asters, brown treeless mountains in the distance, sometimes a few wooden houses with windmill-pumps to water the few cows. On the morning of September 30, we reached the western edge of the American highland, the Sierra Nevada. It was true to its name, since fresh snow covered not only the peaks but also the firs and spruces by the railroad track. The descent would have allowed a beautiful view, if the clever Americans had not encased the entire railroad in wooden sheds for forty miles to protect it from snowstorms. The traveler on the "most beautiful mountain train in the world" sees no more than an ox in a cattle car. Once you are out of the accursed wooden sheds, which fortunately sometimes burn down, a wonderful view briefly opens up from the edge of the lovely wooded valleys out to the fields of California. Soon you see beautiful log houses on the western slopes of the valleys, surrounded by well-tended fruit gardens and vineyards. The vines are grown very low and widely spaced so the plow can loosen the earth between them. After our long famine we obtained a reasonable roast beef and a delicious glass of milk.

From Sacramento, the train followed the clay-colored, navigable river of the same name, passed through a desolate swamp overgrown with reeds, and ran along Suisun Bay, over which the peak of Mt. Diablo completed the horizon. On the giant ferryboat "Solano," the train was carried from Benicia across the Carquinez Strait and continued from Port Costa on the southern shore of San Pablo Bay to Oakland, where we left the train and boarded another ferryboat that took us to San Francisco (with a 4-hour delay and 22 hours later than we had anticipated in Salt Lake City.)

On the way there we had a wonderful view of San Francisco Bay. On the left side, the bright buildings of Columbia University[22] at Berkeley had already appeared. In the west were the picturesque Angel Island, Goat Island,[23] and the fortress of Alcatraz,[24] towered over by the beautifully formed Mount Tamalpais, which is separated by the narrow passage of the

Golden Gate from the southern peninsula covered by the friendly houses of San Francisco.

San Francisco Bay, 100 kilometers long from north to south, could easily harbor all the fleets in the world. The eastern shore of San Francisco is bordered by a row of docks occupied by numerous ships. From the large ferry station, our friends[25] led us to the cable car which took us uphill and down first through the lively Market Street and Sacramento Street and finally to the highest elevation in the city, Lafayette Park.

In the lower city we were most impressed with the activity of the busy population, including numerous Chinese with braided hair, but on the rest of the trip we were surprised by the inviting layout of the streets, planted with dracaena, eucalyptus, pepper bush, and laurel. The two- to three-story houses, mostly built of wood, pleased the eye by their variety of appealing styles and the splendor of their gardens in bloom. The air was fresh as the result of a light autumn rain. A cheerful fireplace in the home of our host warmed our tired limbs. We were already surprised at the contrast between the subtropical vegetation of palms, agave, geraniums, fuchsia, heliotrope, and passion flowers in full bloom – in summer as well as winter – and the need for a warm jacket in the evening and a fireplace in every house. The summer is cool because of the fogs that stream in through the Golden Gate from the cold currents of the Pacific Ocean; in the winter, the same ocean prevents the frost, and the sun and mild rains make this the most pleasant time of year. The moderate climate surprises the visitor not only with the artificially cultivated flowers, but also with the native trees and bushes, cypress, laurel, magnolia, pines, and long-needled firs in the Presidio, which guards the entrance to the Golden Gate and has been transformed into a large botanical garden.

On the day after our arrival, the surgeon-general Dr. Girard led us on a walk through this magnificent park and showed us the fine military hospital, a nicely decorated wooden structure that had been built for the 400 sick and wounded patients transferred to San Francisco from the war in the Philippines. The operating room, kitchen, pantry, and wards were sparkling clean. The diligent care by the nurses bustling confidently to and fro must have made it easier for the patients to forget the rigors of the military campaign. A nice adjoining colony of houses for officers and soldiers were evidence of the comfort that is provided to the American soldier by his government. Of course, the nearby cemetery with numerous white crosses showed that even the best care could not completely hold off the Angels of Death, malaria and dysentery, which claimed more victims than the fatal gunshots of the natives.

While the military hospital was simply a series of one-story barracks connected with covered walkways, and occupied a large surface area, most civilian hospitals in the American cities are tall and massive multi-story buildings, generally founded by private philanthropy or the combined effort of the doctors working there. Even in locations that seem to have ample real estate, the architects prefer to build upward instead of outward. As in the hotels, the transportation is made more efficient by the rapid electric elevators. The operating rooms and supporting areas are often crowded together and sometimes do not allow for sufficient light and air.

As it happens, charitable foundations are abundant in some cities, but completely absent in others, so that some places have an excessive number of the necessary institutions while others lack them. Two universities (Berkeley and Stanford) have been established in the immediate area of San Francisco, which is too many for this region since it is difficult to get enough high-quality teachers and students. The health service in San Francisco, housed in the immense City Hall with its magnificent cupola,[26] is well organized and publishes detailed annual reports. The discovery of some sporadic outbreaks of plague in Chinatown early in 1900 caused some concern and the health officials who identified the plague underwent a lot of rough criticism when they quarantined this area. This was abandoned after several weeks, although there are still cases of plague from time to time among the Chinese and just a few weeks before my visit a White washerwoman had died from it. The official list reported 46 cases of plague between 6 March 1900 and 29 September 1901, of which only one recovered.

The 30-40,000 Chinese in San Francisco live close together in their own section of the city, a Chinese ghetto. The three- to four-story houses have similar façades from the street as the rest of the business district but are different due to their dirtiness, Chinese signs, colorful paper lamps, bizarre woodcarvings of Chinese dragons and gods, and especially their inhabitants. In the main street large shops offer a well-ordered selection of Chinese handicrafts and manufactures. The goldsmiths, watchmakers, and tailors work until late in the night by their flickering oil lamps; the cooks spread a sweet-fatty smell and display an unappetizing selection of smoked and conserved sausages and meats, including suckling pig, dried fish, smoked mussels and snails. The vegetables also make a strange impression, such as strangely shaped melons, pickles, beans, and fruits resembling tomatoes. In the background, a dozen Chinese sat at a round table and expertly used chopsticks to put the steaming food items into small bowls and then into their mouths.

If you visit their houses, you are amazed at the filthiness of the crowded black rooms without windows where they generally spend the night for a dollar a month. The length and breadth of the old rooms are divided into tiny compartments no more than 2 meters long and 1½ meters wide, where the Chinese lie on the floor with their opium pipes and nod briefly when a visitor tosses them a dime. In other huts, they lie in the opium smoke, where they interrupt or finish their otherwise tireless daily work. In front of these dull caves is a walkway, where their unappetizing meal served in iron bowls is being prepared on an open coal stove.

Another interesting feature of Chinatown is the Buddhist temple, colorfully decorated and with several gongs, which you are not allowed to touch so that the gods are not awakened; next to it is a Quaker meeting house, then a meeting hall of the Salvation Army, and finally the Chinese Theater, whose ground floor is full of eagerly attentive Chinese while the foreign guests are placed on the stage right next to the performers. While we were on the stage listening to the long-winded tales of the three actors, of whom one played the role of a woman with a high falsetto voice and little artificial women's shoes, and another carried a primitive hobbyhorse apparently portraying the role of a horse thief, there were gunshots outside in front of the theater. The next morning, we read in the "Chronicle" that an actual event of the "Wild West" had taken place not far from us, in which a Chinese man had been the victim of a revenge killing by an enemy clan.[27] The Chinese strictly maintain their individuality and nationality, even in the melting pot of America. They are prized as irreplaceable house servants, cooks, salespersons, and bootblacks, reliable workers who live completely or partly in Chinatown; when they have done enough work they tend to go back to China and use their passport to send another poor devil to America, since further immigration is not permitted. Even the bodies of Chinese who die are usually returned to China to be buried in their native soil.

Since the Chinese almost exclusively allow only their own doctors to treat them, any sanitary controls are almost impossible. Chinatown is a sanitary danger for San Francisco and the surrounding area. The best evidence for the healthiness of the climate is that even the plague could not produce a real epidemic, even though cases were appearing over an entire year.

[February 12]

Commercial activity has greatly increased in San Francisco due to the war in the Philippines and the disturbances in China.[28] Since uncounted millions of public money flow through the city, it is no surprise that the California salesmen and suppliers have benefitted from overseas military adventures and that the war in the Philippines will not end well.

We made a wonderful excursion through Golden Gate Park to the Cliff House and Sutro Hill. The city created the park out of desolate sand dunes, which ten years ago stretched for three miles to the Pacific Ocean but with extensive irrigation have now been converted into beautiful gardens, with splendid cypress and cedar woods, attractive flowerbeds, ponds with water birds, and enclosures with bison and antelope. The high point of the park for us was the excellent copy of the Weimar Schiller-Goethe Monument on a red granite pedestal donated by the Germans of San Francisco. (*The unveiling was reported at the time in the Frankfurter Zeitung. The Editor.*)

Several times a year, the smooth macadam of the street is sprayed with petroleum instead of water, and thus develops a pleasant dust-free surface. This genuine American method of keeping the streets free of dust has been criticized because it ruins rubber tires and leaves the smell of petroleum for several days. Since rich petroleum deposits were discovered two years ago in southern California, it is replacing coal for burning. In the Cooper Medical College,[29] I was shown a steam kettle apparatus which takes the petroleum from a reservoir through a steam fan into the furnace. The user does not have to do anything except keep the reservoir full. The heating is clean and is said to be 40% more efficient than coal heating.

Golden Gate Park extends to the shore of the Pacific Ocean, where a cliff reaches 100 meters into the roaring waves, on top of which a large restaurant has been built. It is the favorite excursion from San Francisco. An electric and a steam train make numerous trips to transport hundreds of people there to enjoy the waves, the sea lions, and the numerous gulls that inhabit the adjacent cliffs. Nearby is a large bath house with huge swimming pools of heated seawater, which can be inexpensively enjoyed both summer and winter. The neighboring hill has been converted into a zoo decorated with numerous good and bad copies of marble statues. The steam train travels along the edge of the hill bordering the Golden Gate, giving marvelous views across the sea back to the city of San Francisco.

When the cold fog covers the city during the summer, a short trip across the Golden Gate takes the inhabitants into bright sunshine, since the eastern side of the northern peninsula that borders San Francisco Bay is protected by Mount Tamalpais from the cold air currents of the Pacific Ocean. We went there ourselves on October 5, landing in the bay of Sausalito, the site of the California Yacht Club, and took the train to the beautiful Mill Valley. From here a narrow-gauge railway climbs with many turns up the 2500-foot Mount Tamalpais. The view from on top is one of the most beautiful that I have ever seen. To the east is the Bay with picturesque foothills and pretty islands, beyond which are Mount Diablo and further off the blue line of the Sierra Nevada. To the south beyond the Golden Gate the houses of San Francisco disappear into the haze, and to the west[30] the endless Pacific Ocean. This is all bathed in a blue mist that could not be more beautiful even in the Greek islands.

The trip to Monterey in the south was just as rewarding, if somewhat more tiring. It was Sunday, and the few trains were packed with people. We arrived two hours late at 3:00 at the large Hotel Del Monte. This is built of wood in Queen Anne style for 600 guests, situated in the middle of a forest of cypresses and firs, which has been made into a park for a large area around the hotel. Splendid groups of banana trees, Canary Island date palms, and dracaena decorated the protected courtyard of the hotel, along with heliotrope, fuchsia, verbena, and dahlias, among which fluttered numerous butterflies like our Painted Ladies and Hesperia. A large arrangement of cacti, mixed with amaryllis, gladiolus, and California poppies had attracted a hummingbird, who was getting insects from the necks of the flowers. A short walk led to a wonderful avenue of cypress by Monterey Bay, where a large bath house with heated seawater and a flotilla of boats offered a pleasant distraction. A coastal path around the protruding peninsula led thorough a splendid pine woods along the shore, past cliffs inhabited by sea lions, gulls, cormorants, and diving birds, into a picturesque grove of old-growth cypresses. The force of the storm had pressed their tops flat, as if they were trying to shelter on the land. Meter-long pale gray beards of moss swayed from the branches in the wind and enhanced the dark green of the treetops. Many dead trunks stuck up in the air or lay like fallen giants on the ground. Further on, the way led to the Pebble Beach, where agates worn smooth by the waves were being endlessly washed along the shore. In a small hut some Chinese had settled to gather sea mussels (*Haliotis*), whose shells they sell to the traveler for a few cents, while they prepare the contents using sun and smoke as a delicacy for their fellows in Chinatown.

It was difficult to leave such a wonderful place, but we still wanted to visit the famous Yosemite, a deep valley in the Sierras that form the western edge of the American highlands. Unfortunately, there was no direct railway that would cut across from Monterey over the coastal mountains and through the San Joaquin Valley to this National Park. We had to go back to San Francisco and take the ferry to Oakland, followed by a long night journey with a multiple-hour halt in Berenda, to the terminus at Raymond, where the carriage ride into the mountains begins. This became beautiful when we reached the wooded highlands, which displayed all the splendor of an oceanic primeval forest. It consisted mostly of conifers, majestic trunks of the yellow sugar pine (*Pinus ponderosa* and *Lambertiana*) with foot-long cones, and cedars (*Libocedrus*) at the feet of which there was a thick growth of young saplings. Numerous stands of oak added warmth with their yellow-brown foliage, and in the damp valleys the red leaves of the Cornelian cherry (*Cornus florida*) shone brightly in the sun. The undergrowth was formed of evergreen laurel and hazelnut, at higher elevations also rhododendron and azaleas. The mossy covering of our forests was replaced in part by low creeping bushes related to our bearberries or the Christmas roses of Italy. The trunks of numerous giant trees lie undisturbed on the ground, and everywhere you see the traces of repeated forest fires, charred stumps and singed undergrowth, while the tops of the giant trees are still green despite being black on one side. The steep, narrow, and poorly graded road continued upward; twice we went through passes of 6-7,000 feet and descended at a fast gallop in the solidly built stagecoaches pulled by four untiring mountain horses. We spent the first night at Wawona, which lies in the middle of the old forest, has wonderfully refreshing air, and would have rewarded a longer stay.

Wawona is the starting point for Yosemite Valley and also for Mariposa Grove with its giant trees. The road to Yosemite runs by a military camp, constructed of log cabins and tents for about 100 soldiers whose job is to protect the National Park. The narrow road continued with steep turns through wonderful old-growth forest over a 6000-foot mountain to Inspiration Point, which gives an outstanding overview across the deep canyon of the Merced River, which the Indians gave the poetic name "Yosemite" (the great bear). The granite walls climb 1-2,000 meters from the flat bottom of the valley and form mountain peaks partly like domed cathedrals, partly like Gothic towers. Mountain streams, which now in the autumn had little flow, have carved deep channels in the rock walls and created spectacular waterfalls.

The "Bridalveil Falls" was a bit threadbare and the "Virgin's Tears" was just a dark stripe against the cliff, but Yosemite Falls and the Vernal and Nevada Falls were beautifully framed as they plunged vertically over the steep rock walls with white spray. Glacier Point is named for the huge glacier that might have been seen filling the valley here 1000 years ago, like the *Mer de Glace* at Chamonix. Now there were just a few patches of white remaining from the first snowfall of late autumn. To the east a rocky valley forks off and leads on a pretty forest path to Mirror Lake, which is about the size of the *Hintersee* at Berchtesgaden, and reflected the steep cliffs and domes golden in the morning sun; then across the tip of the valley to the Vernal Fall and a well-maintained mule track to the top of the glacier. Yosemite is certainly a wonderful and unique rock valley, but like most of the attractions in America only attained at a high cost in effort and discomfort. You cannot compare it to Chamonix, Zermatt, or the Engadin, because there are no snow-covered peaks, and the mountains are more like the Norwegian granite massifs than the jagged shapes characteristic of our Alps. The Merced River flows through the flat valley floor, with intermittent shallows where the trout like to gather. Occasional fields for a few huts occupied during the summer alternate picturesquely with green meadows and the old forest.

On a walk to Yosemite Falls, at the foot of which I enjoyed seeing a luxuriously blooming scarlet red sage bush, I met three brown-red men from the dwindling Shoshone tribe at the Fresno Camp, who were peacefully cutting wood while their woman[31] sat before their shabby hut and was patching up a pair of old Prussian army trousers, recognizable from their red stripe.

On the way back, the path went over an old glacial moraine with granite walls, which showed traces of erosion. From Artist Point I took a last look at the picturesque valley, whose entrance is guarded by a giant granite dome called El Capitan. We rode back the 25 English miles to Wawona at a rapid gallop and arrived after sunset.

Early in the morning of October 13 we drove to the giant trees; for good reason the Indians had called this wonderful valley "Mariposa Grove" (Butterfly Valley), since numerous butterflies resembling our Silverspots, Painted Ladies, or Camberwell Beauties fluttered in the morning sun on the blossoms of thistles, asters, and labernum. On the way we saw a fire slowly spreading just a few steps from the road in the dry grass and undergrowth. Neither the coachman nor the park rangers who rode by made any move to extinguish the fire, which would have been easy to do at this point with a few shovels of dirt. When we returned, the flames were glowing the same as they had been earlier; we could see that they spread only very slowly with no wind and would only leap to the treetops if they had enough dry brushwood for fuel. The pines and firs we had already seen had been three or four times as large as the greatest trees of our Black Forest, but our first sight of the giant trees far exceeded anything I had ever seen. Just as if a herd of elephants suddenly produced dozens of mammoths, these ancient Wellingtons towered over the giants of the current era of vegetation like the remnants of an antediluvian primeval forest. From a wide gnarly base the red-brown deeply-furrowed trunks reach upward for 100-150 feet before putting out thick branches which project at a right angle, then curve upward with the main trunk like candelabra and extend their bushy crown of needles 300 feet into the sky. John Muir, who knows the most about the giant trees of California, counted 4000 annual rings on a fallen tree with a 25-foot diameter. Trees 30 feet in diameter are not rare, and must be older than the Pyramids of Cheops. Two of these gigantic trees have had tunnels cut to let the road pass through them, so that a four-horse carriage with twelve passengers can gallop through, while the unapproachable treetop remains green, as if unaffected by the puny race of humans who have cut a hole through its base. Almost all the giant trees show signs of charring on the uphill side of their base; some have been struck by lightning and have attempted to replace the fallen crown with picturesque new growth from the side branches. None of these insults can kill these immortal trees. Neither bark beetles nor heart rot ever disturb the red wood of these giants. They reproduce only by seeds, and although they put out enough small hard cones in some years to populate the entire Sierra, you never see saplings by the most traveled paths, which increases the impression of a generation that is dying out. However, Muir maintains that the giant trees have not decreased in the last millennium and that their range has not gotten smaller. In some areas there are plenty of young trees. In addition to the *Wellingtonia* there are also the *Sequoia sempervirens*, which have produced some groves of giant trees in Redwood Canyon at the foot of Tamalpais. With these, numerous sprouts grow up from the roots, and when the old trunk falls due to wood rot, you often can see a circle 15 to 20 feet in diameter bordered by stately young trees that have sprouted from the roots of the old trunk. The giant trees of California are certainly one of the greatest wonders of America, indeed of the world. We cannot overstate our gratitude to the United States that they have taken these under their protection as a national treasure and limit themselves to the rather tasteless practice of labelling the most outstanding examples with the names of American cities, states, and generals.

As we turned our backs on the majestic forest, the sun burned hotly through the dusty chapparal – the thorny thicket that marks the transition to the desolate plain like the *macchia* in Italy. Our coachman, apparently a Spanish-American with sparkling brown eyes and a nice aquiline nose, carried on a charming conversation with the ladies in the carriage, asking them riddles and promising to send them seedlings of the giant trees if they gave him their addresses. As the glowing red sun approached the horizon and the shadows of twilight gave the lonely road an eerie appearance, he told us that the last stagecoach robbery had taken place here the previous year; the bandit had taken all the cash from the gentlemen at gunpoint and apologized to the ladies, when three of the military guards from the National Park rode up smoking cigarettes. The robber let them approach, ordered "hands up," and searched the pockets of these obedient Sons of Mars. After he had taken their valuables, he disappeared without another word into the bushes. It was not like a story of Bret Harte, but was in all the California newspapers and the brave attitude of the park guards was considered appropriate to the situation. We arrived at Raymond tired and covered with dust, where we boarded the Pullman sleeping car and an hour later steamed off to Berenda. We spent the night here in the motionless car, and the next morning the train brought us to Sacramento. The Pullman company uses its sleeping cars in this way as a rolling hotel for a good price.

Sacramento, the capital of California, has a wonderful Capitol Building, whose steps are adorned with a splendid group of marble statues depicting Columbus and Isabella of Castile. Well-maintained parks, shaded avenues of umbrella pines, dracaena, date- and Palmyra palms surround the building. Precisely at one o'clock we boarded the Limited Train, which brought us nonstop to Chicago by way of Nevada, Wyoming, Nebraska, Iowa, and Illinois. We had originally planned to visit Yellowstone Park on the Northern Pacific and to return by the southern route through Los Angeles, Arizona, and New Mexico. But in New York we had heard that the hotels in Yellowstone were already closed by September 15. We had no time or interest in arranging an expedition with tent and cook; we had therefore made the detour to the Great Salt Lake on the way out, but after our unpleasant experiences that I have described with American railroads we decided to return with the one absolutely reliable train. Indeed, we reached Chicago quite punctually on October 17. We continued immediately on the famous Pennsylvania Central Railroad to Washington, where we arrived in the evening of October 18, four hours late, allegedly due to a railroad accident. The trip passed through the famous industrial center of Pittsburgh during the night, and we awoke in the morning in the picturesque, wooded Allegheny Mountains in the Susquehanna Valley. The rail traffic was encumbered by giant freight trains pulling endless cars of coal and coke. The mountains were covered with yellow maples, brown and red oaks, and sumacs. The valleys are similar in many respects to our industrial areas on the Saar.

[February 16]

Washington is a clean, well-designed city, whose broad streets are decorated with trees and at each end offer beautiful perspectives of the monumental buildings or lush parks. The activity on the streets is not like that of New York or Chicago. Thus, Washington is not considered a commercial center. The Capitol with its giant cupola, its large Statuary Hall, and the two wings housing the Senate and the House of Representatives is not only the central point from which all the main streets radiate, but also a worthy representation of the great republic because of its dominant setting and massive appearance. From its large marble terrace, you have an outstanding view over the city, the botanical garden, the great city park adorned with the prominent public buildings and the giant obelisk of white Maryland marble in honor of Washington. The new Library of Congress is an enchanting building. It cost more than 7 million dollars and is designed to hold 5 million volumes, of which 1 million have been collected so far. The reading room is contained in a splendid rotunda adorned with beautiful bronze statues, of which Beethoven is the only German. All the corridors and passages are artistically decorated, which provides an interesting picture of modern American painting and sculpture. The White House, where President Roosevelt just moved in a few days earlier, is in a beautiful garden and seems relatively small compared to the adjoining greenhouses and winter gardens. Toward the southwest of the house are extensive gardens and park grounds, while the War Department is to the west and the Treasury Building with its Corinthian and Doric columns give an excellent setting to the location. Washington has a large Negro and Colored population, which gives its street scenes a unique character. The observer is sometimes especially amused by the brightly adorned Colored beauties and stylish dandies who try to surpass the elegance of the Whites in their top hats and polished shoes.

In the evening, we went to the Columbia Theater, a small but well-appointed house with a very nice appearance. The play was called "The Way of the World," and took place in New York; Central Park, automobile and bicycle, the flirting among four married couples, a child as a necessary evil, ambitious women and men who neglect their families, choice of clothing, all built up a portrayal of modern American life. During the intermission there was some mediocre music. Suddenly, during the playing of some march from the Spanish War, we heard feet stomping, whistles and yells, halloos and cheers. The noise did not abate until a gentleman with a grey moustache went to the front of his box and bowed to the screaming public. A friendly neighbor explained that this was Vice-Admiral Schley, who was under investigation for insubordination at the Battle of Santiago di Cuba. "You will see," he added, "he will win his trial."[32] The slender Admiral conversed earnestly with the ladies and made the impression more of a salon hero than a heroic warrior.

On the way from Washington to New York on October 20 we spent a few hours in Baltimore. Although it was Sunday, colleagues did not mind showing me the extensive hospital facilities of Johns Hopkins University.[33] It is one of the best organized medical schools in America. The original endowment from Hopkins was 3 million dollars, but has been more recently been especially supported by Miss Garrett.[34] The outstanding generosity of American millionaires has no real counterpart in Europe. To be sure, they can more easily make donations because they pay fewer taxes than we do in Germany and because great fortunes can be more quickly accumulated than with us. Since these gifts do not always stem simply from enthusiasm for science, but sometimes are also a not unjustified form of ostentation, so it is understandable that greater emphasis is placed on the external appearances, the reception halls and chapels with ornate stained glass, than on the actual needs of patient care. Thus, I was amazed to find a very poor operating suite at the famous Johns Hopkins Hospital. It was dreadful sight even for a doctor to view the morgue, where during the vacation period of four summer months 300 corpses were being stored at minus 14° C. for the students of the eight medical schools in Baltimore.

The single day that I still had in New York was usefully occupied thanks to my dear friends. I visited the wonderful new St. Luke's Hospital,[35] which is located right next to the superb buildings of Columbia University on a prominent hill by the Hudson. I was particularly interested in the university gymnasium, which, true to the ancient Greek meaning of the word,[36] consists of a giant athletic hall on the upper floor and a huge swimming pool on the lower floor, with baths and showers for the health of the students. I was very interested in two hospitals for cancer patients, the one a large gift of Mrs. Cullum and Mrs. Astor, with monumental construction and all the modern arrangements,[37] the other the New York Skin and Cancer Hospital, a modern inpatient and outpatient facility developed through the voluntary collaborative work of its medical staff.[38]

The hours passed all too quickly, and I regretted that I could devote such limited time to the eastern part of America, for which I have been justly criticized by so many friends. But I had to get back for my lectures on November 1, and I was afraid of imposing on the wonderful hospitality, which can be dangerous to enjoy for too long. So, we boarded the splendid Lloyd steamer *Kaiser Wilhelm der Große* and landed after an excellent crossing of 5 days and 10 hours in Plymouth and a few hours later in Cherbourg.

We had covered 15,000 English miles in 52 days. It may seem senseless to report on a huge country after so brief an exposure. But the trip happened at a very interesting point in time and the first impressions of a strange land are often the most lasting. The contrasts with old Europe are sharpest when you have not yet gotten used to them, and when the journey has required some effort and expense. Any thoughtful person should be extremely interested in keeping the development of this huge land in view and seeing how a masterful people with all the virtues and vices of a young nation creates itself anew from the mixture of all kinds of people. The stream of people that pours into America every year is far greater than in the time of the *Völkerwanderung*,[39] both in numbers and in the distance traveled. The causes are the same: Dissatisfaction with conditions at home, hunger, desire for conquest, a spirit of enterprise, and eagerness for exploration and adventure. Every day, new cities are founded, new lands are settled and growing, faster than during the times of Phoenician or Greek colonization. Americanism quickly assimilates the immigrant, and Germans are not the least of those contributing their strength and refinement. The Americanization of the northern half of the New World can only be compared to the Romanization of the ancient world. Interesting prospects for the future can be considered based on the similarities and also the very different conditions. To the colorful Caucasian mixture with a generous Semitic portion in the large cities can be added in the south the Colored population of several million, which since the abolition of slavery contribute an inexpensive, if not always willing, source of labor. Their equality is only nominal, and creates an embarrassment for the state, which will become stronger as this population becomes more educated and self-aware. An attempt is being made to suppress the Chinese and their immigration. Of the proud original Native Americans, who have only left behind legends and thousands of melodious place names, you only see a few remnants in remote reservations, where they are maintained as rare curiosities by the government like the last American buffaloes in the National Parks.

Original Notes

1. The impressions gathered by the distinguished surgeon of the Ruperto-Carola[40] on his journey through the North American continent last year should be of general interest. Although some of the details are well known, and others have been overtaken by subsequent events, it can still be appreciated as a valuable record of acute observation and objective presentation, especially just now when there is about to be another politically important journey to America.[41] The Editor.

Biographical Sources

Czerny V (edited by Willer W). *Aus meinem Leben*. Heidelberg: Ruperto-Carola, 1967.
Liebermann-Meffert D, Stein HJ, White H. II. Vincenz Czerny (1842-1915): Grand seigneur of oncologic surgery – Life, influence, and work of

the Second Congress President of the ISS/SIC. *World Journal of Surgery* 2000; 24:1589-1598.

Publication Source

Frankfurter Zeitung und Handelsblatt (with the last two words in much smaller type, meaning "and commercial bulletin") was an independent daily newspaper published in Frankfurt. It came under increasing government control starting in 1933 and was finally forced to close in 1943. Today's influential *Frankfurter Allgemeine Zeitung* is not considered a direct successor. Historical issues of the *Frankfurter Zeitung* are available in various libraries and in this case were obtained on microfilm at Harvard University.

Translation Notes

1) September 6, 1901.
2) A park in Paris.
3) Gaius Maecenas (70-8 B.C.) was a patron of the arts under Emperor Augustus.
4) Pavel Tretiakov (1832-1898) was a wealthy Russian art collector who donated his private collection to the state. Despite revolution, war, and political changes, the Tretiakov Gallery is still a major attraction in Moscow.
5) The National Gallery of Art in Washington, D.C., was not founded until 1937.
6) The Légion d'honneur.
7) Theodore Roosevelt actually attended Harvard, not Yale.
8) The mausoleum on the Hudson completed in 1897 and still a major tourist attraction in 1901 was for Ulysses S. Grant, not a general from the Spanish-American War.
9) Paul Wallot (1841-1912) designed the Reichstag building in Berlin. His original plans were repeatedly modified by the Building Commission (and the Kaiser). The glass dome on the rebuilt Reichstag is a popular feature of modern-day Berlin. See Foster N, *Rebuilding the Reichstag*, Woodstock NY 2000.
10) Czerny's autobiography says that "Roswell Park showed me around the new institute supported by the State of New York that

will be dedicated to cancer research." For some reason this was not mentioned in this report.
11) Now the Congress Plaza Hotel.
12) A German city not far from the author's home in Heidelberg.
13) Paul Julius Möbius (1853-1907), grandson of the famous mathematician, was a neurologist who published the controversial book *Über den Physiologischen Schwachsinn des Weibes* (*The Physiologic Feeble-mindedness of Women*) in 1900.
14) William Jackson Palmer (1836-1909) was a principal developer of Colorado Springs, including the Antlers Hotel, Manitou Springs, and Colorado College. His home, Glen Eyrie, can still be visited.
15) The Schneekoppe was at that time the highest mountain in Prussia. Its location is now on the border between Poland and the Czech Republic.
16) Münster am Stein was a spa town on the Nahe river, which flows into the Rhine at Bingen.
17) According to the *Book of Mormon*, "deseret" actually meant "honeybee."
18) The *campagna romana* is the countryside around Rome, a favorite subject of European painters.
19) *Siebenbürgen* (meaning "seven castles") was an area now in central Romania, but then part of the Austro-Hungarian Empire.
20) The Forty-Eighters were those who had fought in the unsuccessful Revolution of 1848, one battle of which occurred in the town of Waghäusel. Many Forty-Eighters fled Germany and emigrated to the United States.
21) The *Railroad Gazette* 1900;32:799 reported on a rear-end collision near Offenbach in Germany that resulted in 9 (later amended to 12) deaths from fire. The train car was a new model "which is entered at the ends like American cars."
22) This must be a misunderstanding. The University of California at Berkeley was never called Columbia University.
23) Now called Yerba Buena Island.
24) The federal penitentiary was not located on Alcatraz until 1934.
25) The author's host in San Francisco was the ophthalmologist Adolph Barkan, who had been his best friend as a university student in Vienna. See *San Francisco Chronicle*, 1 October 1901, p 9, and Barkan H, "Cooper Medical College, founded by Levi Cooper Lane," *Stanford Medical Bulletin* 1954; 12:149-183.
26) The extravagant City Hall collapsed in the earthquake of 1906.

27) "Bullets bring down Yee Kit," *San Francisco Chronicle*, 6 October 1901, p 22.
28) The Boxer Rebellion.
29) A photograph in the Stanford University historical archives (see cover of this volume) documents that the author performed a gastroenterostomy before a large audience at the Cooper Medical College (an institution acquired by Stanford in 1908). It is not clear why he chose to describe the furnace instead.
30) The author actually says "east," but obviously means "west."
31) The author actually uses the English word "squaw," now definitely archaic and generally considered offensive, although it persists in many place names.
32) Admiral Winfield Scott Schley was officially found to have been insubordinate, but was not punished. He appealed the verdict but lost, although he remained a popular hero.
33) The author makes the common mistake of calling it the John Hopkins University.
34) Mary Garrett (1854-1915) endowed the Johns Hopkins Medical School with several conditions, including high standards for admission and graduation, and inclusion of women on the same basis as men.
35) Now the Mount Sinai Morningside Hospital.
36) In German-speaking countries the term *Gymnasium* means a secondary school preparing students for a university education. The original Greek meaning was indeed a place for athletic training.
37) This institution gradually developed into the Memorial Sloan-Kettering Cancer Center.
38) This institution gradually became part of New York University Langone Health.
39) *Völkerwanderung* is the term used by German historians and some others to describe the migration of the Germanic tribes as the Roman Empire declined in Western Europe. Others with a different point of view sometimes use the term "barbarian invasions."
40) The Latin name for the Ruprecht Karl University of Heidelberg, founded 1386.
41) Prince Heinrich, brother of the Kaiser, visited America just after this article was published.

5
Justus Barth (1902)

Justus Barth was born in 1863 in Kristiansand, Norway (until 1905 part of the United Kingdom of Sweden and Norway). He studied medicine at the University of Christiania (renamed Kristiania in 1897 and Oslo in 1925). He first practiced general medicine at the Norwegian resort Hankø Bad, then worked in the Anatomy Department of the university from 1890-1894, resulting in a monograph based on his analysis of skulls from an archeological site. In 1894-95 he spent a year training in obstetrics and gynecology with Max Sänger in Leipzig, Germany, and then opened a private women's clinic in Christiania.

In the summer of 1902, at the age of 39, he traveled to America, and later that year he made the following report.

After returning to Kristiania, he first worked at an obstetrical clinic, and then developed a successful private practice of obstetrics and gynecology. He remained an active outdoorsman until partially disabled by heart disease in the late 1920s. He continued his professional life and artistic interests until his death in 1931.

Spredte indtryk fra en Amerikatur
Norsk Magazin for Lægevidenskaben 1902; 63:333-346

Various impressions from a trip to America
by Justus Barth

Gentlemen!

With the help of a stipend, I had the opportunity this summer to realize a plan that I have long had to travel to America and study a little of American gynecology and surgery.

In the Surgical Association I have already had occasion to mention some of the points that may have more significance to surgeons. This evening, I will allow myself to digress a bit into other questions that may be of more general interest. So, gentlemen, do not expect a scientific lecture here, but just this and that which I encountered on my trip over there.

Here at home, we know very few details about the medical situation in America, and the reports we occasionally get from our Norwegian-American colleagues may be rather one-sided, since the practice of an immigrant Norwegian doctor is not typical in America. I do not think I am wrong to say that our Norwegian colleagues over there have do not have much chance to meet non-immigrant American families – their clientele will be mainly Scandinavians and perhaps Germans, and the dealings our Norwegian colleagues have with the leading American doctors will be rather limited since they have mostly settled in the western states, such as Dakota and Minnesota, where the Scandinavian settlements are most represented. The best-known American doctors, those with an excellent scientific education, are found mainly in the larger cities, especially on the east coast, where there are few Norwegian doctors.

I do not pretend that the few weeks I spent in America allowed me to know America better than the Norwegian doctors who have been working there for years. But since during these weeks I worked exclusively among American doctors, I do think I gained an insight into medical conditions from a different point of view than the usual one of our Norwegian colleagues.

The American is by nature polite and considerate, but if I am not mistaken, he is too nationalistic and considers the immigrant to be somewhat of a parasite. The American doctor – I mean the well-educated one, not the quack or ignoramus – probably also regards the immigrant colleagues with skepticism, and keeps them at a polite distance, as they believe themselves to be superior. And *to a certain extent* they may be correct. It is certainly true that several Scandinavian doctors have achieved the highest scientific positions – here I could mention Hektoen [1] and Fenger in Chicago, for example – but on the other hand in America there is a large number of doctors who are completely up to date, and whose techniques and knowledge are comparable to those of anyone on the other side of the ocean. And it would be strange if that were not the case. It would be strange if America, with all its rich scientific resources, could not produce examples considered among the best of their kind.

I don't know what is actually the common perception of America at home, but what we hear and read in the newspapers about America every day often includes the terms "revolver" or "humbug." Our newspapers like to emphasize this kind of thing. Regarding humbugs, I have no doubt at all that they are widespread among the doctors of America. You get a confirmation of this just by studying the landscape when traveling between New York and Chicago. The most striking observation is the *medical* advertisements. You see huge billboards for "*Omega-oil*," which "cures pain" and all sorts of diseases, but I remember especially "Dr. Pierce's Golden medical discovery," which cures everything from asthma to prolapsed uterus. The advertising posters are the size of a house – most often they literally take up an entire wall or roof of a house or both and can be read from a great distance. And if you read a brochure about these, you get a vivid impression of how the humbug is operated. *Mundus vult decipi*[1] and the Americans *will* have humbugs.

As for the revolver, I never felt it necessary to have something like that. It feels very safe to travel, and in theory I suppose you are better off not having a revolver even if you did encounter robbers, of which there are of course quite a few, for these people would naturally shoot you down faster than you could find your own revolver in your back pocket.

A Norwegian colleague who traveled with me across the Atlantic put his gold coins in his stockings when we got to New York. He must have thought he was a little west of Chicago.

In my opinion, this is just ridiculous if you are not going way out west – I don't understand how you could get robbed on the New York-Chicago train – but my experience is limited, so maybe I shouldn't make this comment – it's just a coincidental digression.

When I say that the common perception of America doesn't go much beyond revolver and humbug – of course, these are the extremes – then I base this also on the surprise expressed by many of my acquaintances when they heard that America was my destination. Was there really anything to learn there? Could the Americans teach *us* something? And so forth.

In fact, you can learn something anywhere if you just keep your eyes open, and it is certainly true that America, which has evolved so brilliantly in many areas, can offer a doctor much that he will not be able to see either in Norway or elsewhere in Europe.

At the big clinics in Europe, we always meet Americans who bring the European teachings home with them. But there are now other social conditions that affect the nation and the doctor.

Obviously, you do not come home from America full of new methods, science is far too international for that, but you can still see different things that have been developed from the sense of practicality that distinguishes the Americans. This mostly applies to instruments and the facilities and management of their hospitals. As far as day-to-day operations, I had the definite impression from the hospitals where I got a little more insight that they are extremely practical and uncomplicated. The most beautiful hospital I saw was the Presbyterian Hospital[2] – a 350-bed institution predominantly constructed of white marble – and here I saw various things that I liked. For example, medication administration in the living rooms, where everything was arranged according to colors: A white patch on the bottle meant 3 times a day, a red one every 2 hours, etc., so it was impossible to make a mistake, and of course the patient's name was written on the bottle.

Most of the hospitals I had the opportunity to visit were themselves exemplary institutions. They are often generously subsidized, and constantly provided with the latest equipment and furnishings – I suppose some excessively rich people like to spend their money *trying out* every new thing. Johns Hopkins Hospital, where I spent most of my time in America, was thus endowed by a single rich man of that name. He gave between 3 and 4 million dollars: about 14 million *kroner*.[3]

The Gynecology Department here had 75 beds. The chief was Prof. Kelly, who had 25 beds at his disposal for private patients – a privilege that I wish our department heads here could also enjoy. In addition to the two Associate Professors, Dr. Cullen and Dr. Russell, there were 7 assistants, all of whom room and board at the hospital; the first assistant, Dr. Hunner, also had some salary. In addition, there were two graphic artists, Mr. Brödel[4] and Mr. Becker, who had the distinction of having illustrated Dr. Kelly's excellent *Gynecology*. These were engaged privately by Dr. Kelly, but the hospital very generously provided them with room and board.

The assistants had a very comfortable time in the hospital. They had large, sunny, well-furnished rooms. In the hospital garden was a large courtyard for tennis and so forth – in the garden, or I should say the park, which was quite large, considerably larger than at the R.-H.,[5] and there were pleasant shady resting places. At mealtimes, they met in a large common dining room with the assistants from the other departments, and the camaraderie was very cordial and pleasant – it was a pleasure to see this. The hospital also had a huge living room with a grand piano, where people gathered for music or other communal entertainment.

I was a very frequent guest at their dining room in the morning between operations and thus had a good opportunity to observe the pleasant tone that prevailed among the young people, among whom there were also some "women doctors." It may perhaps interest our female physicians to hear that their American colleagues were not doing very well. They had the reputation of being conscientious and very good at their profession — they usually pursued some specialty at the hospitals — but when they got into private practice, it was said that they were never very successful. I don't know why that is! It is true that there is no country where women are more protected than in America – in that sense the Americans are a very chivalrous nation – so perhaps this is the psychological explanation why female doctors are not particularly successful in practice – perhaps people are *too* considerate of them and perhaps view them *too* much as the weaker sex.

Johns Hopkins Hospital is a very famous institution in America and Kelly has a very good reputation. Therefore, patients come to him from almost all across America. In any case, it was not rare for patients to come from the Far West, nor was it rare for Kelly to travel west to operate.

Therefore, the case material on the gynecological ward was very abundant – too much for one man, and so the assistants also had a good opportunity to operate. Out of courtesy, I was also invited to operate, and did a Simon-Hegars colpo-perineoplasty[6] and a total vaginal hysterectomy. The assistance was excellent, so the invitation was welcome.

I had the opportunity to see some operative statistics from the department. In the month of May this year they performed 105 gynecological operations, of which 66 were laparotomies – and this I will say – I did not see a single operation where the intervention was unjustified. There was no stretching the diagnoses or indications, everything was serious and distinctly conservative, as I repeatedly was able to observe. On one day I saw the following operations:

1. Vaginal celiotomy for a pelvic abscess.
2. Amputation of cervix with colpoperineorraphy.
3. Ventrofixation of the uterus.
4. Total vaginal hysterectomy – Doyen's method.[7]
5. Total abdominal hysterectomy.

In other words, five major operations, of which four were vaginal or abdominal celiotomies. In between these operations, I saw 3-4 cystoscopies.

Clearly with such material one must have great skill, and therefore it is hardly necessary to mention that Dr. Kelly was the safest and fastest operator I have seen. As a matter of principle, I am not sympathetic to those who operate with a clock in their hands, so to speak, simply trying to keep the time as short as possible. As a rule, it doesn't matter whether an operation lasts 20 or 25 minutes, but it *does* matter whether an operation lasts 1 hour or 2 hours, in that direction time plays a considerable role, and the person who operates fastest, operates best. That is why Kelly stands high in my view, because he was an exceptionally safe and fast operator, who never lost his head and for whom there were never any technical difficulties.[8]

I will not go into specific surgical methods here – as mentioned, I had the opportunity to comment on these in a lecture at the Surgical Association, and they would probably not be of much interest to the majority of those present. I will therefore stick with other topics.

I cannot refrain from talking a little about American hospitality and mentioning my first introduction to Prof. Kelly. I had never met him before, but perhaps 5-6 years ago I had corresponded with him, and he had provided me with an instrument for ureteral catheterization. When I wrote to Kelly about my plans to visit America and asked if he would be working at the time, he replied: I am at home off and on, but when you come, I hope you will go straight to my house and be my guest. This was even greater hospitality than that of the famous old Norwegians. So, when I went to Baltimore I did indeed go straight to Kelly's house. He looked a little surprised when he saw me, and told me later that he had been expecting an elderly gentleman with a grey beard. Well, that came out once. However, Kelly had to travel to Wisconsin the same day for surgery. He had therefore invited some of his assistants and a few other doctors for a little supper. When we had eaten, he said: Go ahead and make yourself comfortable here, my house is open to you, go wherever you want – here is your room with bath, here is my office, where you will find stationery, and here is my library, where I hope you will find what you need. The library was located in a separate building and consisted of several thousand volumes of literature on gynecologic surgery; he had a librarian who was also his private secretary and who was helpful to me in every way.

Then he left, and I was alone in a large 3-story house[9] with a maid and a Negro cook to take care of me. So I lived well and was served a splendid breakfast, lunch, and dinner. The next few days I went over to the hospital. There I found one of the administrators ready and waiting for me, who showed me to the Gynecology Department, where the assistants gave me a hearty welcome that I will never forget. Kelly was gone for 5-6 days. And if it happened that in the morning at the hospital we did not arrange something for the evening, I could be sure that one or the other of the assistants would call me on the telephone. And so I was taken around everywhere in the city, was introduced to clubs, etc. – and as we traveled around, went to restaurants and so forth, I could not even spend 5 cents for a tram ticket; and when this finally became a bit embarrassing for me, and I insisted that now it was my turn to pay, the answer was: "We have the most strict instructions from the Professor not to allow you to pay anything."

So, there I stood and just had to accept it. One fine day, the Acting Professor Cullen, whose work on cancer of the uterus may be familiar to you, comes to me and says: Now we are going up for a walk in the mountains to cool ourselves off a bit. So, we traveled 60-70 miles up into the mountains to a sanatorium that reminded me of Holmenkollen.[10] It was called Buena Vista.[11] And it was indeed nice and cool. We spent a few days up there in lovely surroundings. Again I had no opportunity to pay either for the journey or for the stay.

Allow me to tell you about an observation I made up there which seemed strange on me. There were probably a few hundred people eating together, sitting at 40-50 different tables in a huge dining room. But strangely nobody had a glass of beer or wine. In my naiveté, I asked for a bottle of beer: "It is not served here," was the reply.

I had not understood that it was an abstinence sanatorium. Far from it! But it was not really considered *comme il faut* to drink with food. Whoever wanted to drink was expected to do so in advance in his private room.

Incidentally, there is a lot of drinking in America, especially on the sly. On Sunday morning it was forbidden in some places to serve beer or brandy, but it was never difficult to obtain. On one trip I came to a small town like this, and since it was a hot day I wanted to have a glass of beer. The host said it was forbidden to serve but told me to go down to the cellar. I did so, and came to a door which was closed. When I knocked on the door, it was immediately opened and I entered a saloon where there were a lot of other people calmly drinking their beer, their whiskey, cocktail, or whatever. In other places, I heard you had to go in through a door on which was written "Access prohibited!" then you came to the source. In the bigger cities, you are never far from a saloon, where you can get whatever you want. All in all, America is the land of great contrasts – a lot of drinking and an energetic abstinence movement, immense riches and great poverty, etc. etc. if you want to make comparisons in different areas. However, one thing was quite striking and quite different from what we are used to seeing here: I was out at a public amusement park outside New York called Coney Island. Here there must have been 50,000 people. There were all kinds of amusements, from carousels and roller coasters to theater performances and ballet. Entrance was free everywhere for performances, cinema etc. etc. They figured that you would also sit down and drink your beer – it was the income from beer that supported all the establishments. But among these thousands and thousands of people I did not see a single drunken person. On the whole, I only saw one drunken man in the entire time I was over there – this was quite remarkable!

Anyway, it was not a question of drinking because of the great heat. The first days in New York I walked around with an acquaintance. We had just come from the Atlantic Ocean into this overheated city on the hottest day of the summer. And we naturally went into a saloon and had a cooling glass of beer. But I soon noticed that things were not going well. I felt drowsy, heavy in the head, lethargic, slept poorly, and felt generally unwell. In Baltimore I had hardly any beer or wine, since my host, Dr. Kelly, was an abstainer. Alcoholic beverages were simply not served. And that was fortunate! The people who got sunstroke were usually the ones who drank. And the heat was terrible. In New York over 1000 people died in one week from sunstroke. In Baltimore, which was the hottest city in the United States when I was there, I repeatedly saw both men and horses falling over from sunstroke – they were taken to the shade of a house, given a wet wrap around their heads, and there they lay. Incidentally, the treatment of sunstroke patients was bathing in ice water. If the temperature was above 104° F. = 40° C., they were immediately put into the bath and kept there until the temperature subsided. The temperature was checked every 5 minutes. If the temperature became subnormal, they were given rubs and stimulants. Yes, the heat was bad! For example, when the official temperature at 8:00 A.M. was 105° F. = 40.5° C., then it always rose several degrees by noon. But this was the official temperature at the observatory located at some elevation. Down in the streets between the houses the temperature could be several degrees higher than at the observatory, and there it was rather sultry – between 40 and 50° C. in the shade is pretty warm [2]. Of course, you learned to adjust your suit and went lightly dressed as possible, but the worst was at night in the hot room without any ventilation. Sometimes I had to get up in the middle of the night and get into the bathtub, which fortunately I had nearby; or I took a large sponge, wrung it out in water and put it on my forehead. Then I went back to bed in Adam's costume and without even a sheet over me – you couldn't freeze, since the temperature of the room was higher than the blood temperature. Incidentally, I had no complications from the heat – sometimes I felt a certain sensation of drowsiness and had difficulty keeping my eyes open when I was not busy. I also had a few stomach upsets when I ate too much fruit or drank too much iced tea. This last, however, was my best remedy and I enjoyed it in large quantities. Fairly weak tea with large ice cubes on top, plus sugar and ½ lemon per glass, made an excellent drink, highly intoxicating. Although I would drink about 1½ liters of this at dinner, practically nothing went through the kidneys, everything was sweated out. From a sanitary point of view, it may be doubtful whether iced tea or other ice-cold drinks, lemonades etc. should be recommended. However, they are pleasant, and one must have some kind of liquid to replace the excessive transpiration. It is probably not healthy to drink iced water one moment and then to eat a hot pie – and you can see that the Americans also suffer from this – they have consistently bad teeth and dyspepsia must be very widespread over there. After all, Carlsbad[12] receives a large contingent from America, and the dentists are supposed to be the best in the world.

I have previously mentioned the extreme kindness that Professor Kelly showed me in every way. But it was not enough that he accepted me as a guest in his house and made sure that I got to see everything possible and take part in everything at the hospital; he also took me around on trips into the countryside; I thus assisted him in an operation in a small village, Glen Rock, in Pennsylvania somewhere. But even this was not enough. One fine day he comes to me and says: I have arranged a sporting trip; would you like to join me? We would travel into the country, take a canoe with us, and ride down a river like Indians for a few days, as long as we feel like it – are you in?

This was something that just suited me. We then equipped ourselves for the trip, bought the lightest clothing we could find – we were going to be sitting and paddling in the scorching, tropical sunshine – got some food, and then set off by train with a canoe about 20 feet long. We traveled up to a town, Wilkes-Barre, which is located in the heart of the coal-mining districts of Pennsylvania, and here we put our canoe into the waters of the Susquehanna River, a great stream which arises up in the New England states, and flows into Philadelphia.[13] I can't go into all the details of this trip, which presented such a variety of experiences, but I will briefly mention a few things. We were warned in advance against running the rapids – although that was precisely the highlight of the sport – because the previous year two men from Baltimore had drowned in the same river in the rapids. I myself had no experience in the sport, but I saw that Kelly was already at home here, as we put the canoe on the water and he maneuvered it through the first rapids alone – I saw that he knew what he was doing, and he reassuringly set me up and we headed down the river – an excellent journey with most magnificent varying waves, with indescribably beautiful views, through landscapes that reminded me of Cooper's Indian stories, with riverbanks where the thick woods came right down to the river bank, so that you could only get ashore at certain points where the cattle - or I imagined the wild animals - came down to their watering places. We passed by the town of Rockwell past a stone bridge, said to be the longest in the world with 47 colossal arches;[14] we observed the active animal life, both in the air and in the water: Here flies an osprey, there soars a pair of mighty eagles, here a fish jumps, there a water snake darts, and over there is a river turtle sunning itself on a rock – it plunges with a plop into the water when we cautiously paddle over to catch it. In the evening, when we felt tired and thought we had done enough paddling, we looked for a place to spend the night, and had a selection of all grades, from the rudest village inn to the most luxurious city hotel, which indeed we were fortunate to get for one night. We ate our meals partly on the riverbank, partly at a hotel in some small town, when we had a chance. Everywhere we met friendly people, humorous, cheerful, always keenly interested in our canoeing, which was not common in this part of the country, and always they called out some kind remark or greeting to us as we set off again.

Dr. Kelly, who was a very serious man at home, here became a cheerful, happy sportsman who shouted hurrah when we ran the rapids, and enjoyed himself like a boy – but even here he could be the same serious man as at home, when seriousness was appropriate. I remember clearly the day we had prepared our lunch on the riverbank and were about to eat, when Kelly said: Let us say grace as usual! And then he folded his hands and recited a prayer, while we sat there on the ground in God's natural world – it was a religion that demands respect, that comes from the heart and goes to the heart.

As I said, we had been warned in advance, and we were warned again further down the river about running the rapids – the innkeeper in the hotel where we stayed had almost drowned right by his own house in a rapid. But the river was shallow and seemed relatively harmless, and I trusted in Kelly as an experienced boatman. I sat in the bow; he sat in the stern.

One day we came to a waterfall that consisted of a series of rapids like a terrace.[15] I had butterflies in my stomach as we paddled downstream – but it went well for a couple of the rapids. Suddenly I saw two large rocks in the waterfall. It was impossible to avoid them at the speed we were going. I tried to steer in the middle, into the chute – and it worked – indeed for a moment I was sitting in water, as the wave spilled into the canoe, but we did not capsize, and on we went down the next rapid and the one after that, and then we were through. I turned to tell Kelly: We did well! But when I looked around, he was gone – I was alone in the boat – I had lost him! It alarmed me for a moment, but in the next I saw him sitting up in the waterfall by the two stones at the "Third Cataract," while the foaming wave stood like a fountain around him. Then he pulled himself out, swam for a while, pulled himself through the next rapid and finally down to the bottom rapid, where after several unsuccessful attempts I eventually was able to join him with the canoe. Then we paddled on, but half an hour later Kelly was completely stiff with low back pain, and declared that he could not save himself by swimming, if we happened to capsize; so we paddled over to the shore, and there I had him lie on the warm sand and massaged his back until, to his own great astonishment, he again became supple and relaxed – he gained great respect for "the Swedish massage" after that. He said that up in the waterfall he saw the two rocks I described and thought: Now the canoe will be smashed to pieces! Therefore, he intentionally jumped out to enable me to pass through alone – with excellent results, as you gentlemen have heard. After that we had no further adventures but came home as brown as Indians after a pleasant and memorable trip!

I mentioned that Norwegian-American doctors probably find it difficult to meet real American families. However, if you just have some good introductions, you will get ahead everywhere. I have the definite impression that introductions are important. Any doctor, if he presents his card, can have the opportunity to see the hospitals and their facilities – but I think it will only be in a coldly polite setting.

However, once you have had a good first introduction, then with that assistance you can go on to the next person, who will give you the same cordial reception as the one you came from.

Since I wanted to travel around America a bit, Dr. Kelly wrote to the leading colleagues in the cities where I might go. At home I have a whole collection of letters from America's most famous gynecologists, in response to Kelly's letter of recommendation for the Norwegian doctor. With help of an introduction, I had the opportunity to take a closer look at the Library of Congress in Washington, which is an Italian Renaissance building of white marble that cost the handsome sum of about 24 million kroner. It is estimated to have about 6 million volumes and is furnished with extreme luxury. It has the most beautiful artwork with colored mosaics alternating with oil paintings and the finest sculpture. And all eras and all art forms are represented. Side by side you find a bust of Demosthenes, Goethe, Franklin, Macaulay, or Dante. Then you come to allegories of literature, art, and science, or you find a bronze representation of the art of printing, or the art of writing and history. Americans are the cosmopolitans of the world, despite their tendency to think that America is for Americans – Gentlemen, everyone knows about the Monroe Doctrine![16] However, everywhere you go, you see evidence of their hybrid ancestry. For example: At one of the entrances to Central Park in New York I suddenly encountered Thorvaldsen's well-known self-portrait bust.[17] All nations contribute. – But back to the library, about whose function I had the opportunity gain a little more insight. Everything and everyone is represented here. Colleagues at Johns Hopkins Hospital said that they would make a trip to Washington when they had to do some work. They wrote up their literature at home, then traveled to Washington, and here they could get anything they needed, even if it was quite a small brochure or dissertation, and it would be quickly obtained if it had not been found in advance – and they could buy a round-trip ticket at an office in their own hospital for the moderate price of one dollar.

It is indeed pleasant to work in such conditions!

In New York I was invited to live with Dr. Boldt, a well-known gynecologist. For various reasons I could not make use of this invitation but was a frequent guest in his house and there was no end to his kindness and hospitality.

In Chicago I was kindly received by Dr. Fenger – thanks to Dr. Kelly's letters and his reputation. As you gentlemen know, Prof. Fenger is Danish, and now occupies the university position as a surgeon alongside Senn. Fenger is considered the most scientific surgeon in Chicago, and his knowledge of literature was magnificent. He also keeps up with the Norwegian literature, so it was like being at home.

All in all, American colleagues were exceptionally gracious and accommodating, which I attribute mostly to Kelly's introductions. The work I saw them perform was also completely at the level of what you see in Europe.

I also met some of the Norwegian-American colleagues I have mentioned, and compared with what I have seen before, they seem for the most part to be financially well off. However, there is an undercurrent of homesickness running through their work. From all those I met, I got the impression that their goal was to come home one day, after they have saved enough money for retirement. The psychological explanation for this homesickness is probably that they basically have never adapted to American conditions – they are in a way strangers in the country, and, as I have previously mentioned, this can be further explained because they are almost exclusively working among Scandinavians and have not gained a foothold among Americans who were born here. Their social circles are also very limited – they mainly associate with a few colleagues and the pharmacist – furthermore, they have to associate with a lot of Scandinavians whom they do not like, who are beneath them in terms of education, etc. Compared to the domestic situation that we expect in social relationships, the Americans must feel rather sorry for them – they are longing for the old Norway.

Original Notes

1. Chief of the Institute of Pathologic Anatomy at Rush Medical College, Chicago.
2. An office worker told me that one day he sat in his office in a temperature of 123° F. = 50° C. And he still had to work!

Biographical Sources

F.E.H., "Dr. med Justus Barth," *Norsk Magazin for Lægevidenskaben* 1931; 92:663-664.

Barth J, *Norrønaskaller: Crania antiqua in parte orientali Norvegiae meridionalis inventa,* Christiania, 1896.

Publication Source

The *Norsk Magazin for Lægevidenskaben* (Norwegian Journal of Medical Science) ceased publication in 1938. Digital archived issues are available online through the *Store Norske Lexicon* (Great Norwegian Lexicon).

Translation Notes

1) *Mundus vult decipi, ergo decipiatur*. The world wants to be deceived, so let it be deceived.
2) Now the New York – Presbyterian Hospital.
3) The *krone* (plural *kroner*) was (and still is) the monetary unit of Norway. As stated, it was worth about $0.40 in 1902.
4) See Schultheiss D, Jonas U, "Max Brödel (1870-1941) and Howard A. Kelly (1853-1943) – Urogynecology and the birth of modern medical illustration," *European Journal of Obstetrics & Gynecology*

and Reproductive Biology 1999; 86:113-115.
5) Rikshospitalet, the principal hospital of the Norwegian capital, now part of the University of Oslo.
6) Described by Banga H, "The operation for prolapsus uteri of Simon-Hegar versus that of Bischoff," *American Journal of Obstetrics and Diseases of Women and Children* 1882; 15:554-561.
7) Described by Barbour AHF, "On vaginal hysterectomy by Doyen's method: With six successful cases," *Transactions of the Edinburgh Obstetrical Society* 1897; 22:114-128.
8) Kelly and Barth had both done part of their surgical training with Max Sänger in Leipzig, which may help explain their professional and personal compatibility.
9) Kelly's German wife and their children summered at their elegant second home "Liriodendron" in Bel Air, Maryland. The house is now owned by the county and open to the public.
10) A resort area near Oslo, especially famous for its ski jump.
11) Part of Pen Mar Park, in the mountains on the Pennsylvania-Maryland border. The hotel burned down many years ago, but the park is still there.
12) Famous resort then in the Austro-Hungarian Empire, now Karlovy Vary, Czech Republic.
13) Actually, the Susquehanna arises near Cooperstown, New York (not usually considered part of New England) and flows into Chesapeake Bay, which is essentially its estuary.
14) The Rockville railroad bridge, just north of Harrisburg, had just been completed in early 1902. It is still in use, and is indeed the longest stone masonry arch railroad viaduct ever built.
15) This may have been Conewago Falls, at that time the most notorious rapids on the lower part of the river. It was submerged when the York Haven Dam was built in 1904. See Brubaker J, *Down the Susquehanna to the Chesapeake*, University Park PA, 2002.
16) Following a dispute between Great Britain and Venezuela in 1895, the United States cited the Monroe Doctrine to warn the British and other Europeans not to intervene militarily.
17) Bertel Thorvaldsen was a Danish sculptor. A copy of his self-portrait can still be found near the East 97th Street entrance to Central Park.

6
Francis Munch (1902-1903)

Francis Ernest Munch was born in 1875 in Strassburg, which had been annexed to the German Empire in 1871 along with the rest of Alsace-Lorraine (after the First World War it again became Strasbourg, France). He studied medicine at the University in Strassburg (during which time he spelled his name "Münch"), obtaining his doctoral degree in 1897 with a thesis on the embryology of the external ear. He started a surgical practice in Paris and became an associate editor for the weekly journal *Semaine Médicale*.

In the fall of 1902, at the age of 27, he was sent on a prolonged assignment to America by the journal, and his reports from this tour are given on the following pages.

After his return to Paris, he continued to develop his surgical practice, specializing in ear, nose, and throat surgery, and in 1908 he also became an associate editor for the new *Journal de Chirurgie*. He served with distinction as a medical officer in the French army during the First World War, receiving the *Croix de Guerre* and later the *Legion d'Honneur*.

After the war, he resumed surgical practice and continued as an associate editor of the *Journal de Chirurgie* at least until 1940 (when the journal stopped listing editorial staff on its title page).

He died in 1974.

Lettres d'Amérique
La Semaine Médicale 1902: 22:425-426; 1903: 23:15-16, 33-34, 51-52, 59-60, 74, 90-91, 106-107, 115, 122, 139-140, 146-147, 155-156, 163, 174, 182-183, 192, 202-203, 249-251, 267-268, 296-297, 312-313, 330-331, 338-339, 347-348, 379, 387, 395-396, 411, 420

Letters from America
by Francis Munch

Philadelphia, 12 December 1902

Having left Paris at the end of last August, with an assignment to inform readers of *Semaine Médicale* about current developments of medical science in the United States, I chose as my first stop the city of Boston, the metropolis of New England. The *Harvard University Medical School* of this city has for a long time shared with the *Medical Department* of the *University of Pennsylvania* in Philadelphia the distinction of being the centers of medical culture in the United States. Medical schools have never been rare in this country, where on average there is one doctor for every five hundred inhabitants. But until quite recently, the medical profession here has too often descended to the level of crude empiricism and has been considered mediocre. This reputation was easily explained, not only by the effects of charlatanism but also by the insufficient means of medical education, a situation certainly regrettable, but inevitable in a new country where everything has had to be created under particularly difficult and stressful conditions. We know that considerable growth has occurred in North America during the last twenty or thirty years; along with the progress made in various spheres of human activity, medicine has not failed to keep pace. New centers of medical science have been created, and there is every reason to believe that others will be added to the rapidly growing list. I would like to give my impressions of this daily growth and fruitful activity in the *travel notes* which I will publish in this journal on medical America, of which the present letter is the beginning.

Roentgen rays in therapy

During one of my visits to the *Boston City Hospital* – which is the principal hospital in Boston along with the *Massachusetts General Hospital* – , I had the opportunity to see Dr. Francis H. Williams in the Radiology Department that he leads. Dr. Williams was well prepared for this task as a former student of the *Massachusetts Institute for Technology* [1] and a physician at the Boston City Hospital, and was one of the first in America to take an interest in the therapeutic application of Roentgen rays in medicine. Thanks to his work on this question, he is the undisputed authority on the subject in the United States. I do not intend to speak here of his studies which are widely available in various articles;[1] instead, I will describe some facts about the therapeutic use of Roentgen rays that I observed in his department.

To obtain satisfactory results with Roentgen rays, the choice of the apparatus generating the rays is important. At the hospital, Dr. Williams uses an extremely powerful electrostatic Holtz influence machine; this provides great constancy in the intensity of the light [2], which is very important when it comes to performing a fluoroscopic examination. Indeed, Dr. Williams had originally built his machine for research on the early fluoroscopic diagnosis of pulmonary tuberculosis: we know that in the examination of the thorax, fluoroscopy gives better results than radiography. For the latter, on the other hand, Dr. Williams recognizes that the induction coil has a major advantage over the influence machine, in that it allows the length of the exposure to be reduced.

For the purposes of radiotherapy, he considers the electrostatic machine and the induction coil to be of approximately equal value; in the hospital, he uses exclusively the large electrostatic machine of which we have just spoken.

It is interesting to note that Dr. Williams, despite the thousands of cases subjected to Roentgen rays on his service, has never observed any complications attributable to the effect of these rays. He attributes this result to the precautions which he takes while using the radiographic method. These precautions consist of the following: The tube is enclosed in a box lined with lead; the sheet of lead which forms the cover is perforated with a circular orifice that constitutes a sort of diaphragm from which a pencil-thin beam of active rays escapes. The tube is placed 15 or 20 centimeters from the subject and an aluminum screen is interposed between the tube and the patient down to the floor. In addition, the patient is protected by a screen made of blotting paper and tin sulfide. When treating the face, it is convenient to use a gauze mask coated with white lead.

For radiotherapy, Dr. Williams prefers a low-resistance tube. The sessions last from five to ten minutes depending on the case; they are repeated two or three times a week and continued for a period of time that depends upon the lesion.

Regarding the therapeutic effects of Roentgen rays, I will only briefly mention those obtained in lupus, acne, eczema, psoriasis, etc.; I will pay more attention to those which this method gives in epithelioma of the skin. The treatment is generally curative: The cases shown to me by Dr. Williams – cancroids of the lip and the face – seem absolutely conclusive.

The first effect that is usually noted during the radiographic treatment of a skin cancroid, often from the very first session, is the reduction and then the disappearance of pain. When it is a non-ulcerated tumor, it soon softens; then suppuration sets in, the lesion diminishes in size, and finally only a scar remains, often insignificant in comparison with the initial lesion. In other cases, where the tumor presents as an ulcerated foul-smelling lesion, it suppurates under the influence of radiotherapy, the odor disappears, and the result is the same as in the previous case.

The indications for radiotherapy are not limited to skin cancroids. Any *accessible cancer* may be amenable to this method, whether it is cancer of the tongue, larynx, cervix, or any other area. Even in breast cancer, Dr. Williams believes he can report successes; but on this subject his experiments are still too recent to enable firm conclusions.

Dr. Ellis, whose research I shall mention below, has reported a related experience which is interesting as a physiological experiment. This was an observation of a mammary scirrhous tumor in a forty-five-year-old woman. The breast was covered with a lead shield which had an opening that exposed only the inner half of the tumor. By taking the nipple as a reference point and by delimiting the zone subjected to the cathode rays by a silver nitrate line, it was possible to always place the screen in the same position. However, when the breast was removed after eight sessions of ten minutes each, repeated at two-day intervals, a softening was observed in the half exposed to the Roentgen rays, which on section revealed a cyst filled with sero-purulent fluid. However, the half protected by the lead screen had experienced no such change.

In the evaluation of a new therapeutic method, one certainly cannot be too cautious and must accumulate a great deal of information: In such circumstances, it is often good to be skeptical. This is also the opinion of Dr. M. I. Wilbert, the pharmacist at the *German Hospital*[2] in Philadelphia who is in charge of its radiologic service; Dr. Wilbert is not convinced of the reality of a curative action of the Roentgen rays in cancer; on the other hand, he considers that these rays are capable of rendering real service in cutaneous cancer as an analgesic agent.

On the other hand, Dr. William M. Sweet (of Philadelphia) is convinced of the lasting effectiveness of Roentgen rays in cancers of the skin. He kindly showed me, among other things, photographs from before and after the treatment of a patient suffering from a large epithelioma of the angle of the eye with invasion of the nose and cheek; in this case there was a perfect therapeutic result. The patient had been subjected to eighteen tri-weekly sessions.

A preliminary question had arisen from the start of these therapeutic trials; this was whether the cases treated by the Roentgen rays were truly cancers. It was emphasized that specimens of the tumors had been submitted to the examination of Dr. William T. Councilman, professor of pathological anatomy at Harvard Medical School, or Dr. Frank B. Mallory, assistant professor at the same school, and were confirmed in every case to be epitheliomas.

The macroscopic changes correspond to the histological transformations of the tumor. Dr. A. G. Ellis, assistant chief of autopsies at the *Philadelphia Hospital*,[3] is currently studying this question in the laboratory of Professor W. M. L. Coplin, at the *Jefferson Medical College* in Philadelphia. Dr. Ellis observed relatively pronounced cellular and fibrillar degeneration, sometimes with fatty degeneration. The elastic tissue was always increased, while the number of lymphocytes showed hardly any changes after the treatment. In addition, there is always obliterative endarteritis to a greater or lesser degree in different cases. Moreover, the studies of Dr. Ellis generally prove that when the effect of the Roentgen rays is less apparent than usual there is an epithelioma with advanced keratinization containing numerous Gluge corpuscles.[4]

Even if we accept that radiation therapy is as effective as claimed by its proponents, there is still the question about the permanence of the results. This mode of treatment is still under investigation, too recent in any case to judge the frequency of recurrences. Dr. Williams told me about successes dating back a year. Dr. Sweet's case goes back seven months. But these are still very short follow-up periods in terms of cancer recurrence. Recurrences have sometimes been observed in patients whose treatment had not been completed. It is remarkable, moreover, that even after the cessation of the treatment, the effects continue, and the tumor may disappear completely; effects of this sort would be particularly prone to recidivism. However, even in such cases, it would only be necessary to resume the treatment with the Roentgen rays: The method seems entirely harmless in experienced hands, and nothing prevents application of a new therapeutic trial if the disease recurs.

Before concluding this article, I would like to mention some therapeutic applications of Roentgen rays that I have seen attempted either in Boston or in Philadelphia.

In granular conjunctivitis, Dr. F. L. D. Rust, assistant professor of ophthalmology at *Tufts Medical College* in Boston, has apparently obtained good results by means of radiotherapy; his conclusions are not yet sufficiently firm for me to emphasize them here.

I have mentioned above the analgesic effect of Roentgen rays in cancer. This effect seems to manifest itself also in trigeminal neuralgia. I heard in Philadelphia of very encouraging results obtained in this area. I hasten to add, however, that this is not the standard treatment in Philadelphia for trigeminal neuralgia; indeed, this question will be the subject of a forthcoming letter.

[p. 15]
Baltimore, 28 December 1902

Typhoid fever in some major cities in the United States

It is a commonplace notion that the frequency, as well as the nature, of diseases varies according to the country. The differences observed in this respect between temperate and tropical regions are a striking example of this. However, even between countries located in similar or at least comparable geographical and climatic conditions, such as France and the United States of America, one is surprised at the difference in the characters of certain common affections in the two countries. The frequency and severity of pneumonia in the United States are, from this point of view, very characteristic. Typhoid fever also furnishes a good example of the correctness of this observation; it is difficult to cite exact figures giving an account of this frequency of typhoid[5] in North America. But to give some idea, I will simply point out a fact which struck me at the beginning of my stay in Boston: The service of Dr. Horace D. Arnold, professor at Tufts Medical College in that city and physician at the Boston City Hospital, had *29 typhoid patients* out of 49 patients when I visited him. I might add that in the three American cities whose medical conditions I have studied so far – Boston, Philadelphia, and Baltimore – the situation is the same or worse, and Boston is said to have a fresh water supply meeting all the demands of modern hygiene! A very distinguished colleague from Baltimore, with whom I recently spoke about this epidemiological question, expressed his opinion that the consumption of so-called spring water was at least three times more dangerous in American cities than in Paris, and he was amused at his compatriots who would never drink tap water in Paris for fear of contracting typhoid germs, whereas in their own country they drink without any hesitation water that is certainly much more contaminated with microorganisms.

Treatment of facial neuralgia

I thought it necessary to emphasize these facts, because very often the frequency of a disease in a given country explains the interest which the doctors of that country have in studying it. Also, having seen facial neuralgia among the issues on the agenda in Philadelphia and Baltimore, I had at first thought that this might be explained by a greater frequency of this problem, which would not be surprising since we know that malaria is very common there.[6] However, this is not the case, and facial neuralgia does not seem to be much more frequent here than in France or the rest of Europe; as in France, its origin remains obscure in nine cases out of ten. Thus, we will only consider the treatment of this affliction.

Dr. Charles K. Mills, Clinical Professor of Neurology at the University of Pennsylvania and head of the Neurology Department at the Philadelphia Hospital, treats facial neuralgia with high doses of strychnine; patients in whom this is ineffective or in whom the problem recurs undergo surgical treatment consisting of the section of the sensory root of the Gasserian ganglion. This program, resulting from therapeutic attempts pursued for several years, is implemented as follows:

In a typical case, he starts by giving 2 milligrams of strychnine nitrate twice a day. By increasing the quantity of the drug every day depending on the individual susceptibility of the patient, he arrives at a dose of 15 milligrams per day in about ten days, and may go as high as 30 milligrams if the patient tolerates it. The higher the dose, the better, and it should only be stopped at the maximum amount that the patient can safely take. Once the maximum has been reached, care should be taken not to stop the treatment abruptly, both in order not to provoke acute phenomena of strychnine intoxication and in order to keep the patient, for a prolonged period, under the influence of the therapeutic action. He will then gradually reduce to the initial dose of 4 milligrams per day, and this will complete a first cycle of treatment. It is important to follow this first cycle with several others: The patient, in an average case of *tic douloureux*, must remain under the influence of strychnine for about a year, so that the action of the drug is persistent and puts him at protection from recurrences. One may observe, during the treatment, a certain mithridatism[7] following the prolonged administration of strychnine. It is then possible, in subsequent cycles, to exceed the maximum doses used previously.

When this medical treatment, which corresponds in broad outline to that used by Dr. Dana in New York, does not quickly produce good results, or after initial success is followed by a recurrence, Dr. Mills immediately turns to surgery. This practice is based on the idea that in refractory cases the facial neuralgia arises from a lesion of the Gasserian ganglion. Therefore, this neurologist recommends division of the sensory root of the Gasserian ganglion, which interrupts the nerve conduction between the diseased ganglion and the pain receptors in the brain.

Dr. Mills prefers the osteoplastic method, which enables the large flaps necessary for wide access and also gives much better results than other means of trepanation, with regard to restoration of the region.

Unlike Dr. Mills, Dr. Harvey W. Cushing, "Associate" in Surgery at the Johns Hopkins Medical School in Baltimore, begins with peripheral interventions in cases of neuralgia affecting only one of the branches of the trigeminal; but in recurrent cases, or when all three branches of the fifth nerve are affected from the start, he proceeds to the ablation of the Gasserian ganglion, an operation which I saw him perform once with complete success, in spite of very profuse hemorrhage; in short, by a more radical intervention, he achieved the goal that Dr. Mills aims for, namely a "break in communications" between the brain and the periphery.[8]

In order to access the ganglion, Dr. Cushing at first only made a temporary resection of the zygoma, but now prefers to remove the resected segment completely. Indeed, the atrophy of the masticatory muscles following the destruction of the motor root of the trigeminal – which is inevitable after interventions on the Gasserian ganglion – makes it impossible for the jaws of the operated side to contribute to mastication, which in the long run produces an unsightly prominence of the zygomatic arch if it is preserved; on the contrary, due to the general collapse of the region, the facial asymmetry resulting from the definitive removal of the zygoma is much less apparent.

For the result to be persistent, Dr. Cushing insists on the necessity of a *total extirpation* of the ganglion. In order to ensure ablation *in toto*, he strives to respect the integrity of the ganglion as much as possible during the operation. A histological examination of the specimen is then made: We know that some surgeons have performed an extirpation of a mass with the external appearance of a Gasserian ganglion, but where the histological examination did not demonstrate a single nerve cell.

Despite the current trend toward favoring osteoplastic flaps, Dr. Cushing does not use this procedure, because the trepanation opening can be relatively small due to its low position. Moreover, thanks to this same situation, it is not necessary to elevate the brain very much, an important point, since the cerebral compression, by causing an elevation of the blood pressure, also increases the amount of hemorrhage. This is shown by many recent experiments of Dr. Cushing, the results of which we are now going to describe.

Results found during surgical interventions by the study of blood pressure

When the intracranial pressure is increased, the blood pressure consistently also rises, and always remain higher than the former. In one case where Dr. Cushing had gradually raised the intracranial pressure to 276 millimeters of mercury, he saw the blood pressure rise to 290 millimeters. He considers this increase to be a consequence of anemia of the medulla, which itself results from the high pressure in the cerebrospinal space. It follows from this that any compression exerted on the brain during an intracranial operation will raise the blood pressure and will thus cause more bleeding. These facts demonstrate the inadvisability of temporarily ligating the carotids for an intracranial intervention, as recently recommended by Dr. Crile (see *Semaine Médicale*, 1902, p. 339); it is evident that, in consequence of the bulbar anemia which is its consequence, there will be cerebral compression and abundant hemorrhage. In any case, the practice of temporary ligature of the carotids seems to me very questionable: I will always remember a case from around 1893, where a very experienced doctor, having noticed that simultaneous compression of both carotids produced an attack of Jacksonian epilepsy in one of his patients, repeated the experiment out of interest so often that one day the patient nearly died.

The study of blood pressure can also be useful in other circumstances. We know, in fact, that one of the characteristic features of the condition known as surgical shock is a reduction in blood pressure. By recording the state of this pressure every two minutes during the course of an operation, which is easy using the Riva-Rocci apparatus,[9] one can construct a curve which reflects the variations of this pressure. Dr. Cushing thinks that this graph should replace that of the pulse rate that some surgeons make. He found, in fact, that the blood pressure provides indications on the state of the patient before the pulse rate changes. It is especially in operations on the brain and the abdomen that this method appears useful, by making it possible to detect the condition of the patient at any moment.

Radiography of intracranial tumors

Finally, I would like to describe the application of Roentgen rays to the diagnosis of intracranial tumors in America.

Quite recently, Dr. Church (of Chicago), assisted by Dr. Fuchs, succeeded in obtaining an X-ray showing an image which an operation proved corresponded to a tumor of the cerebellum. For his part, Dr. Mills currently has three observations where he succeeded, with the help of Dr. G. E. Pfahler, in demonstrating by X-ray the location of an intracranial tumor. The first was a large fibrosarcoma which had invaded the parietal lobe and extended over the middle part of the ascending parietal convolution. The second case was an encapsulated spindle-cell sarcoma which was nearly 8 centimeters in diameter. These two patients died a few hours after the intervention. The third observation related to a man operated on for a gumma located in the right motor region; he is currently in good health.

Success in the radiography of an intracranial tumor depends on the duration of the exposure of the plate to the Roentgen rays. An underexposure is as harmful to the good definition of the image as is an overexposure. Under the conditions in which he operates, Dr. Pfahler finds it convenient to place the tube 45 centimeters from the X-ray plate and to run the current for three and a half minutes. The thinning of the cranial vault, common in brain tumors, should to some extent facilitate the success of the procedure. On a test obtained under the desired conditions, we can distinguish the scalp, the two bony tables with the diploë, the frontal and sphenoidal sinuses, the ethmoidal and mastoid cells, the coronal suture, the middle meningeal artery, the contour of the base of the skull, and several sulci which separate the cerebral convolutions.

X-rays are successful in an appreciable number of cases of brain tumors, but not in all, for reasons still undetermined. Cysts and foci of softening, unlike solid or vascular tumors, seem to produce clear areas on radiographic tests.

[p. 33]
New York, 11 January 1903

Diphtheria in Boston and Philadelphia

From the start of my trip to the United States of America, I thought I should not lose sight of certain epidemiological questions on which I hoped to be able to collect interesting facts. In the present letter, I propose to report the information which I was able to obtain concerning diphtheria in Boston and Philadelphia.

For many years, the first of these cities has distinguished itself, on this side of the Atlantic, by the frequency and gravity of diphtheria. However, systematic bacteriologic analyses have been performed only since 1895, so it is only since that time that I could obtain figures accurately expressing the morbidity and mortality from infections due to Löffler's bacillus.[10] In that year – Boston then had a population of about 550,000 – the statistics showed 8 cases of diphtheria per 1,000 inhabitants. In Paris, the same year, there was a proportion of 2 cases per 1,000 inhabitants.

For Boston, the year 1895 was the beginning of a significant improvement from the point of view of sanitary conditions. A special pavilion for infectious diseases was inaugurated that year, as an annex of the Boston City Hospital designated the *South Department* [3]. This department is directed by Dr. John H. McCollom, who kindly showed me around and provided me with some of the information that forms the basis of this article.

One can understand the influence exerted on the sanitary conditions of Boston by the creation of this pavilion if one considers that before the opening of this annex only 10% of the cases of diphtheria were treated in the hospital, whereas since 1895 the proportion of diphtheria cases subjected to nosocomial treatment has gradually risen to more than 50%. Now, it is obvious that in the populous districts of Boston, where diphtheria is most frequent, each patient constitutes a focus of infection from which the disease spreads and radiates, and consequently every diphtheria patient transferred to the hospital removes one of these sources with the dangers it entails. The creation of the *South Department* is one of the factors by which Dr. McCollom explains that in 1899, for example, there were only 5 cases of diphtheria per 1,000 inhabitants in Boston.

Another element to which Dr. McCollom attributes a great deal of importance in this reduction in diphtheria morbidity is the introduction of anti-diphtheria serotherapy. It must be said, however, that in Boston the year 1900 was marked by a considerable recrudescence of diphtheria; this would suggest that the influence of serotherapy on the reduction of diphtheria morbidity in Boston was not as obvious as it might have seemed at first.

The rate of morbidity also seems rather independent of the rate of mortality from diphtheria. The curves that Dr. McCollom has placed before me show a constant decrease in the number of deaths from diphtheria in Boston since 1895. This decline even applies to the year 1900, which was marked by the epidemic that I just mentioned. Diphtheria mortality, in fact, which amounted to 18 deaths per 10,000 inhabitants in 1891, was no more than 5 deaths per 10,000 five years later. Such results are impressive. So, it is no surprise that the man who observed them has a real enthusiasm for the method which he believes to be responsible, and for which he has become a convinced apostle in Boston.

Moreover, Dr. McCollom emphasizes that in serotherapy the serum is not everything: To obtain the desired effect from this means, it is still important to employ it at the appropriate dose, namely the dose needed to curb the disease. It therefore depends on the severity of the infection and varies from patient to patient; it is only reached when the morbid phenomena respond to medication. Generally, Dr. McCollom first injects a dose of serum corresponding to 4,000 antitoxic units [4], a dose which he repeats after six to eight hours, if necessary. In serious cases, he gives the injections of serum more frequently and in larger doses, and it is not uncommon for the same subject to receive from 10,000 to 48,000 units in several frequently repeated sessions. Indeed, this is not the extreme limit for Dr. McCollom; some of his patients have received a total of 80,000 units.

Dr. McCollom's strong faith in the efficacy of diphtheria serum therapy is backed by full and complete confidence in the safety of this therapeutic method. He recognizes that urticaria, eczema, and rheumatoid pains can occur in a certain number of cases after antitoxic injections, but he does not believe that these complications should be considered an obstacle to the use of serotherapy when the patient's life is at stake. He does not attribute to the antitoxic serum the fevers sometimes seen after injection; he maintains that this and other complications, pulmonary for example, may coincide with the injection, but are independent of it. As for albuminuria, Dr. McCollum denies that there is a causal relationship between the serum and nephritis. Having specially examined in this respect 173 cases of diphtheria, he found 99 in which the urinary albumin was absent both before and after the injection of serum; in 33, the quantity of albumin existing before the injection was not modified by it; the use of serotherapy was followed by a reduction in the quantity of albumin in 25 cases; finally, 16 times the albumin appeared or increased after the injection of serum, but since these were serious cases, Dr. McCollom is quite ready to conclude that they were a mere coincidence attributable to an increase in the diphtheria toxin.

The habit of using high doses of antitoxin in diphtheria does seem to be spreading more and more in different countries. I will not speak here of France where the classic data are recorded, among others, in the thesis of Dr. Bayeux. But I will cite England in particular. I remember a clinical lecture given at the *Middlesex Hospital* in London by Dr. William Pasteur, a lesson which I had the opportunity to hear during my stay in London last year. Starting from the principle that the antidiphtheria serum is completely innocuous, Dr. Pasteur thinks that there is no reason for not giving the antitoxin at the outset in high doses. It does sometimes happen that a case, presenting itself initially with all the characteristics of perfect benignity, becomes rapidly aggravated later. If such a patient has been injected from the start with a strong dose of antitoxin, the excess serum acts prophylactically by preventing the more severe phenomena from occurring. Guided by these principles, Dr. Pasteur recommends 6,000 antitoxic units as the normal – or minimum – dose of serum.

I have to say that the chorus of praise for the virtues of anti-diphtheria serum is far from unanimous. Without leaving Europe, one would easily find a number of doctors in Germany who have until now remained skeptical with regard to the efficacy of serotherapy in the treatment of diphtheria. I must admit, however, that on arriving at Philadelphia I hardly expected to find conditions there contrasting so completely with those which had been reported to me in Boston. In the latter city, the evolution of diphtheria epidemics since the advent of anti-diphtheria serotherapy seems to justify the enthusiastic faith of Dr. McCollom, but in the principal city of Pennsylvania the conditions are quite different and likely to leave many doubts.

In Philadelphia, subjects afflicted with infectious diseases are all sent to a special contagious-disease hospital called the *Municipal Hospital*,[11] whose chief physician has for many years been Dr. William M. Welch (who should not be confused with Dr. William H. Welch, Professor of Pathological Anatomy at Johns Hopkins Medical School in Baltimore). I hasten to say that, like Dr. McCollom, Dr. Welch systematically employs high doses of antitoxin, and 6,000 units is a commonly employed initial dose in his department. Despite this, mortality, which was 33% ten years ago, is currently still 20%. We can see that this is far from the brilliant results recorded in Boston where, during the same period of time, the mortality rate fell from 46% to 13.4%. Dr. Welch has remarked, on the other hand, that in Philadelphia the severity of scarlet fever has likewise diminished to some extent during the last few years. We can therefore rightly ask ourselves if this is not one of those attenuations of infectious diseases that we sometimes see and, for lack of being able to give the reason for it, attribute to a "*génie épidémique*,"[12] which is only the observation of a fact and not its explanation.

I will not dwell here on the indications and contraindications of tracheostomy or intubation as practiced in the South Department of Boston City Hospital; intubation is almost exclusively used there. I will add, however, that for Dr. McCollom, the real treatment for diphtheria is neither tracheotomy nor intubation, but the repeated injection of antitoxic serum.

In children who have had to be intubated, it is Dr. McCollom's practice to employ artificial feeding. Alongside rectal feeding, he uses the so-called Casselberry method, where the child is placed on its back, head down, so that the pharynx is on a lower level than the larynx. However, he prefers an esophageal tube. This uses a vulcanized rubber tube, with a *terminal* opening. In accordance with American custom, this tube is gently introduced through the nose. The introduction of food is preceded and followed by a quarter glass of water. The tube must be withdrawn gently, but quickly, otherwise the effort of vomiting can be dangerous, due to the sensitivity of the vagus nerve. The introduction of the tube is not painful; even in children, it is easy the second or third time. Artificial feeding has the advantage of preventing starvation and aspiration pneumonia. Dr. McCollom has also used it successfully in certain cases of post-diphtheria paralysis of the palate.

[p. 51]
New York, 25 January 1903

The treatment of appendicitis in America

So much has been said and written about the treatment of appendicitis that it is difficult, if not impossible, to say anything entirely new or unpublished on this subject. Despite the large number of works devoted to this question, it is still true that in France surgeons are divided into two opposing camps: Some favor an early operation, others proclaim that nothing is more disastrous than hasty intervention. The discussion that has been going on for several months at the *Société de Chirurgie de Paris* bears witness to this divergence of opinions and shows that the question is still evolving. It therefore seemed to me interesting to report on the way in which American surgeons currently view the treatment of appendicitis. Besides, it would be impossible to conceive of a trip devoted to the study of the medical situation in the United States without at least one of the reports that I am responsible for writing being devoted to this affliction, so frequent in this country that it seems to have become truly a "national disease."

It is indeed frequent in America, certainly more frequent than in France. Our American colleagues are very willing to admit that the dietary habits of Americans – hasty ingestion of heavy and indigestible food, often badly prepared and undercooked – may have a lot to do with this.

I will not dwell on what I saw in New York, the city where Dr. McBurney's work originated, as is well known in France, nor in Baltimore where Professor Howard A. Kelly will soon publish a book giving the results of his studies on appendicitis. However, in Boston, where the name of the disease was coined by Dr. Fitz, a physician at Massachusetts General Hospital, we find Dr. Maurice H. Richardson, a surgeon at the same hospital and Assistant Professor at Harvard Medical School, and at Philadelphia Dr. John B. Deaver, surgeon of the German Hospital, both of whom possess considerable authority in the United States on the subject of appendicitis. To show on what vast experience this authority is based, it will suffice to point out that in just one of Dr. Deaver's operating sessions that I observed, I counted 7 cases of appendicitis out of 10 operations performed by this surgeon, and this proportion was not out of the ordinary.

Dr. Deaver believes that the treatment of choice for appendicitis is removal of the diseased organ, performed as soon as possible. It has been said that 80% to 95% of cases can be cured without surgery, using simple medical or expectant treatment. Dr. Deaver only acknowledges this fact as true with respect to a specific attack. However, these recur one or more times in 80% of patients, according to his statistics, so the crisis may resolve without the appendicitis being cured, and one of the subsequent attacks may have a fatal outcome. Indeed, although relapses are less frequent if the first attack was less serious, the benignity of a first attack is not a guarantee of non-recurrence or of the benignity of subsequent attacks. In most cases, the relapse occurs within six months, or at most within a year. The non-operative cure is really definitive only in one-fifth of the patients; therefore the only treatment which is likely to protect the patient from a potentially fatal recurrence is removing the appendix.

From the point of view of when to operate, I must say that American surgeons are almost all of the same opinion: Although some of them give preference to surgery *à froid*,[13] the immense majority advocates and practices early operation as much as possible within the first twenty-four hours, and this radical tendency is accentuated every day. I will add, to clearly show the extent of general agreement in this respect, that the excessive interventionist tendency is even in the process of penetrating very deeply into the opinion of the non-medical public, at least according to certain remarks which have recently been made by a surgeon well placed to know the question thoroughly: It would seem that in America the doctor called to a patient suffering from appendicitis who does not advise immediate intervention runs a great risk to his reputation and his customers. Dr. Joseph Price (of Philadelphia) compares appendicitis to a fire: Just as firefighters are called in not to watch the fire, but to fight it without delay, so appendicitis requires not temporization, but immediate operation.

If the agreement is almost complete to consider immediate appendectomy as the intervention of choice, the reasons which convinced the various surgeons are a little different. Some, like Dr. Richardson, believe that in a case of appendicitis characterized by sudden, spontaneous pain on palpation, with vomiting, abdominal tympany and rapid pulse, there is a lesion to treat according to the same principles as a penetrating gunshot wound, that is, because in both eventualities there is threat of general peritonitis from intestinal perforation. For others, it is the insidious course that the disease often follows, the impossibility of foreseeing the outcome of a case presenting itself even with all the characteristics of benignity, which have made them interventionists. Appendicitis, says Dr. Deaver, is like typhoid fever: You never know how it will develop or how it will end.

When a patient cannot be operated on in the first hours of the crisis – either because the surgeon was called too late, or for any other reason – surgery *à froid* is used; it is interesting to note that the Americans then say that they operate "in the interval between attacks." This phrase shows how deeply rooted the belief in the frequency of recidivism is, for it has thus passed into everyday language.

It is when you see the patient for the first time on the third to fifth day that you might temporize in some cases with relative safety. At this time of the crisis, it is too late for an early intervention, too early for an operation *à froid*. However, even then, Dr. Richardson favors active intervention; however, he takes the greatest care not to break the still weak peritoneal adhesions which are in the process of forming, thus avoiding infection of the major serous cavity. It is appendicitis operated on during this period which provides the worst results; however, surgeons who wait for the formation of pus before deciding to intervene generally operate on cases that have been evolving for three, four, or five days, that is to say in the worst possible conditions.

While considering early intervention as an axiom, Dr. Deaver nevertheless recognizes a certain number of contraindications to it, such as advanced Bright's disease,[14] diabetes, or advanced tuberculosis. He also refuses to operate when, in diffuse septic peritonitis from perforation of the appendix, the patient does not seem able to withstand the intervention.

In cases where the operation is contraindicated, the medical treatment that Dr. Deaver uses consists essentially in the administration of a purgative. This practice would have the effect of relieving the intestine of irritating masses both by their stagnation and by the virulence of the microbes they contain. In addition, the peristaltic movements stimulated by purgation rid the appendix of microbes, fecal concretions, etc., which it may contain. For this purpose, Dr. Deaver prescribes castor oil, which has the advantage of not causing hypersecretion of the intestinal mucosa. However, when the patient cannot tolerate this drug, he replaces it with a saline purgative or preferably with calomel (at a dose of 5 to 10 milligrams repeated every fifteen minutes up to 100 milligrams), along with a little bicarbonate of soda. The purgative can be replaced by an ordinary warm enema with a teaspoonful of turpentine. However, for the purgation to produce its maximum effect, it is important that it be administered as soon as possible and in a dose sufficient to induce one or more abundant stools. A convinced partisan of the purgative in appendicitis, Dr. Deaver is also a resolute opponent of opium, which he accuses of masking the symptoms of the disease. In his opinion, the only beneficial effect of opium in appendicitis is to ease the pain; however, a bowel evacuation obtained with the aid of a purgative would give the same result at much less cost.

Contrary to Dr. Deaver, Dr. Richardson fears the administration of a purgative, because it may provoke vomiting and thus weaken the patient. Also, if the appendix is perforated, the increase in peristaltic movements may flush more infectious material into the peritoneal cavity.

From the point of view of the technique of the operation, which must consist of an appendectomy and not of a simple drainage of an abscess, there is hardly any need to dwell at length here: It is essentially the same in the United States as in France. Most American surgeons use McBurney's transmuscular incision in simple cases without abscess; some make an incision analogous in principle to that of Jalaguier,[15] here called Kammerer. When there is a purulent collection, preference is generally given to an incision – variable depending on the case – leading directly to the purulent focus and providing a sufficient opening by its dimensions.

As for peritoneal adhesions, they are most often respected by the surgeon who sees in them a protective barrier preventing pus from entering the peritoneal space. Dr. Richardson also thinks it is exceptional for cases to have more than one abscess cavity.

In what precedes, I have tried to present the ideas currently prevalent in the United States on the treatment of appendicitis: As we see, the tendencies towards early intervention have only been strengthened and gained ground there. In Europe, meanwhile, an opposite evolution has been taking place; in Germany first, following Dr. Sonnenburg, as Dr. de Quervain showed in this journal (see *Semaine Médicale*, 1900, p. 191), surgery *à froid* has recruited new partisans every day, and in France, Dr. Auguste Broca has defended the same ideas. Contrary opinions have therefore simultaneously emerged in the two hemispheres; I thought it was interesting to point this out.

[p. 59]
New York, 1 February 1903

The treatment of malignant tumors in New York

In this letter I will describe the practice of New York surgeons with respect to the treatment of cancer.

Dr. William Bradley Coley is especially concerned with this question in New York. He is well placed for such a study as a surgeon at the *General Memorial Hospital* (formerly *New York Cancer Hospital*),[16] and has had a particular interest in the therapy of malignant tumors for several years.

The starting point of this surgeon's research was the inoculation of inoperable tumors with virulent cultures of streptococcus. Having observed a few cases of death following the erysipelas thus provoked, Dr. Coley gave up the microbial cultures to inject only their recently prepared toxins, the virulence of which he augments by adding toxins of *Bacillus prodigiosus*.[17] The effectiveness of this treatment seems to depend, in large part, on the histological nature of the tumor. Carcinomas are rarely affected: At most their growth seems retarded by injections of erysipelas toxins. For sarcomas of the spindle-cell variety, the toxins exert a curative action in about half of the cases, whereas sarcomas of the round-cell variety are cured in only about 5% of patients; finally, melanotic sarcoma is even more resistant than epithelioma to the therapy recommended by Dr. Coley.

In general, after a month of ongoing treatment (daily injections), we can judge the results to be expected. If after this lapse of time he does not notice any real improvement in the patient's condition, Dr. Coley thinks there is no advantage in prolonging the experiment and regards the case as beyond the resources of this method. When, on the contrary, the patient derives some benefit from the treatment, the daily injections of toxins in moderate doses are continued until the tumor has entirely disappeared. In a certain number of subjects this cure is complete and definitive, and Dr. Coley has seen some in whom it has been maintained for several years. Sometimes, the recurrence occurs after a relatively long delay; the initial lesion may remain healed, the recurrence being the result of a metastasis.

Among the patients whom Dr. Coley was good enough to show me in his radiotherapy laboratory at the General Memorial Hospital was a young boy with a large osteosarcoma of the thigh. The tumor has almost disappeared, but the patient is beginning to show signs that suggest the existence of lung metastases. It was the same in other cases which Dr. Coley has observed.

Despite the good results that this surgeon has obtained for several years from his method, it still does not seem to him to have stood the test of time enough to replace surgical excision where possible. Thus, Dr. Coley only practices and recommends injection of toxins for recurrences and inoperable tumors.

It is difficult to explain how the toxins affect sarcoma. Dr. Coley believes that it is mainly the character of malignancy of the tumor which is influenced. One of his cases where the cure persisted for several years involved a superficial sarcoma of the buttock which, under the influence of the treatment, was reduced to a nodule recognized as being of a fibrous nature after excision and microscopic examination.

These attempts to treat sarcoma are interesting because radiotherapy, while it seems to have a certain value when it comes to epithelial neoplasms, is not very effective in the treatment of sarcoma. Dr. F. H. Williams (of Boston), whose work on the radiotherapy of cancer I have previously mentioned (see *Semaine Médicale*, 1902, p. 425-426), has little confidence in this method of treating sarcoma.

Dr. Coley has for some time been employing Roentgen rays in conjunction with erysipelas toxins in the treatment of sarcomatous tumors. He has been able to obtain favorable results in some cases of this kind [5]. Indeed, he has seen very extensive or even inoperable sarcomas disappear entirely, as if the tissues were actually melting away, and with a cosmetic result far superior to that which a surgical intervention would have procured. In certain cases, Dr. Coley even believes that he has obtained better effects from the Roentgen rays than from the use of toxins. These are patients in whom the latter had been ineffective, whereas radiotherapy brought about an improvement or a cure.

I add, however, that all New York surgeons do not share Dr. Coley's opinion on the comparative value of these two therapeutic agents. Thus, for example, Dr. Howard Lilienthal, surgeon at the *Mount Sinai Hospital*, has much more confidence in toxins than in Roentgen rays. In this respect, he was kind enough to show me a patient with a large osteosarcoma of the right scapula, which was easy to appreciate by examining a plaster cast taken before the institution of any treatment. Most of this tumor has now disappeared. Although, in this particular case, the toxins and the radiotherapy were employed simultaneously, Dr. Lilienthal believes, based on the results which he has obtained in previous cases, that he can attribute this improvement to the use of the toxins. In order to be sure of the fact, he will interrupt the radiotherapy treatment and only continue the injections of toxins.

From the point of view of the permanence of therapeutic success in cancer radiotherapy, Dr. Coley has so far personally observed five recurrences in cases which he had considered cured. The future will show if, with progress in technique, it is possible to avoid the recurrence of disease, or if in fact the observed cures were simply due to chance.

Dr. Turnure, who created a radiotherapy department at the *Roosevelt Hospital*,[18] affiliated with the *Columbia Medical College* in New York, has also tried Roentgen rays in the treatment of sarcoma. The improvement in his patients was only transient, and after a momentary pause the neoplasm soon resumed its progression. Quite different were the results in cases of epithelial tumors. Superficial epitheliomas, in fact, generally gave him success. In one case, however, in which the cancer of the lip recurred three weeks after extirpation of the tumor, the neoplasm appeared little influenced by the

Roentgen rays. In order to make the treatment more effective, Dr. Turnure increased the duration of the sessions and decreased the distance from the tube. The neoplasm nevertheless continued to progress, and the lower lip soon became the site of an extensive ulcer. In cancer of the tongue, parotid, and breast, Dr. Turnure does not believe in the effectiveness of radiotherapy; most of the patients he has treated in this way have shown no appreciable improvement even after prolonged therapy for several weeks. In a case of breast cancer, the Roentgen rays even seemed to accelerate the neoplastic process and hasten the formation of chest wall cancer. In another case of the same kind, on the contrary, a very superficial recurrence, occurring in the operative scar, disappeared entirely under the influence of the treatment and has not reappeared for four months. I add that Dr. Turnure recognizes the analgesic action of the Roentgen rays, but thinks that this effect is solely due to the psychological effect on the patient due to the novelty of the therapeutic agent in question.

From the above, it can be seen that, in general, surgeons in New York are rather skeptical with regard to the effectiveness of radiotherapy against malignant tumors. After having pointed out, in my first letter, the enthusiasm which reigns in Boston and Philadelphia, it was interesting to contrast it with this skepticism of New York, in order to thus give a complete picture of current ideas about radiotherapy for cancer in the eastern United States.

[p. 74]
Cleveland, 15 February 1903

Surgical treatment of cholelithiasis

In one of my previous letters, I described the principles which guide American surgeons today in the treatment of appendicitis (see *Semaine Médicale*, 1903, p.51); these principles seem, at the present time, to have "crystallized" in a form, if not definitive, at least fairly stable: It seems that the evolution of ideas in this respect has reached a point where it will continue for some time. There is another abdominal condition which seems to arouse at present in the American surgical world an interest equal to that aroused by appendicitis, namely cholelithiasis and its operative treatment.

Better known than appendicitis in its pathology – and for a very long time – this condition has until recent years remained almost exclusively confined to the medical field, and the surgeon has only rarely been called upon to intervene. Now, in the United States, there is a tendency to treat cholelithiasis episodes essentially according to the same principles as acute appendicitis: The question is actually still in the process of evolution and there is not yet a set of definite principles as there is for appendicitis; aggressive interventionists are far from having won unanimous support, as is the case for appendicitis, but there is a powerful movement in favor of operative intervention, and it very clear to an observer that it is currently going through phases analogous in all respects to those for the treatment of appendicitis.

Certainly, we are not yet at the point of taking advantage of any laparotomy to remove the gallbladder incidentally – as I have seen done many times for the appendix – and thus rid the patient of an unnecessary organ that may become a source of danger at some point. It is no less true that the removal of the gallbladder tends more and more to be considered as the operation of choice for all episodes caused by the presence of stones in the extra-hepatic bile ducts.

The reasons which are likely to lead to adopting the principle of surgical intervention in such a case are exactly modeled on those which determine the action to be taken in appendicitis: There too a purely medical treatment, that is to say expectant treatment, sometimes makes it possible to overcome the crisis: But even if the episodes are momentarily averted, there is no cure strictly speaking, since at any moment a new attack can occur, which might be fatal.

Dr. John B. Deaver, surgeon of the German Hospital in Philadelphia, whose practice I have already had occasion to describe with respect to the treatment of appendicitis, is again among the leaders of the movement. This surgeon starts from the point of view that one cannot establish in advance what will be the progress of the disease in a given case, because one is in the presence of a purulent collection contained within an abdominal organ, and that it is never possible to predict what will become of this pus sequestered in a closed space. For each attack which ends favorably, without operative intervention, there are others where everything suggests a benign evolution, but result, like many unfortunate cases of appendicitis, in a perforation of the organ, with generalized purulent peritonitis. To this insecurity, Dr. Deaver opposes the benignity of an operation performed at an opportune moment, a benignity comparable to that of early appendectomy. Thus, he has made it a rule to intervene whenever he had to deal with infectious episodes of the gallbladder.

Moreover, Dr. Deaver is willing to operate on patients in whom it is only a question of purely mechanical episodes, attributable simply to the migration of a calculus. On the one hand, in fact, it may happen that the calculus falls back into the gallbladder, and, on the other hand, it is by no means proven that, once the biliary colic is over, the gallbladder is empty and does not contain any other calculi. In addition, it seems highly probable that large stones do not follow the natural pathways of bile excretion, but are eliminated by an intestinal fistula. To extract the calculus, in such a case, is to protect the patient from the dangers which may result from an ascending infection of the biliary tract; and we know that recovery is exceptional in suppurative cholangitis. The simple migration of the stone can also lead to an obstruction of the bile duct [6].[19] Choledochotomy now does not have as bad a prognosis as it once did, but it nevertheless entails a mortality comparable to that of acute appendicitis with purulent peritonitis.

Dr. Deaver further believes – and this opinion is shared by Dr. Howard Lilienthal, surgeon at Mount Sinai Hospital in New York – that cholelithiasis creates very favorable conditions for the development of cancer of the bile ducts; not to mention hemorrhagic pancreatitis, which Dr. Opie has devoted himself to studying for several years in the pathological anatomy laboratory of the Johns Hopkins Medical School. This disease always has a fatal outcome, and Dr. Opie believes the cause is usually obstruction of the duct of Wirsung by gallstones.

Once the appropriateness of the intervention has been accepted, the proper timing must be established. Here again, American surgeons tend to follow the same course of action for biliary surgery that they have adopted in their operations on the diseased appendix: They advocate an early operation. Intervention at the start of the attack should be safer for the same reasons invoked in appendicitis: The absence of pus in the peritoneal cavity and the ability to avoid subsequent peritoneal adhesions with all the sequelae – pain, obstruction, etc. – that they entail. Although this solution has currently rallied the majority of surgeons, it does not yet have all the votes, in particular the medical votes.

The choice of procedure varies according to the operators. Dr. Deaver considers cholecystectomy to be the standard operation for cholelithiasis and hydrops of the gallbladder; however, when this surgeon encounters an empyema of the gallbladder, he resorts to cholecystostomy, which allows regular drainage of the purulent pocket. This last intervention, which once was used exclusively in biliary surgery, corresponds to opening and draining abscesses of the iliac fossa: In both cases, the operation is incomplete, since it leaves the true focus of the infection intact. This is why Dr. Lilienthal performs cholecystectomy just as he performs appendectomy for appendicitis.

Among the surgeons whose operations I had the opportunity to follow during my travels through the United States, Dr. Lilienthal seemed to me the most radical. Comparing the gallbladder to the appendix as completely as possible, he removes the gallbladder as the operation of choice. From a functional point of view, this excision seems to him an example where any inconvenience due to loss of the physiological role of the gallbladder does not seem important enough to contraindicate cholecystectomy. On the other hand, it eliminates the difficulties resulting from drainage of an infected gallbladder; it also avoids producing adhesions of the gallbladder to the abdominal wall, adhesions which can be the starting point of painful symptoms due to traction on the liver. Cholecystectomy would be the ideal operation whenever one could intervene before the development of cholecystitis, the formation of adhesions, and the appearance of jaundice.

Contrary to Dr. Lilienthal, some American surgeons, including Dr. Deaver, as I have just said, see cholecystectomy as an exceptional operation, rarely indicated.

From the point of view of operative technique, I will simply make a few particular points.

The incision which is always employed here crosses the rectus abdominis muscle; this uniformity contrasts with the multiplicity of incisions in use for appendicitis operations.

In Cleveland, Dr. George W. Crile, surgeon at Lakeside Hospital and St. Alexis Hospital,[20] uses special retractors to expose the deeply located bile ducts. These retractors are wide strips of nickel-plated copper, flexible as desired, somewhat analogous to those used in operations on the brain and the base of the skull; they illuminate the operating field very well, reflecting the light into the depth of the wound.

To avoid the fairly common oozing of blood from the liver, or at least to diminish its intensity, Dr. Deaver usually has his patients take 500 milligrams of calcium chloride, three times a day; if there is postoperative bleeding on the bandages, he will increase the dose of this drug up to 4 grams every four hours.

Finally, I would point out that to bring the edges of the cutaneous wound closer together, Dr. Lilienthal has given up on skin sutures after abdominal surgery: He replaces them with sterilized strips of rubber, about one centimeter wide, covered with an adhesive zinc oxide plaster. The resulting scar is firm and resistant; after a few months it widens, apparently without losing its solidity. This healing process has the advantage of protecting against any complication from infection of the stitches.

[p. 90]
Chicago, 22 February 1903

Operative asepsis in the United States

Since the works of Pasteur, Lister, and the modern school, there is universal agreement on the need to follow the rules of asepsis and antisepsis in any operative intervention. However, the physician who has traveled a little and been able to study *in person* the practice followed in this respect in the different countries, is struck to see that the theoretically immutable principles are applied in a variable way from one country to another; for each country, a certain average is established which can be considered as characteristic of this country.

In support of this viewpoint, I will quote the opinion of a Swiss colleague, who frequented Swiss and German hospitals for many years, then followed the services of Paris for a time, and finally settled in London. In a conversation I had with him in London last year, this doctor, well placed to judge in such a matter, expressed his astonishment at seeing that in Paris the rules of asepsis were less rigorous than with his first teachers, and his further astonishment on his arrival in England to find asepsis in an embryonic phase in Lister's own country [7]. It goes without saying that these are quite general comparisons, and it will suffice to point out hospitals like *St. Thomas' Hospital* and the *London Hospital* to show that, even in London, operative asepsis is not ignored everywhere.

If I emphasize the differences with which antisepsis is handled in the various European countries, it is because it seems to me interesting to indicate the present state of the question in America, or at least in the eastern part of the United States which I have just visited. The four principal centers of the American East are, going from north to south, Boston, New York, Philadelphia, and Baltimore. I will say immediately that in these four cities the rules of asepsis are applied with much greater rigor than in Europe; I would even add that the American surgeon willingly emphasizes questions of operative asepsis; it is a point on which he thinks he is superior to his European colleagues, and he doesn't hesitate to say so!

The first condition to be satisfied in terms of asepsis is to have an operating room that meets the requirements of modern surgery. In this regard, I would first like to note that it is absolutely exceptional in the United States to see an intervention, whatever it may be, carried out in the patient's home. The prejudice against the hospital is as unknown here as it is widespread in the Old World; the first thought that the American has, when he is unwell, is to be transported to a hospital: In addition to a ward service, he knows that he will find there, if he wishes, paying rooms with all the desirable comforts [8].

The operating rooms in most hospitals are nearly all capable of meeting the most stringent requirements. In this connection, I would point out that the habit of having special rooms for aseptic operations, and others for infected patients, is tending more and more to disappear, because of the frequent difficulty of knowing in advance whether a given case falls into one category or the other. The main goal is to make the rooms as easy to clean as possible. Those of Dr. Roswell Park at the *Buffalo General Hospital*, those of Dr. E. Laplace at the *Medico-Chirurgical College* [21] of Philadelphia, for example, are equipped with special devices allowing the whole room to be flooded, simply by opening some water outlets located at its upper part.

On the other hand, more and more attempts are being made to keep accidents requiring emergency surgery away from the hospital. Not only are most hospitals provided with a special service dedicated to these cases, but efforts are currently being made to separate the emergency services completely by assigning them to separate hospitals that are appropriately organized and equipped, and which deserve better than the name of *relief station* that is generally given to them.

One of the precautions to which the greatest importance is attached here is to exclude the nurses responsible for the service of the wards from any involvement in surgical operations. We do not see in the United States, as is done so commonly in France, the ward supervisor coming to "pass the instruments" when we operate on "her" patient. Special nurses are assigned to the operating rooms here. Often – always in large hospitals – a nursing school is attached to the hospital; thus, it is the students of this school who in turn take care of the operating rooms under the constant and effective supervision of a qualified nurse who knows this department thoroughly. It follows that the preparations intended to ensure operative asepsis are carried out with the greatest care, and that the nurse who is responsible for them is a competent person and always the same. It seems like an excellent method.

On the sterilization of instruments, dressings, etc., I have little to say: Sterilization is done essentially in the same way as in Europe, and the devices used for this purpose are original or European models. I will simply mention a process employed in Boston to soften the gauze, which consists in soaking it in a 5% solution of glycerine, before sterilization in a dry oven. I have rarely seen natural sponges used, except in Baltimore by Dr. Howard A. Kelly, Professor of Gynecology at the *Johns Hopkins Medical School*.

Drains of rubber are generally employed [9]: For the abdominal cavity, they frequently use glass tubes surrounded by aseptic or iodoform gauze in the

United States. A form of drain particularly used in Boston and Philadelphia for the drainage of the peritoneum is the *cigarette drain*, consisting of a wick of gauze wrapped in a thin sheet of rubber, as the tobacco in a cigarette is surrounded by a sheet of paper. The advantage of this drain is the ease with which it is removed from the wound without causing any pain. Mainly used for drainage of the abdominal cavity, it is also used in otology, for example by Dr. Fred Jack, otologist at *the Eye and Ear Infirmary* in Boston (a special ward of the *Massachusetts General Hospital* in that city), for the drainage of the mastoid cavities after their trepanation.

For sutures and ligatures, silk is much less widespread here than in Europe; catgut of varying sizes accounts for most of the cost of sutures and ligatures, and if special materials, such as kangaroo tendon or horsehair (the latter in Chicago) enjoy a certain vogue, it seems to me that this is only a local or individual fad. *Crin de Florence* [22] is generally used for suturing the skin, alone or reinforced by a catgut overlock.

In the United States, catgut is commercially delivered completely sterilized, but it is the rule in almost all hospitals to give it a second sterilization. The processes used for this purpose are quite variable and give catguts of very unequal quality. I had the opportunity to note several which seemed to me to meet the two main desiderata in such a matter: Solidity and asepsis of the thread.

At *Boston City Hospital*, the process employed is due to the hospital pharmacist, Mr. Greenleaf R. Tucker. The catgut, rolled up on glass spools, is first immersed for twelve to twenty-four hours in aniline oil, then heated in this liquid at 120° for a quarter of an hour. The coils are then transported in an alcohol bath where they are left for several hours, until the aniline is completely extracted. The material is stored in alcohol with or without added 5% glycerine.

At Philadelphia, the catgut intended for the service of Dr. W. W. Keen, Professor of Surgery at the *Jefferson Medical College*, is prepared in the following manner: One begins by degreasing it by leaving it in ether for forty-eight hours; then it is immersed for a variable time in a solution containing 1 gram of bichloride of mercury for 150 grams of alcohol at 95°, and acidified by the addition of 5 grams of tartaric acid. The duration of the stay of the catgut in this antiseptic differs according to the gauge of the thread: The fine catgut is maintained there from five to seven minutes, the average catgut from ten minutes to a quarter of an hour, the strongest catgut from twenty to thirty minutes; the thread is then preserved in 95% alcohol to which is added one drop of a one-thirtieth solution of palladium chloride per 125 grams of liquid; it is important not to exceed this proportion, in order to avoid the formation of a precipitate which would entrain all of the palladium. This mode of sterilization seemed to me to give a remarkably solid and flexible catgut.

The following procedure, to which Dr. N. Senn, professor of surgery at the *Rush Medical College* of Chicago, has used for some time, is distinguished by its simplicity; the catgut which it furnishes is also very strong, although it seemed to me less strong than that which is sterilized by Dr. Keen's process. Dr. Senn's process consists of simply immersing the catgut, wound on glass coils, in a solution containing 1% iodine and adding a little potassium iodide; after remaining eight days in this liquid, the catgut is ready to use; according to Dr. Senn's experiments, it no longer contains any pyogenic germs.

The preparation of the patient and the asepsis of the surgeon and his assistants take place here essentially under the same conditions as in France. Since a long discussion about operating gloves took place at the *Société de Chirurgie de Paris* in 1900 – a discussion reported in this journal – I will say a few words on this topic. From what I have seen so far, the use of rubber gloves, both for the surgeon and for his assistants, is quite universal in the United States; it is unusual to see an operation performed without the hands being protected in this way. To show the confidence that American surgeons have in this precaution, I will relate the opinion of Dr. George E. Brewer, Assistant Professor of Surgery at the *Columbia Medical College* in New York: This surgeon believes that the rubber gloves have enabled him to gradually reduce from 40% to 5 or 6% the proportion of post-operative infections in his department at the *City Hospital* of Blackwell Island,[23] one of the two large municipal hospitals in New York.

[p. 106]
Chicago, 8 March 1903

Typhoid fever in the United States

In an earlier letter, I already mentioned the considerable frequency of typhoid fever in the United States (see *Semaine Médicale*, 1903, p. 15). I was judging then from what I had seen in Boston, Philadelphia, and Baltimore, and I can now add that in New York it is much the same as in these three other cities. I was curious to know what situation I would find after leaving the coast of the Atlantic Ocean and heading towards the interior of the continent. Well, I must say that the hygienic conditions there are even more deplorable than in the American East: In the hospitals of Buffalo, Cleveland, and Chicago, it is no longer just rows of beds that are occupied by typhoid patients, entire wards and entire departments are devoted to them. It should also be noted that I visited Buffalo, Cleveland, and Chicago in February and March, that is to say at the time of year when cases of typhoid fever are least numerous, whereas I was in Boston and Philadelphia at the very moment of the autumn upsurge which each year marks the peak of the epidemic [10].

We can imagine the extreme care with which the Anglo-Saxon installs and supervises everything that comes within the purview of the plumber (which he calls the *plumbing*) – indeed everything in his home having to do with hygiene – so this great frequency of typhoid fever is an unexpected finding. Therefore, it seemed interesting to discover what could be the origin of such excessive morbidity. In the following lines, I will record the observations that I made in this regard and the information that was provided to me by various American colleagues.

First of all, it seems obvious that the nature of the drinking water plays the greatest role in the frequency of typhoid fever. This is a consideration not only when we draw a parallel between the state of things in America to that which prevails in the principal European cities, but also when we compare American cities with each other.

In this respect, we can divide the urban areas of the United States into two groups (I am currently only considering the American cities that I have just mentioned, since they are the only ones that I have visited so far and of which I know the situation *firsthand*): The first group includes the cities which are spread out along the Atlantic Coast – Boston, New York, Philadelphia, and Baltimore; the second, the cities on the Great Lakes, namely Buffalo, Cleveland, and Chicago.

The former draw their drinking water from the rivers by which they are located, and it is easy to imagine that this water might be contaminated because of habitations located upstream. The towns classified in the second group, on the contrary, draw their drinking water from the Great Lakes by which they are built. This seems to be a process infinitely superior to the previous one, because these lakes are, by their size, truly small inland seas: Lake Michigan, for example, on the shores of which Chicago is located, measures 580 kilometers long by 175 kilometers wide, and its depth reaches 275 meters. It is therefore likely that by moving far enough from the shore, drinking water would be found which could in practice be considered pure, for it is difficult to imagine that shipping on these lakes, as active as it is supposed to be, could appreciably contaminate such an immense quantity of water.

The fact is that the various water intakes that Chicago has successively established on Lake Michigan, after having been originally placed at 1,500 meters from the shore, have gradually been pushed back to nearly 7 kilometers. This distance would probably have been sufficient if the lake, in addition to supplying the town with drinking water, was not at the same time the outlet for contaminated water. It was nice work, and a credit to those who knew how to do it, to reverse the course of the little Chicago River, which gave its name to the city it flows through – a real American Bièvre[24] which is little more than an open sewer – so that the lake currently flows into it instead of receiving it. However, other sewers still exist which empty into the lake, and when certain winds prevail, the water from these sewers is driven into the water intakes which supply the city, and immediately the municipal pipes fill with sewage water. Since these winds prevail on average one day out of six, it can be said that the water supplied for consumption to Chicago's two million inhabitants is simply sewage water at least one day a week.

This being the case, it is a rule that samples are taken daily from the various water intakes in the lake and that they are subjected to immediate bacteriologic analyses. Given the time needed for the water to reach the outlet to the consumer's tap, there is time to warn the population of the need to boil and filter the water supplied to them. Such, at least, is the theory; but, in practice, one can wonder whether the frequent repetition of the fact is not of a nature to provoke an indifference within the population, resulting from a sort of habituation to danger. Dr. W. K. Jaques, who is in charge of the water surveillance service at the Chicago City Hall, and who was good enough to show me the functioning of this service, does not himself seem very convinced that the periodical notices which he is required to publish are effective. Moreover, it is difficult to imagine that the pathogenic germs disappear from the water pipes as soon as the sewage water no longer enters them: It is likely that the water remains polluted for several days and one must fear that it will never be as pure as it should be.

Having taken Chicago as an example, I find it hardly useful to go into details about Buffalo, Cleveland, or other towns on the lakes. The conditions there are essentially the same: The sewers contaminate the lakes from which these cities are supplied with drinking water.

Another question is whether it is possible to prevent water pollution, or whether it is better to purify it [11]. This is the second solution adopted by all the American cities that have made attempts in this area. Boston has built huge sand filters through which water passes before being delivered for consumption; Philadelphia is doing the same; the city of Albany, located on the Hudson upstream from New York, has seen its mortality from typhoid fever drop very low since its drinking water has been filtered through sandbars before passing through the municipal pipes.

Since typhoid fever is very common in the United States, as I have just shown, one might suppose that the treatment of this disease constitutes an important question there. However, this subject is far from being high on the agenda and arousing the same interest as appendicitis or gallbladder disease. It is among the matters least discussed at the moment on this side of the Atlantic; in general, we agree on the fundamental point, namely the necessity of hydrotherapeutic treatment; as for the way in which this is applied, it sometimes differs from one doctor to another, but especially from one hospital to another. I have even found here, in the matter of hydrotherapy of typhoid fever, more variety than in any of the other countries which I have previously visited.

Accustomed to seeing typhoid patients treated in Europe with baths at a temperature of 18° to 32°, I was not a little surprised to notice, during my visit to London last year, that the bath was not in common use in this city for the treatment of typhoid fever. According to my personal observations, as well as according to the information provided to me by Dr. Lees, physician of *St. Mary's Hospital* and of the *Great Ormond Street Hospital* in London, the bath is only used in one of the twelve major London hospitals, namely at *Middlesex Hospital*. In other hospitals, it is replaced by cold lotions, which are considered easier to practice and just as effective.

I found a similar idea in Boston: There too bathing is considered inconvenient. Here also, in mild cases, it is replaced by cold lotions repeated every three or four hours. In moderate or serious cases, they use a procedure which seemed to me original enough to deserve reporting here in some detail, such as I have seen it applied in the service of Dr. H. Arnold, physician at *Boston City Hospital*. The patient is completely undressed and wrapped in gauze previously soaked in very hot water, at a temperature higher than that of the body, i.e. approximately 40° C. The patient is stretched out on his bed with his wet wrap, and a nurse creates a current of air using a fan which she directs to the immediate vicinity of the subject; the rapid evaporation which is thus determined is so intense that the temperature gradually falls by several degrees. This is the "fan treatment." This being the case, and given the large number of typhoid patients, a process based on the same principle was soon developed that enabled "work on a large scale," using a mechanical device. Everybody knows this little 4-wing propeller driven by electricity, called an *electric fan* in English, that is used to create a current of air in overheated rooms. As you might imagine, to pass from the hand fan to the electric fan there was only a small step, and this step was quickly taken in the manufacturing country *par excellence* which is the United States; therefore at present, when typhoid patients are numerous in a hospital ward in Boston, they are prepared as just described, by wrapping them in very hot wet gauze, and then an electric fan is placed in such a way that the beds are in its ventilation zone, and the device is operated. By this means, a drop in temperature of 1° to 1.5° is obtained.

The fan treatment is unique to Boston; I have not seen it employed in any other American city. In Philadelphia, as in Boston, lotions are used only in mild cases. Thus Dr. John H. Musser, professor of clinical medicine at the University of Pennsylvania, and physician of the *Philadelphia Hospital* and of the *Presbyterian Hospital*, never gives lotions when the temperature exceeds 39.5°; then he always uses baths, which he believes to be much more effective and as simple to administer as lotions. Such is also the practice of most other physicians in Philadelphia, as well as that which Professor Osler follows in his department at the *Johns Hopkins Hospital* in Baltimore. As for the temperature of the bath, there is general agreement to gradually reduce it from one bath to another, the first being around 30° and the following being cooled according to the individual susceptibility of the patient.

In closing, I would like to point out that the epidemics of typhoid observed in the United States vary considerably in their character. For example, during the epidemics of recent years, diarrhea has become an increasingly rare symptom and, in the current epidemic, constipation is the rule. Similarly, decubiti are now rare. Moreover, morbidity and mortality seem to follow fairly independent curves: This is how, during the epidemic observed this year in Philadelphia, mortality remained low despite high morbidity, according to what Dr. Musser told me, while last year "the patients were dropping like flies." Finally, it is appropriate to mention the particular characteristics which the affliction assumes according to the origin of the patient: In subjects of Italian origin, splenomegaly is always much more considerable and slower to resolve than in other patients; it is quite possible that, in these cases, we are dealing with a diseased organ due to a previous malarial infection and, for this reason, reacting in a different way to the Eberthian bacillus.[25]

[p. 115]
Chicago, 15 March 1903

Radiation Therapy in Chicago

On several occasions already I have drawn attention to the interest aroused in the United States by the therapeutic applications of the Roentgen rays: There is hardly a town of any importance which does not have its radiotherapy laboratory. It seems, however, that this mode of treatment is especially favored in three centers, which are Boston, Philadelphia, and Chicago; in New York, on the contrary, this method is used less, as I have described in connection with the treatment of malignant tumors as it is practiced in that city. To complete the information previously furnished on Boston and Philadelphia, I will now set forth what I learned on this subject in Chicago, particularly from the information kindly supplied to me by Dr. W. Allen Pusey, who abandoned dermatology for radiotherapy three years ago and who is currently preparing a book on this subject.[26]

From a technical point of view, I will only point out that Dr. Pusey takes his electric power from the industrial current distributed in Chicago for lighting. He usually converts it into a low voltage current (about 35 volts); rarely he uses a voltage of 110 volts.

In the case of cancroid, for example an epithelioma of the lip, the surgeon's scalpel is often as effective as the Roentgen rays. But the superiority of the rays is apparent for skin cancers which have become inoperable due to their size. Dr. Pusey was kind enough to show me, among other things, the records of a large epithelioma that had invaded the skin over the entire extent of the forehead and the eyelids, as well as the greater part of the nose, and had caused the destruction of the left eye. It was one of those inoperable cases which, euphemistically, the official statistics of Great Britain still designate at the present time under the name of rodent ulcer, and which are actually just well-differentiated epitheliomas of the skin. As evidenced by a series of photographs taken during the course of the treatment, this vast ulcer, under the influence of the Roentgen rays, rapidly desiccated; after four months, it has now been entirely replaced by skin, thin and fragile to be sure, but healthy and of good quality. The treatment will be continued to avoid recurrence.

Despite these brilliant results, we cannot, of course, consider radiotherapy as a panacea. It even seems that if the first attempts made in this direction did not attract much attention, it is partly due to the fact that their authors somewhat exaggerated the value of the method. Hence, as a reaction in the opposite direction, an effort has been made to establish, with particular care, the restrictions that must be applied in the indications for radiation therapy. With this in mind, Dr. Pusey insists on the uselessness of radiotherapy in deeply located cancers, such as stomach cancer. He does not even believe in its effectiveness for all epitheliomas classified among so-called accessible cancers; in cancer of the uterus, for example, he has never obtained definite improvement by radiation; only the pain seemed to be influenced. However, when the patients are seen early enough for the surgical operation to be carried out successfully, Dr. Pusey is at present trying radiotherapeutic applications with a view to combatting recurrences in the vaginal scar.

In breast cancer, on the other hand, radiotherapy seems likely to provide results, if not absolutely regular and constant, at least very satisfactory, even in inoperable cases. Several Chicago surgeons, notably Doctors A. J. Ochsner, surgeon at the *Augustana Hospital*,[27] and L. L. McArthur, surgeon at *St. Luke's Hospital*,[28] routinely submit their patients to prolonged radiotherapy treatment after the removal of the cancerous breast and axillary dissection, with the aim of thus protecting them from a later recurrence. In this respect, it is interesting to note that the cathode rays exert *no* action on metastases in the lymph nodes or elsewhere. It is also because of metastases that these patients sometimes die, especially from spinal metastases.

As a corollary to the information given on New York, I will add that, in the treatment of sarcoma, I have seen several very good results obtained by Dr. Pusey.

We hear relatively little about radiotherapy for tuberculosis of the skin in the United States. The reason is, according to what Dr. Pusey told me, that lupus – lupus vulgaris even more than lupus erythematosus – constitutes in this country a disease that we rarely see in Europe. This is a point of medical geography for which I have been unable to find a plausible explanation.

In the different forms of leukemia, it would also seem that radiotherapy could render service, to judge by the successes which this method has given to Dr. Pusey. Dr. Nicholas Senn, professor of surgery at *Rush Medical College*, University of Chicago, and surgeon at the *Presbyterian Hospital*,[29] also reportedly saw complete recovery in a very advanced case of Hodgkin's Disease.

Dr. Pusey studied the histological modifications which occur in the tissues under the action of Roentgen rays, research of which he kindly communicated the results to me, including microscopic preparations. It seems to me all the more interesting to make known here the conclusions reached by Dr. Pusey, as there is up to a certain point – as we shall see – discrepancy between these results and those obtained by Dr. Ellis in Philadelphia (see *Semaine Médicale*, 1902, p. 426).

To ascertain the effect exerted on cancerous tissues by cathode rays, Dr. Pusey excised specimens of tumor at different periods of radiotherapy treatment and subjected them to histological examination. He thus convinced himself that only the neoplastic parts are affected by the Roentgen rays, while these have no action on the surrounding healthy parts.

Chronologically, the first changes appear on the periphery of cancer cell clusters. Then the destructive process gradually invades deeper and deeper layers. The cancerous elements degenerate gradually, but this degeneration is of a particular nature. Usually, indeed, in necrobiosis, the cellular body retains its shape more or less perfectly; the nucleus is the first to be altered and the histochemical reagents determine in the cell a general diffuse coloration. On the contrary, under the influence of Roentgen rays, the cell and the nucleus first lose their shape, the nuclear chromatin diffusing into the cellular protoplasm where it forms blocks which resemble those formed by mucin. The blood vessels are the site of active obliterating endarteritis, and the degree of degeneration of the cancerous cells is directly related to the progress of the occlusion of the vascular lumen. Finally, the neoplastic cells seem to be destroyed by virtue of a true cytolysis leading to their total resorption. In the scar obtained after healing, Dr. Pusey found only a layer of normal connective tissue, a layer covered with a thick epithelial stratum, the papillae of the dermis having disappeared. At this stage, there is no longer any trace of neoplastic tissue.

For Dr. Pusey, the cathode rays act primarily on the epithelial cells themselves, the alterations which supervene in the latter greatly preceding the appearance of the vascular lesions. He is even willing to admit that these changes occur in all tissues, neoplastic or normal, but with varying speed and intensity. It is only at final period that the modifications of the local circulation intervene in the restorative process.

We know that the therapeutic application of Roentgen rays is sometimes accompanied by more or less extensive burns which constitute one of the most unfortunate complications, in that they create wounds that easily become infected, suppurating and sometimes oozing for many months, and even more so in that they make it necessary to suspend the treatment and thus to delay an intervention which it would often be urgent to pursue in an active way. These burns have been explained by the most diverse causes; some have even gone so far as to say that they do not result from the cathode rays themselves, but to certain completely foreign elements. Such is not the opinion of Dr. Pusey, who, with the aim of forming an opinion on this significant practical issue, undertook experiments from which appear to show that the burns observed in radiotherapy are indeed attributable to the Roentgen rays.

By placing a guinea pig on a strip of lead and covering the anterior part of the animal with a strip of the same metal three quarters of a millimeter thick, the posterior part being protected by an aluminum plate half a millimeter thick, Dr. Pusey protects the animal from any electrical influence, as well as from any radiation for which lead or aluminum would not be permeable. Prepared in this way, the guinea pig is exposed for an hour and a half to a powerful Crooks tube, the cathode of which is 12 centimeters away. Ten days later, a burn accompanied by hair loss appeared in the area which had been covered with aluminum, while the rest of the animal had been perfectly protected by the lead shield.

The lesions produced in this experiment, which was repeated several times with the same result, cannot be attributed to electric waves, since the guinea pig is insulated by a kind of grounded metallic envelope. Furthermore, there can be no question of an effect of the ultraviolet rays of the spectrum, which some blame for the burns observed in radiological applications, since these radiations do not pass through either lead or aluminum. By exclusion, Dr. Pusey thus manages to deduce from his research that only the Roentgen rays have the properties belonging to the physical agent which causes the burns in question.

Moreover, clinical observations seem entirely favorable to this view; if, in fact, one surrounds a determined zone with sheets of lead, the burn is strictly circumscribed to the unprotected part, the limit of which is never exceeded by the lesion. The fact that electric discharges may cause a dermatitis analogous to that produced by Roentgen rays in no way proves that in both cases the same agent is the cause of the lesion: The effect is the same whether or not the lead shield is grounded, the parts which are hidden by the screen remaining unscathed in one case as in the other; consequently, electrical phenomena cannot be invoked in the pathogenesis of radiation dermatitis [12].

As to knowing *how* the cathode rays act, Dr. Pusey thinks that it is the actinic properties of these rays which must be incriminated in this case. These properties are very analogous to the actinic properties of light. Indeed, like certain luminous radiations – the ultraviolet part of the spectrum – the Roentgen rays are invisible, determine in certain substances fluorescent effects which make them perceptible to the sight, act in a similar way on silver salts and cause identical inflammatory lesions in the skin and subcutaneous tissues. We see that there is there between the luminous rays and the cathode rays a series of points of contact which allow us to think, in conformity with the views of Dr. Pusey, of the actinic nature of the radiological action.

[p. 122]
St. Paul, 22 March 1903

Diphtheria in Chicago
In an earlier letter, I described the present state of the question of

serotherapy treatment of diphtheria using the information furnished to me in Boston and Philadelphia (see *Semaine Médicale*, 1903, p. 33). I do not intend to return to this subject in each city that I visit during my trip to the United States; this would be a thankless and tedious task, since the information thus collected would most often not result in sufficiently large figures to allow general conclusions. It seemed to me, however, that there would be some interest in pointing out the data communicated to me in this respect in Chicago, the more so as the chief of the municipal office of hygiene of that city, Dr. Arthur R. Reynolds, was particularly concerned with anti-diphtheria serotherapy from the beginning.

Without going into details here on the public health services in America, their functioning, their attributes, their duties, their rights, etc., I wish to indicate the role of these institutions in the fight against diphtheria. Starting from this point of view that the surest process to prevent the propagation of the pathogenic agent and to fight its action effectively consists in ensuring the bacteriological diagnosis as early as possible, they have created, in each city of the United States, with the municipal office of hygiene, a special service in charge of bacteriologic examinations of the district. To make things easier, they give practitioners a strong paper envelope containing a tube to be inoculated, as well as an instrument of variable model to perform the inoculation. In Chicago, the tube has been replaced by a small aluminum box containing Löffler's medium, hermetically sealed with a flat rubber ring and sterilized after having been prepared in this way. This box has the advantage over the glass tube of being unbreakable; moreover, because of its smaller dimensions, it can easily be placed in the vest pocket: In this way, it is maintained at body temperature, which is the most favorable to the development of the culture. This is thus set in motion as soon as the inoculation is done, hence the possibility of often saving a few hours on the time necessary to obtain a bacteriological analysis result. The containers are preferably made of aluminum because they deteriorate less rapidly in air than when they are made of tin. As for the culture medium they contain, it keeps there in good condition for a period of two months, according to Dr. W. K. Jaques, in charge of the bacteriological analysis department at the Chicago sanitation office.

The instrument used for taking the culture varies according to the towns, from the classic platinum wire to the most rudimentary instrument. In Chicago, it is a wooden stick with a cotton tip, contained in a special envelope with a wooden tongue depressor. These two instruments, sterilized beforehand, are intended to be burned after use, in accordance with the instructions on the envelope. It also contains detailed information on how to inoculate the culture medium.

The envelopes containing the various necessary documents are deposited by the hygiene office in the pharmacies of the city and are held there *free of charge* for the doctors; of course, the bacteriologic analysis is also free of charge. If I emphasize this gratuity, it is because it ensures the bacteriological examination of *all* cases of diphtheria. It is conceivable, in fact, that given the facilities which result from such an organization, the bacteriologist is available for all suspected cases, even for those which are only mildly suspicious. From another point of view, it seems legitimate to admit that in the towns where such a service functions on a regular basis, the municipal statistics indicate the *totality* of the cases of diphtheria which have presented themselves. The statistics of diphtheria morbidity established before the organization of this system offer, on the contrary, only relative guarantees of accuracy.

In Chicago, this service dates from October 1895; in other words, its creation is contemporaneous with the advent of anti-diphtheria serotherapy. It is also conceivable that if in this city we want to study the influence of serotherapy on morbidity and mortality from diphtheria, the comparison of the two periods – before and since – is based only on uncertain elements, because the uncertainty of statistics going back to the pre-serotherapeutic era.

Another difficulty arises, for a comparison of this kind, in a city like Chicago: We do not know the exact population, since the censuses are carried out in the United States only every ten years. Chicago, which in 1890 had a population of 1,100,000 inhabitants, saw this population rise by 600,000 during the ten-year period which elapsed from 1890 to 1900. In the presence of such a rapid increase, it is obvious that taking the average annual increase – equal, in this particular case, to 60,000 individuals – as the basis of the calculations, the results obtained are not very exact. This is a cause of error which does not affect the cities of the American East – Boston, Philadelphia – which, however rapid their growth, are considerably outdistanced in this respect by Chicago. Nevertheless, it is the only procedure available for forming an approximate idea of the influence of serotherapy on diphtheria in Chicago.

If we consider the five-year period extending from 1890 to 1895, we find that there were in Chicago during these five years 7,411 deaths from diphtheria, that is an average of 1,482 per year. For the next five-year period, which began in October 1895 (the period to which systematic bacteriological examinations date back, as well as the application of diphtheria antitoxin), there were 4,309 deaths from diphtheria, or 862 on average per year. Taking into account the overall population increase occurring during the two periods, we arrive at a rate of 11 deaths per 10,000 inhabitants in each of the years from 1890 to 1895, this rate falling to 5 deaths per 10,000 during the next five-year period.

If we now consider the percentage of deaths in relation to cases diagnosed with diphtheria, we obtain an even more marked difference: In fact, case mortality, which was 35% on average for each of the years of the first group, dropped to 7% for those of the second.

Such findings are very striking. So we should not be surprised at Chicago's enthusiasm for the antitoxic treatment of diphtheria. In this respect, this city can compete with Boston: The American East and West are approaching each other. It remains to be seen how the corresponding figures will look over a longer period.

[p. 139]
Denver, 5 April 1903

Surgical anesthesia by cocaine injection into nerve trunks

Local anesthesia using cocaine is well known in America but little used. At least I have very rarely had the opportunity to see intradermal or subcutaneous injection practiced, and I do not think that this method enjoys great favor in the United States. As for spinal anesthesia, I have not yet seen it performed anywhere; I have even observed a determined resistance among American surgeons to the introduction of this mode of anesthesia into general practice. However, I have heard that spinal anesthesia is commonly used in San Francisco by Professor Huntington. Having not yet extended my trip to California, I have not been able to verify this.

There is another mode of cocaine anesthesia that I want to describe today, whose use is not widely known but is tending to spread somewhat over here. This involves injection of a weak sterile solution of cocaine into nerve trunks, which I saw practiced especially in Cleveland by Dr. G. W. Crile. This "blocks" the nerve impulse and prevents it from spreading beyond the point where the cocaine was injected. The result is a veritable *physiological division* of the nerve, an experimental phenomenon of which Dr. Crile makes a frequent clinical application. While, in fact, general anesthesia only suppresses pain and voluntary motor activity, the intra-truncal injection of cocaine also annihilates the spinal reflexes. To obtain this result, it suffices to "block" the nerve with cocaine and then one can then manipulate its peripheral segment without in any way affecting the entire nervous system. It is thus possible, during an operation involving important nerve trunks, to prevent the group of respiratory and cardiovascular reflexes commonly referred to as surgical shock.

The injection is performed using a Pravaz syringe[30] loaded with a 1% solution of cocaine. If we want to obtain an immediate effect on a large trunk, we must make several punctures close to each other in the thickness of the nerve. In general, such a precaution is not necessary, since cocaine diffuses very rapidly into the nervous substance. Usually it suffices to make the cocaine penetrate under the nerve sheath. The time necessary for the complete interruption of nerve transmission under these conditions is not greatly lengthened, and on the other hand one can avoid damaging the nerve fibers. In fact, the integrity of the nerve fiber matters little, since the intra-truncal cocainization is only a temporary section of the nerve trunk. The nerve remains "blocked" for a variable time, then the function is restored and the nerve impulse circulates freely again, without there being any degeneration or inflammation of the nerve.

For Dr. Crile, intra-truncal cocainization has the main advantage of attenuating the severity of operative shock. This surgeon has been using the method in question for several years already, particularly in operations on the limbs [13], and he uses it almost routinely along with a light general anesthesia. When, for some reason, general anesthesia is contraindicated, he does not hesitate to operate with the sole aid of intra-truncal cocainization.

Dr. Crile currently has several observations of leg amputations carried out without general anesthesia, after having simply blocked with cocaine the three main nerve trunks which innervate the lower limb: The lateral femoral cutaneous nerve, whose superficial situation makes it easily accessible; the femoral nerve, which is found near the femoral artery, and the sciatic nerve, which is punctured at the level of the gluteal fold. The intra-truncal cocainization of these three nerves constitutes a true physiological amputation, after which it is easy to carry out the removal of the limb without the patient noticing it, except for the noise that the saw makes on the bone.

When the operation involves the region innervated by the ulnar nerve, it is easy to block this nerve as it passes through the epitrochlear groove. To do this, two injections are enough, the first subcutaneous which prepares the way, and the second pushed more deeply into the very substance of the nerve trunk. After about ten minutes, one can note the existence of complete anesthesia in the distribution of the ulnar nerve, allowing the performance of any operation (amputation, resection) without causing the slightest pain. Sensitivity usually remains abolished for about half an hour. Sometimes, Dr. Crile has seen the return of sensitivity accompanied by a rather pronounced burning sensation in the zone innervated by the ulnar, a sensation which disappears after a few days without leaving a trace.

We know the fairly high mortality of shoulder disarticulation. Starting from the idea that the danger inherent in this operation is essentially due to the shock resulting from the seriousness of an operation usually performed on debilitated subjects, Dr. Crile has adopted an operative approach which frees him from general anesthesia, decreases surgical shock, and partially eliminates hemorrhage. These indications are fulfilled, on the one hand, by the cocainization of the nerve trunks, on the other by the temporary occlusion of the arteries, following the process of Dr. Crile, which this journal described a short time ago (see *Semaine Médicale,* 1902, p. 339) [14].

Here is how our colleague proceeds: Under local anesthesia, an incision is made, corresponding to the lower third of the posterior edge of the sternomastoid muscle and descending inferiorly to the level of the clavicle. He then proceeds to the dissection of the planes; if care is taken to prevent the blood from obscuring the operative field, the nerve fibers are visualized through the connective tissue and can be cocainized as they arise; moreover, they become less numerous as one advances deeper. By pushing the omohyoid muscle downwards, the trapezius behind, the anterior scalene forward, he exposes the brachial plexus and below this plexus the arch of the subclavian artery. He begins by injecting the sheath which surrounds the entire plexus (a 0.5% cocaine solution is sufficient for this), then gradually penetrates more deeply and ends up with an interstitial injection into the very substance of the trunks that make up the plexus.

Sensitivity and motility are then totally abolished in the territory to which the terminal branches of the brachial plexus are distributed. The subclavian artery is then occluded with Dr. Crile's clamp, and the operation can be completed without causing pain and without losing an appreciable quantity of blood. Dr. Crile has used this operative procedure on old people, consumptives, etc., and he has always obtained satisfactory results.

In scapulothoracic amputation, the same surgeon combines intra-truncal cocainization of the brachial plexus with general anesthesia. In this case, the cocainization of the nerves has no other purpose than to attenuate the gravity of the operative shock.

Having had the opportunity to see Dr. Crile in Cleveland using this method, Dr. Harvey Cushing (of Baltimore) had the idea of applying it to the radical cure of inguinal hernia. It suffices, in fact, to inject the few nerves which distribute themselves to the inguinal region to numb all this region and thus render the operation absolutely painless. I will not currently describe the precise technique of this intervention, since it will find its natural place in future correspondence about the treatment of hernia in the

United States.

The intra-truncal injection of cocaine can also render service by inhibiting certain reflexes, such as those which follow the vagal route, as Dr. Crile was good enough to demonstrate to me during an operation which I observed. This was a branchiogenic carcinoma extending to the entire right lateral region of the neck, in a man in his sixties. The tumor had invaded the carotid and the vagus and it was impossible to free these organs. Under these conditions, Dr. Crile, having blocked the vagus at the lower end of the tumor, was able to section it at this level without seeing any respiratory or cardiac effects. A hemostat placed on an arterial branch in the upper corner of the wound inadvertently pinched the upper end of the vagus, causing the sudden cessation of breathing. It was sufficient to remove the unfortunate forceps and make an interstitial injection into the nerve to see breathing re-establish spontaneously.

The injection of cocaine according to the procedure which we have just described does not have a purely local action, since this action affects the whole distribution zone of the blocked nerve. *Intra-truncal* by its nature, it is therefore *regional* in its effects, and thus deserves a special place. A distinction should also be made between the mode of application of cocaine and the effect of this application: if the local application of cocaine is generally intended only to obtain anesthesia, it nevertheless allows, in certain case, to abolish reflexivity at the same time. Thus, by simple topical application to the supraglottic mucous membrane of the larynx, one can prevent a fatal syncope due to cardiopulmonary arrest, such as one sees occurring reflexively in operations on the larynx (like laryngectomy, or even just when introducing the Trendelenburg cannula.[31] So, Dr. Crile has made it a rule to begin any intralaryngeal intervention, however minimal it may be, by applying a 1% solution of cocaine to the mucous membrane of the larynx.

[p. 146]
Saint Louis, 12 April 1903

Autoplastic procedure for removal of lip cancers[32]

Among the multiple procedures which have been advocated to avoid as much as possible the deformity caused by the removal of a cancer of the lip, the one which is most commonly employed consists of a wedge excision, because it presents the advantage of a simple and fast execution. However, the coaptation of the edges of the wound often causes considerable tension in the tissues and the scar, due to the size of the defect that the intervention generally leaves at the level of the operated lip; hence the need to have recourse in certain cases to a secondary autoplasty to remedy the insufficiency of such a result. In order to obtain a satisfactory effect from the outset and in all cases, Dr. W. W. Grant (of Denver) has adopted, for the ablation of cancers of the lip, a process different from those which are ordinarily used [15]. Here is what it consists of:

If, to take an example, it is a tumor of the lower lip, which is the usual case, we first create, in completely healthy tissue on each side of the lesion, a vertical incision including the entire thickness of the lip. The lower end of the two vertical incisions is then joined by a horizontal incision which passes below the level of the tumor. The part of the lip which has been excised in this way and which contains the neoplasm thus has a rectangular shape. To fill in the loss of substance resulting from this excision, Dr. Grant makes two additional incisions, each starting from one of the lower angles of the wound, where the horizontal incision meets each of the two vertical incisions. Directed downwards and outwards, these complementary incisions determine with the vertical incisions two triangular flaps that are always easy to bring together when the complementary incisions are of sufficient length: For this, one must not be afraid of going beyond the edge of the lower jaw and extending onto the neck. More often than not, such a practice is indicated, on one side at least, in order to remove the lymphatic metastases which are located in the carotid chain. To bring the two triangular flaps together, we start by suturing them on the midline, then we join the lower border of the flap to the skin of the chin. The result is a sort of inverted Y, with an inferior sinus and including the chin in the opening of its branches. When the cancer is in the midline, the Y has a symmetrical shape. When the tumor is closer to one of the labial commissures, the Y is irregular and its branches are of unequal length.

For the upper lip, the operation is done in a similar way; there is therefore no reason to dwell on it.

With this method, the incisions rarely extend beyond the mobile parts of the lips and cheeks. Also, the flaps are usually easy to bring into their new position without resorting to extensive undermining of the lower jaw.

The results obtained by this procedure are generally superior to those obtained by wedge excision, both aesthetically and surgically. Indeed, by placing the incisions in completely healthy tissue, a smaller extent of the lip has been sacrificed, so that the mouth is less constricted. It is also less distorted, and the lip sag that is so often seen with traditional methods does not occur or is not as pronounced. It also results that speech is less impaired. Furthermore, the tension of the tissues is much less, so that it is not necessary to use relaxing incisions or to require secondary operations to relieve dangerous tension.

In the case of an early cancer which not very large, and if the patient has a large mouth, Dr. Grant does not perform the operation which we have just described, but simply performs a wedge-shaped excision.

Suspension apparatus for rhinoplasty[33]

Recent attempts to inject paraffin under the skin of the dorsum of the nose with a view to restoring this organ to its normal form demonstrate, after so many others, the difficulties presented by a restoration of this kind. I had occasion to see, in Denver, a device which Dr. Grant uses for this purpose. The simplicity of this apparatus and the good results which it has given in the hands of its author lead me to speak of it here.

The principle of the method consists in using a kind of bridge passing above the nose, resting at its ends on the skeleton of the face and to which the skeleton of the nose is temporarily *suspended* by a silver wire. The instrument used for this purpose consists essentially of a flat metal rod, curved in two places. It has a series of holes in its middle part which allow the silver wire to be fixed. At each end of this rod is fitted a hardened rubber plate, intended to rest on the zygoma, the shape of which it follows as exactly as possible. Ribbons passing above and below the ear hold the device in place. The whole forms a sort of metallic hoop resting on the malar bones and passing, above the nose, at a certain distance from the skin. Whether it is then a fracture or a caries of the bones of the nose, one begins by replacing the different bony parts in their normal situation with the help of an appropriate operation. Then, having put the device in place, the loop of a silver wire is attached to it, which then crosses the bones of the nose to come out on the opposite side and go to attach, by its other end, to the metal band of the apparatus, which thus constitutes a real temporary nasal prosthetic apparatus.

This device is left in place for a variable period according to the length of time necessary to obtain a sufficient consolidation of the parts, which requires, in general, only a week, according to Dr. Grant.

The process employed by this surgeon obviously cannot be suitable for cases where the entire bony skeleton of the nose has been destroyed. But in less extensive destructions, it seems likely to render real service. The pressure of the plates on the malar bone is supported without any inconvenience due to the large surface along which this pressure takes place, as well as the precise adaptation of the plates to the malar region. In addition, it is a much less serious intervention than introducing a permanent prosthetic device under the skin.

[p. 155]
Saint Louis, 12 April 1903

Breast cancer treatment in the United States

During my trip, I have often had the opportunity to observe procedures for breast cancer. The operation that I saw generally carried out involved the systematic ablation of the pectoral muscles and the dissection of the supraclavicular fossa: This large excision is, it is true, known to European surgeons, but it does not seem that they have used it as frequently as their colleagues in America. Here, the current in favor of this intervention, radical from the outset, started in Baltimore by Dr. W. S. Halsted, Professor of Surgery at the *Johns Hopkins Medical School* and surgeon at the hospital of the same name. Here is how our colleague proceeds:[34]

The incision he uses, instead of having the usual racket shape, circles round the breast; from its inner and upper edge a secondary incision runs upwards and outwards towards the apex of the axilla. This results in a triangular flap with an external base and whose apex is at the meeting point of the two incisions. This flap, once dissected from its subcutaneous fatty layer, so as to contain only the thickness of the skin, is tilted outwards. Then he divides the sterno-costal attachments of the pectoralis major muscle, and penetrates with the scalpel between the sterno-costal portion and the clavicular portion of this muscle, which he separates up to the level of the Lisfranc tubercle.[35] There, he makes an additional incision, perpendicular to the original incision, dividing at the same time the skin and the clavicular portion of the pectoralis major and extending to the clavicle, to lay bare the axillary vessels at the apex of the axilla. He then repeats the incision which separates the two portions of the pectoralis major, and extends it as far as the humerus, cutting the insertion of the sterno-costal portion of the muscle near the bone. Then he divides the pectoralis minor in the middle of its length and detaches the mass circumscribed by the previous incisions from the base by which it adheres to the deep planes. Originally, Dr. Halsted limited himself to removing the fibrous layer which separates the two pectoral muscles. Currently, he prefers to complete the operation by also sacrificing the muscle belly of the pectoralis minor. The rib cage is thus exposed; it is stripped with the greatest care of all the loose and fatty cellular tissue which covers it and which is often infiltrated by neoplastic spindles, continuing this dissection to the level of the coracoid insertion of the pectoralis minor, above and below this muscle. This done, the axillary vein and its ramifications are freed from the sheath that surrounds them, proceeding from top to bottom. It is rarely necessary to denude the axillary artery. After freeing up this mass of tissue, the glandular tissue in front of the subscapularis, teres major, and latissimus dorsi muscles is removed. A final stroke of the scalpel, carried out from the inside out along the base of the triangular flap dissected at the start of the operation, is then sufficient to remove the diseased breast with its attachments.

To dissect out the supraclavicular fossa, which immediately follows, Dr. Halsted makes a vertical incision, parallel to the posterior border of the sternomastoid muscle. By retracting the muscle at this level, one easily reaches the venous angle of Pirogoff[36] where the subclavian and internal jugular veins meet. It is from this point that we start to dissect the supraclavicular fossa. In order to enlarge the operative field, it is advisable to section the intermediate tendon of the omohyoid muscle; traction on the two muscular bellies gives better exposure and facilitates the operation.

We can see that this is a radical process, since the operation includes – whatever the size of the tumor itself – the removal of the mammary gland in its entirety, with the skin that encloses it, the sterno-costal portion of the pectoralis major muscle and the pectoralis minor muscle, and finally a recess of the axilla and supraclavicular fossa. Dr. Halsted was not originally as radical as he is now. He did not at first dissect out the supraclavicular fossa in a systematic way, only exploring it when palpation revealed enlarged lymph nodes there. The experience acquired by the histological examination of these lymph nodes proved to him, however, that it is true for the supraclavicular fossa as well as for the axilla: One often finds lymph node metastases which were not previously suspected, either because the infiltrated lymph nodes were too small, or because they were too deeply located; in general, it can be said that the supraclavicular nodes are affected in one third of breast cancers at the time of operation. This seems to be reason enough to justify supraclavicular dissection in all cases, suspicious or not. It must be practiced even if it is recognized at the time of the operation – a rare occurrence – that the axillary lymph nodes are unaffected. The state of the supraclavicular fossa is, in fact, completely independent of that of the axilla, and we are by no means entitled to infer one from the other.

To perform this exploration, Dr. Halsted has currently abandoned the temporary division or resection of the clavicle. A simple division does not give enough exposure and resection is unnecessary: Simply by lifting the shoulder, one obtains enough room through the costo-clavicular space that the manipulations necessary for the dissection of this space can be easily performed. Dr. Halsted therefore limits himself, as we have just described, with a supraclavicular incision. One can either leave the adipo-cellular tissue of the supraclavicular fossa in continuity with that of the subclavicular region and release it through the costo-clavicular space, or remove it separately, taking care in either case to resect the tissue connecting the two regions, which is always suspicious.

In general, Dr. Halsted recommends removing *en bloc* all the parts intended to be removed: Breast, muscles, and cellulo-adipose extensions. By breaking up this mass, there is a risk of omitting the clearing out of suspect areas; moreover, by sectioning tissues liable to be invaded by the neoplastic infiltration or to serve as routes for its propagation, one opens up the lymphatics and runs the risk of inoculating regions which are still unaffected.

To cover the extensive loss of substance resulting from this intervention, Dr. Halsted brings the edges of the wound together with a purse-string suture. This only passes through the base of the external triangular flap. This flap itself serves to cover the axillary fossa. No drain is necessary. In the center of the wound there generally remains a surface which can be allowed to heal by granulation; however, Dr. Halsted prefers to cover it from the outset with the help of Thiersch grafts.[37]

Since this process may leave something to be desired, Dr. J. Collins Warren, professor of surgery at *Harvard Medical School* and surgeon at the *Massachusetts General Hospital* in Boston, has substituted another way of doing it: With the help of an autoplastic flap, it restores the cutaneous plane in a very satisfactory way.

The skin incision as practiced by Dr. Warren differs somewhat from that of Dr. Halsted. It originates at the top of the axilla, descends along the anterior edge of this region following the outer edge of the pectoralis major muscle and circumscribes the breast below. A second incision starts from the middle of the front edge of the axilla and goes around the breast on its internal side to join the first incision below this organ. This results in a pear-shaped or racket-shaped incision, which eliminates Dr. Halsted's triangular flap. It is completed later by the additional incision that the Baltimore surgeon also makes and which, going from the upper edge of the wound towards the clavicle, exposes the axillary vessels and their sheath. Extended beyond the clavicle, this auxiliary incision uncovers the axillary fossa when Dr. Warren dissects it out, which he does not do routinely.

In order not to repeat myself, I will not follow here in all its details the procedure of Dr. Warren; it differs essentially from that of Dr. Halsted, apart from the cutaneous incision, only in the mode of closing the wound. Here is how Dr. Warren proceeds:

From the middle of the lower edge of the wound, he makes an incision at right angles which includes the skin and describes a rounded line. Depending on whether the curve presents its convexity upwards or downwards, there results a lower or upper flap. Usually the lower flap is preferable; in some cases, it is useful to trace two flaps, lower and upper. By detaching them from the chest wall, these flaps are mobilized enough to bring them closer to the inner edge of the wound. This immediately results in a wound covered everywhere with skin, a condition favorable to healing by first intention. Usually, Dr. Warren interposes between the edges of the wound a wick of gauze which is withdrawn at the end of twenty-four hours. When the flaps have been well traced, this procedure gives an excellent result, without any tension in the flaps or the scar, as I had the opportunity to ascertain for myself in a patient undergoing the operation which Dr. Warren was good enough to have me observe, and whom I saw again a fortnight later.

The results furnished by these radical processes of amputation of the breast are very encouraging. Nearly half of those operated on pass the third year without complications, and half of these still seem free from a recurrence. Of course, it must be recognized that these are only patients initially considered "operable."

This is moreover only the percentage for the intervention: it cannot give an idea of the prognosis of breast cancer in itself, since many cases are too advanced at the time of presentation to benefit from any intervention. I add that, in these apparently desperate cases, Dr. Robert Abbe, surgeon of *St. Luke's Hospital*[38] in New York, has sometimes performed ovariotomy with very impressive results. But as this operation was advocated for this purpose and performed for the first time in England by G. Th. Beatson (of Glasgow), I need not dwell upon it in these articles exclusively devoted to medicine in America.

[p. 163]
New Orleans, 26 April 1903

The radical cure of inguinal hernia in the United States

Macewen's procedure was, for many years, adopted by the majority of American surgeons for the radical cure of inguinal hernia, almost to the exclusion of all other methods. At present, however, it has been completely abandoned in the United States for the more recent procedure of Bassini, and it is the latter which is commonly practiced by the American surgeons whom I had the opportunity to see operate. There would therefore be no need to describe the interventions in use in the United States for the radical cure of inguinal hernia, except that several surgeons in this country have made various modifications to the method of Bassini which, while not changing the general approach, add some particular characteristics which I think are interesting to point out.

New York has a hospital, half of which is exclusively devoted to the treatment of hernias. It is the *Hospital for Ruptured and Crippled*,[39] whose hernia department is under the direction of Drs. W. T. Bull and W. B. Coley. The method employed on this service represents in its broad outlines the operation of Bassini; it differs, however, in a few technical details due to Dr. Coley.

As in the process of Bassini, the operation performed by Drs. Bull and Coley has the main goal of repairing the inguinal canal, for which a deep layer is formed using the conjoint tendon of the internal oblique and transverse muscles, which are sutured against the femoral arch, the spermatic cord running in front of this tendon, and behind the aponeurosis of the external oblique muscle. But starting from the idea that the Bassini repair has a weak point at the internal inguinal ring, where the spermatic cord enters the inguinal canal, Dr. Coley generally places an additional suture immediately above this opening, comprising the entire thickness of the internal oblique muscle and attaching this muscle to the femoral arch. As a result, at the location where the cord crosses the musculo-aponeurotic plane of the abdominal wall, it is enclosed between two sutures, one of which has just been mentioned and the other is the highest of the five or six separate points which fix the conjoined tendon against the femoral arch, thus reconstituting the deep plane of the inguinal canal.

This is the principal modification made by this surgeon to the original technique of Bassini. We know that the latter always insisted on the absolute necessity of using non-absorbable sutures for the deep layer, to ensure the solidity of the posterior wall of the canal in a satisfactory manner; he still uses heavy silk for this purpose today. However, the experience of surgeons at the Hospital for Ruptured and Crippled would tend to prove that it is unnecessary to use non-absorbable sutures. Furthermore, Drs. Bull and Coley consider that such a practice has many disadvantages; they have observed that even three years and more after the operation one can still see complications arising from deep sutures of silk, horsehair, or silver wire, even though the surgical wound had healed by first intention. According to the New York surgeons, these late suture abscesses are much more frequent than is usually admitted. On the other hand, it is certain that catgut, the resorption of which begins from the fifth to the eighth day, could not be a satisfactory suture material for an operation such as the radical cure of an inguinal hernia. What is needed is a thread that lasts for three or four weeks and then disappears spontaneously. A material fulfilling these conditions is obtained by treating catgut or kangaroo tendon with chromic acid. It is particularly the kangaroo tendon thus prepared that is given preference at the hernia hospital, and I would add that this practice, without being general in the United States, is nevertheless followed by a large number of American surgeons, even those who do not use this thread as a common suture, for example, Dr. Deaver in Philadelphia.

Dr. Coley also modifies the Bassini operation in women: Instead of placing the round ligament – which in women corresponds anatomically to the spermatic cord in men – above the conjoined tendon, he covers it with this tendon, the walls of the canal (conjoint tendon and aponeurosis of the oblique muscle) being treated as in men and sutured separately. This practice seems rational, if one considers that the round ligament is much smaller than the spermatic cord and consequently requires much less separation of the constituent elements of the musculo-aponeurotic plane of the abdominal wall.

The process used by Dr. Deaver in Philadelphia differs from that adopted by Drs. Bull and Coley only in that this surgeon, reminiscent of Macewen's procedure, instead of excising the sac, forms a kind of plug from it which he lodges at the level of the internal inguinal ring.

The procedure which Dr. Halsted practices at the *Johns Hopkins Hospital* of Baltimore differs in certain essential characteristics from the method of Bassini. After having isolated the spermatic cord, Dr. Halsted excises the veins of the spermatic plexus, with the exception of one or two trunks which he retains. He then resects the sac. The suture of the musculo-aponeurotic plane of the abdominal wall is done with silver thread and in a single layer. The spermatic cord is placed above this layer; the cord is thus found immediately underlying the skin, which is closed with an intradermal suture of silver thread. For a long time, Dr. Halsted has been in the habit of extending upwards and inwards the incision of the aponeurosis of the external oblique by which one enters the inguinal canal. The notch thus made in the musculo-aponeurotic plane of the abdominal wall exceeded the level of the internal inguinal ring by 2 centimeters and involved the external and internal oblique muscles, the transverse, and the transversalis fascia. He would then pass the cord through the upper corner of this notch. But he has now abandoned this practice because it does not seem to him to give results superior to those obtained without the extension.

Dr. Halsted attaches great importance to the resection of the veins of the cord: For him, it is one of the conditions of success, judged by the permanence of the result. It would seem, however, that this venous resection results in atrophy of the testis in a certain number of cases, of which Professor Keen (of Philadelphia) estimates the proportion at 1%. According to Dr. Keen, the preservation of these same veins may lead to a recurrence of the hernia. The alternatives therefore seem to be a problem, since one must choose between two equally unfortunate eventualities: Atrophy of the testicle or recurrence. However, based on recent observations, Dr. Halsted believes that the testicular atrophy that occurs in some of the subjects operated on according to his method may be attributed not to the resection of the venous plexus, but to the displacement of the cord and its subcutaneous situation.

The conjoint tendon sometimes presents a particularly pronounced congenital weakness, so that even after it has been brought closer to the femoral arch, the abdominal wall still seems too weak to protect against a recurrence of the hernia. In such cases, Dr. Bloodgood, a lecturer at *Johns Hopkins Medical School* in Baltimore, uses the lower portion of the rectus abdominis muscle to strengthen the wall. For this purpose, he lifts the upper inner lip of the incision along which he has split the aponeurosis of the external oblique muscle; he then easily recognizes the outer edge of the rectus abdominis; on this edge, he incises the sheath of the muscle which immediately herniates through the orifice thus made in its sheath. Then Dr. Bloodgood, drawing the muscle down and out, secures it against the femoral arch by staggered silver thread sutures from the origin of the muscle at the pubic spine, to the level of the internal inguinal orifice. This muscle flap seems to have provided lasting results in cases with a rather poor prognosis.

It remains for me to add a few words of the practice of Dr. Harvey Cushing (of Baltimore), to which I have already alluded in an earlier correspondence (see *Semaine Médicale*, 1903, p. 140). This is less a particular procedure for the radical cure of the inguinal hernia than a method of regional anesthesia applicable to this intervention. This method also finds its indication in any other operation on the inguinal region, such as celiotomy for strangulated hernia, especially in old people and debilitated subjects. It is based on the fact that, since the iliohypogastric, ilioinguinal, and genitofemoral nerves supply sensory innervation to the inguinal region, it suffices to inject these three nerve trunks with cocaine before their penetration into this region to prevent any sensation from the peripheral territory to which they are distributed to be transmitted to the brain and perceived by it.[40]

Generally, Dr. Cushing gives a subcutaneous injection of 5 milligrams of morphine one hour before the operation and repeats the injection at the start of the operation. Local anesthesia is then ensured, using intradermal injections of 1% cocaine, along the line chosen for the incision of the skin. The section of the subcutaneous tissue is not painful, and it is therefore unnecessary to anesthetize the fatty panniculus. One can therefore penetrate straight away with the scalpel as far as the aponeurosis of the greater oblique, at least in the upper angle of the wound: In the lower angle, in fact, one finds, running in the deep layer of fat, branches of the ilioinguinal nerve, as well as some unimportant small veins, and these may be painful if divided. If, therefore, the inguinal canal is opened in the upper part of the wound, by incising the aponeurosis of the external oblique, the iliohypogastric nerve is uncovered above, and below it the ilioinguinal nerve and the genital branch of the genitofemoral nerve. By "blocking" these nerves with 1% cocaine injections into the nerve trunks, it is easy to anesthetize the entire operating area. The peritoneum is not sensitive, and manipulation of the intestine is painful only if the intestinal walls are stretched. The muscle, on the contrary, always has sensation; thus it is important, if the operation is carried out according to the process of Halsted, to assure its anesthesia before incising it.

[p. 174]
New Orleans 3 May 1903

The causes of surgical shock

We frequently observe, either clinically in humans, or experimentally in animals, that certain subjects react poorly to an intervention which may be very minimal in itself. This fact is explained by the hypothesis of a particular state that is given the name of *surgical shock* or more simply *shock*. This can also appear in the absence of any specific cause; it may follow a violent nervous shock, such as that which results from an intense trauma, from a major hemorrhage, or from a violent fright. Anesthesia is also a factor that may create the state of shock. Cases are known where minor operations performed under chloroform or ether were followed by death in a short time. In cases of this kind, it is especially necessary to consider functional disorders and toxins which result from the administration of the drug, in addition to the well-known effect of the anesthetic as a cellular poison.

The effects which arise from these last two categories of organic disturbances being less well elucidated than those which are attributable to the intoxication of the cell, Dr. Fenton B. Turck (of Chicago) has made them the subject of prolonged research, which casts an interesting light on the mechanisms by which surgical shock is produced; also it seemed interesting to report these studies recorded in the documents which Dr. Turck was good enough to communicate to me.[41] This will serve as an introduction to the treatment of surgical shock, which will be the subject of a subsequent letter.

The failure of blood pressure and respiration that is usually described cannot, on its own, satisfactorily account for the shock which results from the excessive administration of an anesthetic agent. It is also important to consider the toxins that appear in the blood serum. If, in fact, normal animals are injected with serum from animals in a state of shock, syncope occurs with stertorous breathing and a rapid drop in blood pressure. It must be concluded that the injected serum contained toxic substances capable of provoking a state of shock in the new animal. These poisons are either elaborated in the blood, or they are simply retained poisons preexisting in the normal state of the blood. There are reasons to think that these two hypotheses each contain a part of truth. We know, in fact, that acetonuria has been observed in normal individuals after prolonged anesthesia, which indicates the presence of abnormal substances in the circulation; on the other hand, a delay in the elimination of methylene blue has been reported under identical circumstances, which testifies to a slowing down in the metabolism, manifested by a delay in the excretion.

Dr. Turck has made a number of experiments to establish the reason for this abnormal metabolism. For this, he added chloroform and ether to blood and kept the mixture in an oven until the chloroform and ether had completely evaporated. If then we place in this liquid a disc of egg-white, we see the disc melt and disappear as the albumin is digested. By repeating this same experiment with normal blood, without chloroform or ether added, the albumin disc is hardly attacked by pancreatin. It therefore seems that in the first case a substance was produced which interfered with the antitoxic action which has been attributed to the blood since the well-known research of Dr. Bordet.

The blood serum of animals in which a state of shock has been induced by anesthesia also exhibits very marked hemolytic properties. If, in fact, we collect the blood of an animal in such a condition by bleeding it white, we find that this blood has a great tendency to hemolyze. We cause the same state to appear in the serum of another animal by injecting it with the serum of the first.

To demonstrate this phenomenon more precisely, Dr. Turck keeps a dog under chloroform for five hours. At the end of this period of time, the serum of the experimental animal already contains 15% hemoglobin. By adding it to new blood, after centrifugation, a serum containing up to 50% hemoglobin is obtained. This effect seems, moreover, to be quite strong, for only a small quantity of the first serum is needed to bring about an intense hemolysis of the new blood. In one case, for example, where a dog was kept under narcosis for six hours, 15 cubic millimeters sufficed to cause the hemolysis of 4 cc of normal blood.

The serum of an animal in a state of shock also has agglutinating properties, which moreover vary in their intensity according to the duration of anesthesia. Thus, in an experiment in which Dr. Turck added to a drop of normal blood the serum of an animal which had been chloroformed for three hours, the agglutination was immediate. It was still so after four and five consecutive dilutions, the narcosis having been prolonged for six hours.

As for the tendency to coagulation which manifests itself in the blood after a long anesthesia, it has been observed many times in the clinic. Thus, there is no need to emphasize it here other than to recall it.

It follows from the experiments related above that shock is accompanied by the appearance, in the blood, of toxins which are normally absent. The presence of these substances explains the fatal effect, at non-lethal doses, of injections of staphylococci or colon bacilli in animals under the influence of prolonged anesthesia. The isolated action, either of the microbe or of the anesthetic agent, is insufficient to cause death; but by bringing these two factors together, the resulting cumulative effect causes the animal to perish.

Apart from these different changes which occur in the blood of a subject in a state of shock, it is important to take into account that the gastrointestinal disorders which are normally accompanied by general anesthesia also give rise to poisons which penetrate rapidly into the circulation and which, through this intermediary, will exert their deleterious action on the organism. The fact itself has been known to clinicians for a long time, but the mechanism has hardly been studied so far.

Now, if a dog with a gastric fistula is administered chloroform or ether with the aid of a tracheostomy cannula or, which is simpler and produces the same effect, inhalations are practiced by the natural routes after having carefully blocked the esophagus, it is noted by the gastric fistula that the gastric juice first becomes hyperchlorhydric, then the proportion of hydrochloric acid and ferments decreases, and finally the stomach mucosa secretes an abundant quantity of mucus, demonstrating the irritation of this mucosa. By macerating in water the gastric mucosa of a dog subjected to anesthesia for two or three hours, we obtain a liquid in which we can isolate by distillation the chloroform or the ether used for narcosis. The anesthetic was probably brought to the stomach walls by the circulatory route and exerted there an effect analogous to that determined by the local application of silver nitrate, tannin, or mustard, as evidenced in the works published in 1894 by Dr. Turck and confirmed since then in St. Petersburg by Professor Pavlov and his school.

The gastric mucosa is not, moreover, the only layer of the digestive tract where the anesthetic is found. This can also be detected in the intestinal mucosa, as well as in the gastrointestinal muscle. This last fact explains the disorders of gastric motility which add to those of secretion. One easily obtains the characteristic reactions of chloroform or ether after the distillation of the liquid of maceration of the coats of the stomach or the intestine, even when the anesthesia has lasted only one hour. But the quantities thus found increase in direct proportion to the duration of anesthesia. Moreover, the anesthetic does not disappear quickly from the mucous membranes: Several hours after the end of the anesthetic, appreciable quantities are still detected in the internal membranes of the stomach.

The sluggishness of the gastrointestinal muscle resulting both from the local inactivation by the anesthetic and from its effect on the vasomotor center accounts for the visceral congestion which is common after prolonged anesthesia. It is from these vascular disturbances that in turn arises the distention of the digestive tract, as Dr. Turck proved by the following experiment: If we place ligatures on the cardia and the pylorus and evacuate the gases from the stomach by a gastric fistula, we see these gases reproducing immediately, not because of fermentation, which cannot happen under the given circumstances, but as a result of the gases of the blood which are released in the stomach. It is evident that the resulting meteorism reacts in its turn on the circulatory disturbances which have determined it, and thus a kind of vicious circle is established between the splanchnic circulation and the development of gastrointestinal gases. These are conditions that highly favor the increase in the toxicity of the gastric chyme and the overgrowth of the stomach flora.

The experiments of Dr. Turck which we have just described therefore show that shock is not due solely to a paralysis of the vasomotor center, but also to gastrointestinal auto-intoxication. Hematological changes also account for a certain number of phenomena, thus testifying to the complexity of a syndrome which does not consist of simple nervous exhaustion.

[p. 182]
Washington, 10 May 1903

Treatment of surgical shock in the United States

Today I plan to present the essential features of the treatment of surgical shock as it is practiced in the United States. I certainly do not intend to exhaust the question. It would be tedious, in fact, to dwell on the therapeutic means employed both in America and in Europe, especially in France: I will therefore content myself with emphasizing the points which seem to differ from the practice of European surgeons. I have already had occasion, in previous letters, to touch on certain aspects of this subject, for example the use of the Riva-Rocci apparatus by Dr. Harvey Cushing (of Baltimore), which should be considered as belonging to the preventive treatment of shock (see *Semaine Médicale*, 1903, p.16). On the other hand, I will speak in some detail about the procedures implemented in Cleveland by Dr. George W. Crile, especially since these processes, new and still unpublished, seemed particularly interesting.[42]

In the United States, strychnine is the remedy *par excellence* for the treatment of surgical shock. It is agreed that it acts as a cardiovascular tonic reinforcing the action of the heart and increasing the amplitude of the arterial pulsations. When dealing with confirmed postoperative shock, Dr. John B. Deaver (of Philadelphia) administers 1 milligram of strychnine every hour. When during an operation the assistant in charge of anesthesia notices that the pulse is beginning to weaken, he almost always uses strychnine. Confidence in the efficacy of this drug is so great that many surgeons have it administered as a preventive measure, before any operation during which they fear seeing the development of shock; they routinely give 2 or 3 milligrams of strychnine by subcutaneous injection, one hour before the operation.

We can therefore say that in America strychnine occupies in the treatment of surgical shock essentially the place assigned in France to caffeine for cases of this kind. Indeed, caffeine is almost never used here in such cases.

Atropine is also frequently used on this side of the ocean in the treatment of surgical shock, giving serious competition to strychnine. The beneficial effects that we recognize in atropine, in these cases, would result less from its influence on the vagus than from its action on the vasomotor system. By preventing vasodilatation when it does not yet exist, or by causing vasoconstriction when the vascular walls are relaxed, atropine would ensure normal tone in the circulatory system; the blood, instead of stagnating, would thus be carried towards the brain and the other essential organs. Atropine is considered by our American colleagues as the most effective vasomotor stimulant in shock. As such, it is commonly used in many conditions accompanied by vascular hypotonicity, such as pneumonia, pulmonary edema, nephrotic syndrome, typhoid fever, etc., that is in the cases for which the school of Nancy has advocated and popularized the use of ergotine in France. Atropine is most often administered by subcutaneous injection, combined with strychnine. The proportion commonly adopted in case of emergency is 10 milligrams of strychnine and 1 milligram of atropine [16].

Digitalis is given by many surgeons in extreme cases of shock, because of its powerful cardiotonic action. They do not hesitate to administer up to 1.5 grams by hypodermic injection.

Whiskey plays an important role in the treatment of surgical shock. This is no surprise to those who know the importance attributed to this *eau-de-vie* in the American therapeutic arsenal. Indeed, we can say that whiskey is the national remedy in the United States just as appendicitis is the national disease there, and it is hardly possible to conceive of any treatment here that does not involve whiskey. I would add that this alcoholic beverage is administered not only by mouth, but also as an enema or subcutaneous injection.

Without going into the details of the therapy implemented by the various American surgeons, I will also point out that the subcutaneous injections of salt water, while being used quite frequently, notably at the Johns Hopkins Hospital in Baltimore, are much less commonly used in the United States than in France. I will add in this connection that Dr. Deaver, finding the practice of these injections inconvenient and their action slow to appear, has abolished the use of them in his department of the *German Hospital* of Philadelphia; he replaces them, according to the gravity of the case and the urgency which it presents, either by small enemas, or by intravenous injections.

Such, in general, is the classic treatment for surgical shock in America. It is quite uniform throughout the country and varies relatively little from one hospital to another. But must we conclude that it is well founded? This is what remains for us to examine now.

In the course of his studies in surgical physiology, to which my letters have already drawn attention on several occasions, Dr. G. W. Crile (of Cleveland) submitted the different terms of this classic treatment to the test of the laboratory, these are his findings:

With regard first to strychnine, Dr. Crile, in numerous experiments, has never seen a rise in blood pressure in a dog in a state of shock after the administration of a *therapeutic* dose of this drug. A rise in blood pressure only occurs when strychnine is given in such quantity that it results in actual poisoning and generalized seizures. The question therefore arises as to whether the increase in blood pressure is not due to the convulsions, the muscular contractions which accompany them giving rise to an intense production of calories. However, if the animal is curarized beforehand, the convulsions are suppressed, but a rise in the blood pressure curve is nonetheless seen. We must therefore conclude that the convulsions have nothing to do with the phenomenon. Nor is it a question of excitation of the myocardium by strychnine, since this substance raises the pressure even in a curarized dog to which the two vagus nerves and the two accelerating nerves of the heart have been severed. Strychnine therefore acts essentially on the vasomotor system.

This action persists for a period of time that can vary from thirty minutes to several hours depending on the individual. If a second dose of strychnine is injected into the animal after the effect of the first has faded, it is found that its action is notably less than that of the first dose, and after having repeated the experiment two, three or four times, the administration of strychnine remains unable to raise the blood pressure. Furthermore, the curve is now as low as in an animal which is in a deep state of shock, and no external excitation – neither an electrical excitation of the sciatic, nor a burning of the paw – is able to raise it. In other words, the administration of strychnine, which is harmless but ineffective in normal therapeutic doses, in large doses provokes a state of shock analogous in all respects to that observed after major surgical or other trauma. This observation therefore provides the means of experimentally creating a state of shock by simple poisoning with strychnine. It also shows that the administration of this alkaloid, useless at normal doses for the patient in a state of shock, becomes dangerous at high doses, because the shock resulting from strychnine intoxication is then added to the original problem.

The action of most of the other stimulants of the nervous system usually employed against surgical shock – alcohol, trinitrin, amyl nitrite, etc. – is analogous to that of strychnine, according to the experiments of Dr. Crile. These experiments would be tedious to describe in detail after what we have just said about strychnine, but show that these drugs do more harm than good when they are employed in sufficient doses to have any effect on blood pressure. As for digitalis, Dr. Crile does not attribute any value to it, this medicine being less active when the blood pressure is low.

I will dwell a little longer on the researches of Dr. Crile concerning the value of injections of a physiological solution of sodium chloride. In experiments where moderate hemorrhage causes only a moderate drop in arterial pressure, it is quickly brought back to normal by the introduction of saline solution into the general circulation. But when the fall in blood pressure results from an exhaustion of the nervous system due to major trauma, that is to say when there is a state of shock, the injections of saline solution do not raise the blood pressure unless the nerve centers are not yet entirely exhausted, and their efficiency is then inversely proportional to the gravity of the shock. If it is very deep, the action of saline solution will be absolutely nil. Moreover, even when following physiological injections there is a rise in blood pressure, it hardly exceeds normal, because of the rapidity with which the liquid introduced into the body is eliminated, especially through the gastrointestinal tract. In addition, the strength and frequency of heartbeats then decrease and blood pressure is brought back to its normal level by peripheral vasodilation. As it is on the state of this peripheral resistance that the vascular tension depends, it is conceivable that, in deep shock, where this resistance has disappeared, saline solution, whatever the quantity injected and the speed of the injection, is unable to restore blood pressure to normal. But when the shock is partly due to the accumulation, in the veins, of blood which circulates badly, or if it is consecutive to a major hemorrhage, the injection of saline solution can be of service, because of the integrity of the peripheral resistance. In certain cases where this resistance has disappeared, it can be artificially made to reappear by administering adrenaline, which then acts in the same way as in the treatment of apparent death (see *Semaine Médicale*, 1903, p. 86). In any case, and whatever the effectiveness of saline injections in the treatment of profuse hemorrhage, as far as surgical shock is concerned, they would only respond, according to Dr. Crile's research, to very limited extent. In major trauma, for example, one easily manages to obtain a full pulse by injections of saline solution, but this pulse is easily crushed under the finger, because the arterial wall lacks tone, and it disappears as quickly as it came, as the peripheral resistance fails.

It is because of the severity of the loss of peripheral resistance in shock that Dr. Crile has attempted to create it artificially with the aid of a sort of "pneumatic garment." This garment, which laces up on the sides, goes down to the ankle and goes up to the waist. It consists of three pneumatic rubber chambers, one for each of the lower limbs and one for the abdomen. Each of these compartments can be inflated separately using an ordinary bicycle pump. When operating on the abdomen, the abdominal piece is folded over the thighs to leave the operating field free.[43]

Dr. Crile puts this garment on all the patients in whom he fears that shock will occur during the operation. An assistant takes the blood pressure at regular and frequent intervals using the Riva-Rocci device. As soon as he notices that the blood pressure drops below 100 or 90 millimeters of mercury [17], he begins to fill the pneumatic trousers with air. One then immediately sees the mercury rise in the manometer; the blood rushes to the heart and the brain; the face, which was pale, takes on a rosy tint, and this rosy tint henceforth persists, contrary to what is observed after the administration of strychnine and the other substances usually employed in similar cases. A sufficient quantity of air is introduced into the compartments of the pneumatic trousers to bring the blood pressure back to a good average. Once this is done, all one has to do is maintain the blood pressure at a constant level, by letting out air or by insufflating new quantities, as the case may be.

Dr. Crile has been using the pneumatic trousers consistently for about a year. At his instigation, Dr. G. E. Brewer, surgeon of the *Roosevelt Hospital* in New York, also uses it, and he told me that this surgeon has found them useful.

In conclusion, the pneumatic trousers and the injections of cocaine into the nerve trunks are the only therapeutic means that Dr. Crile uses for surgical shock, thus eliminating all the procedures usually implemented for this purpose.

[p. 192]
New York, May 24, 1903

The smallpox parasite

The smallpox parasite is like cancer: From time to time, almost periodically, an author announces that he has discovered the pathogenic agent of one or other of these diseases. Until now, however, none of these supposed discoveries has withstood serious criticism, and scientific scrutiny has quickly disposed of these often youthful endeavors. After so many disappointments, it is not surprising that our minds have become skeptical when it comes to discovery of the smallpox parasite. I believe, however, that I should mention here the work carried out on this subject by Dr. W. T. Councilman, Professor of Pathological Anatomy at the *Harvard University Medical School* and chief of the autopsy service at the *Boston City Hospital*. This was the subject of his report to the "Congress of American Physicians and Surgeons," which I have just attended in Washington, and it is no exaggeration to say that this communication was the "high point" of the Congress. The great reputation which Dr. Councilman enjoys in the United States and the consummate experience which he has acquired in matters of pathological anatomy and bacteriology gave his conclusions particular weight. I should add that Dr. W. H. Welch, Professor of Pathological Anatomy at the *Johns Hopkins Medical School* in Baltimore, having subjected the Dr. Councilman's research to a rigorous analysis, declared himself to be entirely in agreement with his colleague from Boston and supported his conclusions wholeheartedly. It therefore seemed interesting to me to report on this work, the accuracy of which will of course have to be corroborated by the test of time.

If sections of the skin are made at the level of smallpox lesions which have not yet reached the vesicle stage, one finds amorphous corpuscles lodged in the interior of the epithelial cells of the deep layers of the epidermis, whose diameter varies from 1 to 4 µ and which are located in vacuoles. As the corpuscle grows, the vacuoles also increase in size and around the corpuscle a clear space forms which also extends around the nucleus of the cell. Little by little, we see granules appear in the meshes of a network. The largest of these corpuscles – some are larger than the cellular nucleus itself – present extensions reminiscent of ameboid movements. No individualized nucleus can be distinguished in these elements, but it is possible that they possess a nucleus in the diffuse state, represented by the meshes of the network containing the granules. At this stage of its development, the corpuscle is segmented into a number of small globular bodies of about 1 µ in diameter. Anatomically, the cutaneous lesion which corresponds to this stage in the evolution of the corpuscle is the vesicle.

The nuclei of the epithelial cells containing the corpuscles described by Dr. Councilman appear normal at this stage; at least they do not yet present any of the elements which soon make their appearance in the form of small round or oval corpuscles, at the rate of one or more per nucleus. These corpuscles, as they enlarge, take on the appearance of a central vacuole, the contour of which has a considerable affinity for the coloring reagents, which is surrounded by a crown of smaller vacuoles. However, first the nucleus and then the protoplasm of the cell containing the inclusion degenerate, thus setting free the corpuscle which had developed in the nucleus of the cell. Once the vacuolation of the intranuclear corpuscle has reached a certain degree of development, one sees appearing in the clear spaces with which the corpuscle is stuffed with small rounded elements. After a certain time, these group together in clusters surrounded by a halo which is probably only the residue of the intranuclear corpuscle which gave them birth.

The elements described by Dr. Councilman would represent, for this anatomic pathologist, the evolutionary phases of the organism which may be the true pathogenic agent of smallpox. There would therefore be two stages to be distinguished in the evolutionary cycle, one traversed in the protoplasmic body of the deep epidermal cells, the other in the interior of the nucleus of these same cells. The former would be the *intracellular* stage, the latter the *intranuclear* stage. The granulations appearing in the vacuoles of the intracellular period would be nothing other than spores then passing into the nucleus to continue their evolution there. In the intranuclear stage there seem to exist sexual elements: Certain large corpuscles would represent macrogametes or female elements, small corpuscles coloring in an intense way would be microgametes or male elements.

By inoculating the corneas of rabbits with variola pus, Dr. Councilman obtained corpuscles analogous in all points to those which he met with in the first or intracellular stage of the element which he regards as the small-pox parasite. The same elements were found after the simple vaccination of the rabbit. Dr. Councilman thus arrived at the concept that the vaccine corresponds to the partial evolution of the same micro-organism which, by going through a complete cycle, causes smallpox. A number of experiments support this view. A smallpox spore which, when inoculated into a calf, gives only vaccinia, only goes through the intracellular cycle; after this passage through the calf, the spore in question would no longer cause smallpox in subjects otherwise capable of contracting this disease.

We know that, unlike the calf and the rabbit, the monkey can have actual smallpox: After having inoculated it with smallpox pus, Dr. Councilman found in this animal the two evolutionary stages, intra-cellular and intra-nuclear, which he had recognized in humans.

From what I have just said, we see that the parasite to which Dr. Councilman attributes a determining function in the etiology of smallpox, goes through two successive evolutionary cycles, one asexual, the other sexual. When the parasite stops at its first asexual stage, it gives rise to the cowpox. Because it is the same pathogenic agent, this would explain the nosographic unity of smallpox and vaccinia, the latter being only an attenuated form of the former. However, we see that there are still many unknowns in the problem, and before it is definitively resolved, many related questions will have to be solved.

[p. 202]
Washington, 17 May 1903

In the past three weeks, I have attended a whole series of American medical meetings in New Orleans and in Washington. These are quite specific meetings, some of which only include one or two sessions. I could say many things about them which might be of some interest to the readers of a French journal; because, in many ways, these Congresses are different from those we are used to seeing in Europe. However, to fully understand the purpose pursued by the American meetings, the way they are organized, the results they produce and are likely to produce, it is important to have previously explored related questions, such as the practice and teaching of medicine in the United States, matters which I propose to deal with later. I will therefore reserve the right to speak in due course about American medical meetings. For the moment, I will simply say that, among the subjects which have given rise to my previous letters, several relate to questions whose current state I have already had reported on based on the information I gathered during my trip. Among these is the question of radiotherapy, to which a whole morning was devoted at the Washington Congress; having discussed this subject in previous letters, it does not seem useful to return to it now: I found there the same enthusiasms, the same skepticisms, the same antagonisms that I have already described. I will say the same of cholelithiasis; as I indicated, cholecystectomy is daily gaining favor with American surgeons. Dr. W. J. Mayo (of Rochester) expressed the general feeling on this point by saying that "cholecystectomy is the operation of the future." Other questions have not yet been dealt with in my correspondence; what I shall have to say about them will find its natural place in the articles which I propose to devote to them, using information which I have gathered previously in the course of my journey. So I will not dwell on it now.

I must add, however, that during these three weeks of meetings, I hardly heard a word about appendicitis. I emphasize this fact because it is characteristic: It shows – as I said a while ago – that on this side of the Atlantic the treatment of appendicitis is a settled matter.

Operative treatment of uterine retrodeviations

There is another question which has hardly been discussed in these different meetings, although American surgeons seem to be taking a certain interest in it at the present time. In any case, I think it is an interesting technical matter apparently in the process of evolution. I refer to the operative treatment of uterine retrodeviations, and will describe today the practice of American gynecologists.

Assuredly, the evolution of ideas on this point is slow and progressive, and the advocates of hysteropexy always find themselves in the presence of partisans for shortening the round ligaments. But it is obvious that neither of the two camps believes that they have said the last word in the matter of operative treatment of uterine retroflexion: On both sides, they are above all working to improve the techniques originally employed.

Dr. Howard A. Kelly, who was one of the early champions of hysteropexy [18], is still one of the most fervent supporters of this operation, which he always uses when the non-operative treatment of retroflexion is insufficient or impracticable. He frequently even performs it as a preventive measure, or as an incidental procedure at the end of a laparotomy.

Dr. Kelly has gradually but noticeably changed his original procedure. Instead of opposing the anterior surface of the uterus to the posterior surface of the anterior abdominal wall, he now attaches the posterior surface of the uterine fundus to the anterior abdominal peritoneum. To bring the uterus into this position, it is placed in a forced anteflexion; it is therefore not a question of a simple correction, but of an actual overcorrection of the faulty position that one seeks to remedy. This anomaly is only temporary. Indeed, Dr. Kelly has verified by bimanual palpation that after a certain number of weeks the uterus returns to a perfectly normal situation and conformation.

This is because the fundus of the uterus does not contract a surface adhesion with the abdominal wall; only a few bands are formed joining the visceral layer of the peritoneum to its parietal layer. And these attachments, under the influence of the weight of the abdominal organs which rest on the uterus, lengthen sufficiently to allow the latter to resume its normal situation, although not enough to reproduce the retroflexion. Having had occasion on several occasions to reopen the abdomen in cases where he had performed a hysteropexy following these principles, Dr. Kelly found adhesions varying in length from 4 to 5 centimeters. These adhesions, unlike those obtained by the usual methods, do not present any disadvantages during the course of pregnancy or at the time of delivery. Here are the details of the process Dr. Kelly is currently using:

The abdomen is opened by a midline laparotomy with its lower end two centimeters from the pubic symphysis; the hand is introduced into the abdominal cavity and slides over the bladder, then over the anterior surface of the retroflexed uterus until reaching the bottom of this organ on the pelvic floor. Along the way, any peritoneal adhesions which may be retaining the uterus in its abnormal position are dissected away; these adhesions are divided between two ligatures if they are more resistant. At this time, the ovaries and Fallopian tubes are inspected. When the condition of these organs makes their removal indicated, this operation is immediately carried out, thus replacing the hysteropexy by an abdominal hysterectomy. Otherwise, the uterine fundus is brought into the abdominal wound, and the organ is placed in anteflexion such that its posterior part is anterior. A needle threaded with silk then penetrates from inside to outside a good centimeter from the edge of the peritoneum, which it includes for a length of about two centimeters. It then travels from outside to inside in the uterus a finger's breadth below and behind a line which joins the two Fallopian tubes and comes out about a centimeter further. It is important that the suture include, in addition to the uterine serosa, a certain thickness of the muscular wall of the organ. Finally, the thread is passed through the abdominal peritoneum on the other side so as to ensure the symmetry of the suture, which is tied immediately. Although the hysteropexy is now performed, Dr. Kelly usually places a second stitch one centimeter above the first. This second point, by increasing the anteflexion of the uterus, puts a greater part of the posterior surface of this organ in contact with the abdominal wall and serves to "relieve" the first point of suture. It is exceptional for more than two sutures to be required.

The adhesions thus produced, in the opinion of many surgeons, are likely to cause painful symptoms. I must say, in this connection, that, in general, peritoneal adhesions, even of insignificant appearance, are ordinarily feared in the United States, as much because of the pain as because of the incidents of obstruction which they are likely to cause. Many surgeons are quick to reopen the abdomen to resect adhesions resulting from previous operations (appendicitis, etc.) or from any other causes (peritoneal plaques from chronic tuberculous peritonitis). This explains the resistance that hysteropexy meets with many American gynecologists who give preference to procedures aimed at shortening the round ligaments. I add that hysteropexy is hardly practiced except along the Atlantic coast; I heard no more of it once I left the eastern United States.

The original Alquié-Alexander procedure[44] is still employed by a number of surgeons, such as Dr. Mayo (of Rochester) and Dr. Ochsner (of Chicago). I will only point out that Dr. Mayo insists on the necessity of stripping off the peritoneal sheath from the round ligament as far as possible, before attaching it to the femoral arch: it is the length thus stripped of peritoneum that produces the shortening. By pushing this denudation far enough, it often happens that the peritoneum is perforated. This produces involuntarily the operation recommended by Dr. Goldspohn (of Chicago) which consists, as we know, of an intraperitoneal shortening of the round ligaments (see *Semaine Médicale*, 1899, p. 276). This also leads to the process of pleating proposed by Dr. A. Palmer Dudley (of New York), and on which there is no need to dwell here, since it has been published previously.

These procedures constitute the natural transition to another group of operations, also intraperitoneal, which I saw performed by Dr. J. M. Baldy during my stay in Philadelphia. Here is how this surgeon proceeded during the operation I observed:

After performing a midline laparotomy, he divided the round ligaments flush with the uterus, first placing a ligature on the round ligament stumps that remained attached to the uterine *cornu*. To make the internal extremity of the round ligaments mobile, Dr. Baldy then divided, over a length of about 3 centimeters, the *mesos* which constitutes the anterior wing of the broad ligament. Then, using hemostats, he collapsed the broad ligaments into the angle formed by the lateral edge of the uterus and the Fallopian tube. This orifice must be made as close as possible to the edge of the uterus without there being any reason to fear complications due to the venous plexuses which are at this level, because they have been dissected off with a blunt instrument. The round ligaments, having passed through the hole thus made in the broad ligament, were fastened together by a silk overlocking suture. This resulted in a sort of sling embracing the uterus by its posterior surface and drawing it forward towards the symphysis. In order that this traction be exerted in the desired direction, it is important to fix the sling by a suture to the fundus of the uterus as high as possible, over the whole width of the posterior surface of the organ.

Dr. Baldy varies this operation according to the different cases. It is obvious, in fact, that such a considerable shortening as that which results from the process of which we have just spoken is not suitable for all the retrodeviations and could possibly create complications because of the tension which it causes. In cases of this kind, Dr. Baldy, instead of forming the sling of which we have spoken, limits himself to fixing the extremity of the round ligaments to the posterior surface of the uterine *cornu*. The level of implantation of the sling or isolated ligaments varied in Dr. Baldy's early operations; currently, this surgeon believes that the highest implantations, on the uterine fundus, give the best results.

This procedure has not so far appeared to create any difficulties during gestation or at the time of childbirth. Nor has it been observed to interfere in any way with normal bladder function. It can only be reproached for giving an irregular position to the ovaries which are lifted, but it seems that no inconvenience results from this.

[p. 249]
San Francisco, 21 June 1903

Stomach surgery in the United States

It is only in recent times that surgeons in the United States have begun to take an interest in the treatment of stomach disorders, and it may be said that if in America the operative treatment of appendicitis was yesterday's question, just as cholelithiasis is today's question, operative intervention in diseases of the stomach is probably tomorrow's question. I had the opportunity to show in my previous correspondence that the majority of American surgeons are currently in agreement on the course of action to be taken for appendicitis and that, for cholelithiasis, we begin to see in what direction this agreement will doubtless be established in the relatively near future; on the contrary, as far as surgery of the stomach is concerned, we are still at the beginning phase of trial and error. Curiously, and contrary to what usually happens, the leadership in this area comes from West and Northwest, not from the Atlantic coast.[45] I can particularly name Dr. William J. Mayo, surgeon at *St. Mary's Hospital* in Rochester, Minnesota, and Dr. A. J. Ochsner, surgeon at the *Augustana Hospital* in Chicago, as dealing especially with operations on the stomach. It is primarily the practice currently adopted by these two surgeons that I will describe in the following lines.

Among the non-cancerous conditions of the stomach, ulcers and the complications which arise from them (hemorrhages, perforations, pyloric stenosis, total or partial gastric distension) most often provide the indication for surgery. The tendency is to intervene as early as possible. It is thus that Dr. Ochsner has made it a rule to operate on all cases of gastric ulcer in which medical treatment does not give a complete and permanent cure, or in which signs of pyloric obstruction appear. Such a course of action, according to this surgeon, protects against future complications at the cost of a much less serious operation than that which is necessary once these complications have appeared. It is therefore, to use the expression of American surgeons, the treatment of the ulcer "in the interval between attacks" that our colleague from Chicago advocates and implements.

Of the various procedures performed for non-cancerous conditions of the stomach, gastrojejunostomy is undoubtedly the procedure most commonly used by American surgeons. It is thus that out of 169 operations performed under similar conditions by Dr. Mayo, and recorded by him in a series that this surgeon communicated to the Washington Congress which I just attended, gastrojejunostomy appears 87 times, that is to say in about half of the cases. From the point of view of operative technique, Dr. Mayo attaches great importance to the choice of the location where the anastomosis between the stomach and the intestine should be made. For him, in fact, the essential thing is to place the gastrointestinal anastomosis at the most inferior part of the stomach wall. It is only on this condition that it would be possible to effectively ensure the drainage of this reservoir, the main goal of the intervention, and to prevent the stagnation of part of the stomach contents in the pocket which tends to form below the visceral anastomosis. Indeed, the production of such a pocket is the usual, if not the only, source of persistent post-operative vomiting occurring after gastroenterostomy. Dr. Mayo thinks that when the von Hacker operation is performed – in which the loop of intestine, entering through an artificial orifice in the transverse mesocolon into the retro-gastric serous space known as the lesser omental bursa, is attached to the posterior surface of the stomach – this anastomosis is always placed correctly in the low position, owing to the local constraints, and it is to this circumstance that he attributes the superiority of the results obtained by the majority of surgeons with von Hacker's procedure. Dr. Mayo himself is careful to establish the gastrojejunal anastomosis at the most inferior part of the stomach, but otherwise can use the anterior or posterior approach with equally good results; what currently guides him in choosing the course to follow is primarily the length of the transverse mesocolon.

Dr. Ochsner, who has accepted the ideas expressed by Dr. Mayo, also insists on the advantage of making the anastomosis at the most inferior part of the stomach. Having no longer seen the vomiting which frequently appears following the establishment of a gastroenterostomy and which is usually attributed to a vicious circle, since he placed the anastomosis as low as possible, he is willing to admit that this vomiting is indeed usually due to the fact that the anastomosis is not in a good position; he considers that it is sufficient to ensure perfect drainage of the gastric contents in the intestine to suppress the post-operative vomiting in question.

As for how the gastrointestinal anastomosis is performed, suturing by hand with the straight needle is still the most common method. On the subject of mechanical procedures, I would say that Murphy's metallic button is in very common use, and certain surgeons, such as Dr. Mayo, use it in a systematic and exclusive fashion. I will add, however, that from what I have heard the Murphy button is now much less frequently used than it once was, and the indications for its use seem likely to become more limited. This would be an area where Europe has preceded America: We know that in France, for example, the Murphy button is no longer applied except in special cases. As for the bone bobbin recommended by Dr. Mayo Robson (of Leeds), I heard a great deal about it in the United States, but I have never seen it used. I therefore believe that I can conclude that its use is not very frequent there.

On the other hand, the elastic ligature method of Dr. Th. A. McGraw (of Detroit), seems to me at present in the process of supplanting the Murphy button;[46] I saw it used on my first visits to American hospitals – notably at the *Massachusetts General Hospital* in Boston, where I observed a gastroenterostomy performed by Dr. J. Collins Warren – and I found it everywhere in the course of my travels across the United States, in the northwest, in New Orleans, and finally here, in San Francisco. This process having been described by its author, it will be enough for me to point out the popularity it enjoys with American surgeons and the excellent results it seems to have given in their hands. It seems that this process is recommended above all for the ease and rapidity of its execution, the solidity of the anastomosis, and the permanence of the opening which would not tend to shrink progressively, as with certain other methods.

Unlike McGraw's process, that advocated by Dr. G. Ryerson Fowler (of Brooklyn) is quite complicated. However, it does not seem to me destined to become widely used, despite the good results that its author has obtained from it. It essentially consists of a double anastomosis of the intestine, first to the stomach, then to the jejunum, the lumen of the intermediate intestinal loop between these two anastomoses being occluded using a silver wire ligation to prevent biliary and pancreatic secretions from flowing back into the stomach.

The procedure of gastroduodenostomy described in the middle of last year by Dr John M. T. Finney (of Baltimore) as a *pyloroplasty*, although it is still on trial and has not yet stood the test of time, has a number of supporters.[47] Dr. Mayo, for example, has performed it more than 25 times. He thinks that Finney's procedure is likely to render service in cases of pyloric obstruction where the dilatation of the stomach is not excessive and where the pyloric lesions are not very extensive. The procedure in question would then make it possible to carry out a detailed examination of the pyloric region of the stomach and could easily be completed by the excision of an ulcer in a juxta-pyloric location. When the dilatation of the stomach is very considerable, Dr. Mayo considers the procedure of Finney as contraindicated unless it is combined with the operation of Beyea (shortening of the lesser omentum); in general, the Rochester surgeon then gives preference to simple gastrojejunostomy. As for the usefulness of Finney's procedure in cases of simple ulcers not complicated by pyloric stricture, this is a question still under study and which, *a priori*, does not seem to me to have to be resolved in the affirmative: It is conceivable, in fact, that the passage of food and stomach contents at the level of the ulcer does not constitute a favorable condition for healing.

With regard to cancerous tumors of the stomach, in particular of the pylorus, the operation usually performed in the United States is gastroenterostomy. The technique followed in these cases differs too little from that used in France for me to dwell on this subject. I will only say that, here again, both Dr. Mayo and Dr. Ochsner emphasize the importance of placing the anastomosis at the most inferior point of the stomach.

In a certain number of cases, Dr. Mayo has attempted to perform a subtotal gastrectomy, recalling in many respects, as we will see and as I pointed out to this surgeon during my visit to Rochester, the operation described in France by Dr. Cunéo as early as 1900. The part of the stomach resected by Dr. Mayo is located to the right and below a line joining the level where the left gastroepiploic artery joins the greater curvature. A sort of "dome" is thus preserved, consisting essentially of the large fundus of the stomach. This process would present no drawback from the point of view of recurrence, the portion of the organ left in place being only rarely affected by stomach cancer — except in cases of neoplasm at the cardia — because of the poorly developed lymphatic system. In addition, the blood supply to the "stomach dome" would be ensured in its right part because of the cardiac branches of the left gastric artery, and in its left part because of the short gastric vessels which arise from the splenic artery or its ramifications. The advantage of a subtotal gastrectomy over a total resection of the stomach is not so much in the greater benignity of the operation – the latter appearing to present about the same seriousness in both cases – as in the advantage that there would be to keep part of the stomach to facilitate the joining of the intestine with the esophagus.

Here is the exact technique adopted by Dr. Mayo:

The left gastric artery being tied beforehand at the level where it reaches the lesser curvature of the stomach, he places, between this point and the pylorus, and as close as possible to the liver, a ligature around the lesser omentum *en masse*. A section of the lesser omentum passing flush with the ligature makes it possible to extirpate almost all of this serous fold and gives great mobility to the pyloric end of the stomach; this mobility greatly facilitates subsequent maneuvers. The right extremity of the greater omentum is then tied, the duodenum is sectioned between two clamps and the duodenum is immediately closed off *definitively* by a procedure similar to that employed by Dr. Mayo for the occlusion of the appendix in appendectomy (see *Semaine Médicale*, 1903, p. 119). Then he completes the ligation of the greater omentum and ties off the left gastro-epiploic artery. The stomach is clamped with a strong forceps and a catgut suture is placed in the furrow created by the clamp. This done, cautery separates the "dome" of the stomach from the part of the organ to be resected which because of the clamp can be done without appreciable hemorrhage and without opening the viscus. All that remains is to reinforce the occlusion of this gastric remnant with a certain number of stitches, and to create an anastomosis between it and the jejunum, which completes the gastrectomy.

Sometimes, Dr. Mayo has noted that the intestine tends to kink at the level of the anastomosis: The jejunum is drawn to the left and superiorly for a length of 35 to 40 centimeters, and there is consequently an accumulation of biliary and pancreatic secretions in the segment of the jejunum located upstream of the anastomosis; the strength of the traction exerted under these conditions is sufficient in certain cases to bring about a disruption of the anastomosis; this is the mechanism to which Dr. Mayo attributes the two deaths he has observed following his operation. Therefore, he now routinely completes the subtotal gastrectomy with a jejuno-jejunostomy which allows the free flow of liquids which accumulate upstream of the gastroenterostomy.

We see that the operation recommended and practiced by Dr. Mayo resembles that of Cunéo in that, in both cases, the resection involves the whole of the lesser curvature. It is essentially about the greater curvature that there is a difference of opinion. *A priori*, it is evident that by retaining a larger portion of the greater curvature, Dr. Cunéo greatly facilitates the establishment of the gastrointestinal anastomosis, the functioning of which is also accomplished with greater ease, so that the complementary entero-enteric anastomosis practiced by Dr. Mayo becomes unnecessary. However, the Rochester surgeon would have, in a certain number of cases, encountered lymph nodes invaded by the neoplasm along the greater curvature, at a point which remains outside the area resected by Dr. Cunéo. It remains to be seen whether, in these facts, these were not too advanced cases for an intervention as serious as a subtotal gastrectomy to still be justified. This is a point that only experience at the patient's bedside can settle.

[p. 267]
Defense against yellow fever in the Gulf of Mexico

The vast surface covered by the territory of the United States may be subdivided into a number of natural regions, often markedly differing from each other. The distinction which has been established for a long time between the North and the South is one of the most obvious and most clearly accentuated; it is found everywhere and at every step, and it also asserts itself in the epidemiologic area. Most infectious diseases behave very differently depending on whether they affect an inhabitant of the Northern States or an individual living in the South.

Take, for example, typhoid fever. I had previously had the opportunity to emphasize the special characteristics of those affected by typhoid in the United States, and to show how often it presents itself there in an attenuated form, especially in recent years (see *Semaine Médicale*, 1903, pp. 15 and 106). I had also pointed out in this connection that, despite the enormous morbidity due to Eberth's bacillus, it seemed that the lethality was decreasing and the disease was becoming more benign.

Now, in the South - I have studied New Orleans in particular, but the same remark generally applies to all the states of the South - it is curious to note that typhoid seems rather to follow an opposite course, namely increasing. Whereas a few years ago, the diagnosis was often uncertain, now typhoid fever has evolved in New Orleans to present the classic picture of a serious and well characterized disease. I discussed this question with Dr. E. M. Dupaquier – a former student of the Faculty of Medicine of Paris, practicing in New Orleans – who has been very impressed by these developments that have occurred in Louisiana; he attributes them to a double importation, on the one hand by the increasing contact with the North and West of the United States and on the other hand by European immigration, especially Sicilian, which has also been growing for some time.

This explanation seems quite plausible, if one considers the behavior in the South of most of the endemic and epidemic infections raging in the North. It follows, in fact, from all the information that was given to me on the spot, from several sources, that measles, scarlet fever, diphtheria, etc., evolve in the South with a remarkable benignity. The cases are generally sporadic, and a serious epidemic is almost never observed, either by the number of individuals struck, or by the severity of the attacks. It is as if the subtropical climate of Louisiana were contrary to the development of contagion, which is the determining factor of these diseases.

It is quite different with essentially tropical epidemic diseases, such as plague, cholera, and especially yellow fever. It is easy in the North to stop the extension of these diseases, but it is difficult to control them in the South. This explains the almost draconian measures enacted by the southern states to protect themselves from the introduction of these afflictions on their territory, which generally takes place by sea.

Plague and cholera come especially into account for the ports of the Pacific coast: We know, in fact, that both of these diseases have their center in Asia. On the contrary, yellow fever has its main focus in Central America – continental and insular – and is therefore an ongoing risk for the American ports located on the Gulf of Mexico. It is therefore easy to conceive of the interest that these ports have in the defense against an invasion of yellow fever, especially the largest of them, New Orleans.

The measures to be adopted depend on the ideas one has about the mode of transmission. Now, these very ideas are being radically modified, under the influence of the work carried out since 1898, the date of the American occupation of the island of Cuba, where yellow fever existed in an endemic state. This is what emerges clearly from the often impassioned discussions on this subject, which I had the opportunity to observe at various meetings in New Orleans. As this debate focuses on the question of the mode of transmission of yellow fever and prophylaxis against this infectious disease, it seems interesting to describe it briefly.

The controversy in New Orleans, always lively, often bitter and vehement, was between Dr. Edmond Souchon, president of the Louisiana Board of Health, and Dr. J. M. Lindsley, health officer of the United States Medical Corps maritime hospitals.

It was a question of whether the boats coming from the island of Cuba, in particular from Havana, capital of the island, do or do not constitute a danger for New Orleans. Dr. Souchon said yes, Dr. Lindsley said no. The choice that is made has important consequences.

To accept Dr. Lindsley's thesis is, in effect, to grant all ships from Cuba free access on arrival in New Orleans, and to abolish all the precautionary measures currently in use. But if the theory on which Dr. Lindsley bases himself is incorrect, it will expose the entire region to yellow fever; for if this disease gains a foothold in New Orleans it will almost certainly produce an epidemic as serious as it is widespread: The epidemic of 1878 cost more than 4,000 lives.

To adopt instead the views of Dr. Souchon would be to maintain prohibitionist regulations which create a considerable obstacle and barrier to trade. These regulations – the last is of September 2, 1902 – require first a complete disinfection of the vessel, including the clothing and luggage of the passengers, as well as the cargo, at the last stopover; and a second disinfection at the entrance to the Mississippi, at the quarantine station established by the State of Louisiana, requiring at least five full days between the two disinfections: When the vessel has remained at sea less than five days after the first disinfection, the unloading of the cargo is permitted, but the passengers are held in quarantine until the end of the fifth day.

This double disinfection is justified because they have sometimes seen the occurrence, on vessels not infected at the start and presenting no suspected case at the time of arrival, of typical and undisputed cases of yellow fever after arrival at the port. Dr. Souchon, who has collected some facts on this subject, thinks that the appearance of the disease is due in such an occurrence to the fact that during the maneuvers carried out to disinfect for the first time, some agent is set in motion or in circulation, which was previously latent. On the other hand, they have never seen a case of yellow fever declare itself after the regulatory incubation period which follows the second disinfection.

The arguments on which Dr. Lindsley relies to request the abolition of these quarantine measures with regard to ships from Cuba are entirely based on the research carried out in Havana by Reed, Carroll and others. According to this work, only one particular mosquito, the *Stegomyia fasciata*,[48] is capable of transmitting the agent of yellow fever to man. Destroying this mosquito is therefore equivalent to eliminating the possibility of the transmission of yellow fever to humans. It is thanks to the systematic destruction of mosquitoes in Havana that yellow fever is said to have been eradicated, and there is currently not a single case. At least that is the official statement. I must add that, during the discussion of the question before the Medical Society of the State of Louisiana, I heard several colleagues – notably Drs. Jones, Perkins, Stewart – question this allegation.

Be that as it may, it is obvious that, if we accept that Cuba is henceforth free from yellow fever, the abolition of quarantine measures is desirable and the double disinfection of the boat becomes as useless as the detention of passengers.

Where the question becomes complicated is when we consider the various states bordering the Gulf of Mexico. Indeed, two of them, Florida and Mississippi, have now granted free passage to all vessels coming from Cuba. Louisiana, Texas, and Alabama, on the contrary, continue to maintain their prophylactic measures [19]. We can therefore see how easy it must be to circumvent the regulations of these three states. It is true that the latter maintain special health inspectors on their land borders responsible for preventing fraud, but one can doubt the effectiveness of such a measure. In reality, the importance of the health coalition of the three states lies above all in the fact that the main ports on the coast – New Orleans, Galveston, and Mobile – are on their territory, while Florida or Mississippi can offer ships only limited resources from a maritime point of view.

In conclusion, I would say that the general impression of those of our colleagues in New Orleans who have followed the discussions on the quarantine to be imposed on ships coming from Cuba from their inception, is that the views of the partisans of the mosquito theory gain more adherents every day, and that on the contrary the rigor of the measures imposed by the Louisiana Board of Health is becoming more and more relaxed. Already many concessions have been made; others will follow, according to some rumors. It would be a question, in fact, of granting free practice to those coming from Cuba if within a year a new epidemic of yellow fever does not break out on this island.

This fact would have general importance, because it would show that it is possible to combat this formidable disease effectively; it would also indicate the procedure that should be adopted to arrive at such a result. This is a point which is not without interest for the inhabitants of old Europe, since today, with the ease of transoceanic relations, distances are no longer an obstacle to the spread of infectious agents.

[p. 296]
Prostatectomy in the United States

On several occasions already, in my letters devoted to the present state of surgery in the United States, I have had the opportunity to describe the interest of our American colleagues in questions of operative technique and on the improvements that can be made. The question of surgical treatment of prostatic hypertrophy is further evidence of this. Until a few years ago this was a virtually unknown chapter of surgery in America, and bladder catheterization was considered the last word in the treatment of prostatic hypertrophy. Since then, however, doubts have arisen as to the value or even the safety of such therapy, and it is fair to say that palliative treatment by the catheter has now been totally abandoned, if not by all of our American colleagues, at least by those in the vanguard of surgical progress. They are currently in agreement that the rational treatment of this condition consists in an early removal of the hypertrophied gland. But the agreement breaks down when it comes to determining the best way to proceed with prostatectomy. Let us say right now that a trend seems to be taking shape which would make perineal prostatectomy the standard operation, with suprapubic route being reserved for special cases where perineal intervention is contraindicated because of certain special conditions.

Thus Dr. James E. Moore, Chief Surgeon of *Northwestern Hospital* in Minneapolis and Professor of Clinical Surgery at the University of Minnesota is one of the most convinced supporters of the standard operation, but in many cases does not hesitate to give up the perineal route in favor of the suprapubic route. This surgeon estimates that the progress of the technique will make it possible in the not distant future to use the perineal prostatectomy in a larger proportion of cases than today.

The studies made by Dr. Moore on the procedures for removing the prostate began with observations which he made while performing massage of this organ through the rectum. He noticed that in cases where the prostate is not palpable through the rectum, introducing a probe into the bladder and directing the beak downwards and backwards made the prostate accessible in all its parts by a hand placed in the rectum. However, to operate by the suprapubic route, one is obliged to open the bladder, sometimes even to make several openings in it. Each of these incisions made on a hollow organ with septic and virulent content is unnecessary, since the cystitis accompanying prostatic hypertrophy has a natural tendency to clear after the removal of the hypertrophied gland; it is dangerous, because opening the infectious focus in the bladder is likely to become the starting point of a generalized and potentially fatal infection.

As to the possibility of keeping the prostatic urethra intact by adopting the suprapubic route – as Dr. Freyer, for example, has proposed in connection with the procedure which he popularized in England – Dr. Moore thinks that this is wishful thinking, because of the intimate connections that the gland has to the urethral wall at the level where the ejaculatory and prostatic ducts enter the urethra.

Although clinical experience has shown that a large area of the prostatic urethra can be sacrificed without significantly compromising the normal functioning of the bladder during urination, it would be advantageous to retain much of the urethral wall, because the greater the loss of substance, the greater the tendency to stricture. Now, Dr. Moore considers that intervening via the perineal route provides the best chance of sparing the urethra. Moreover, in accordance with the ideas expressed and defended by Dr. John B. Murphy (of Chicago), Dr. Moore thinks that it is never useful to practice the ablation of the glandular bridge which unites the two lobes of the prostate gland where the ejaculatory and prostatic ducts run, because the area in question is never the location of hypertrophy. The so-called median lobe or valve of Mercier is always an extension of one of the lateral lobes of the prostate and undergoes the fate of that lobe when it is removed.

An important argument of Dr. Moore in favor of the perineal route is the greater facility for drainage. In the suprapubic operation, drainage can only be done in the opposite direction to gravity, which allows the persistence of purulent collections in the bladder. This is an important fact, since after suprapubic prostatectomy one is often obliged to make an additional perineal incision simply to ensure effective drainage.

The main contraindication admitted by Dr. Moore is a soft and friable or very vascular state of the prostate in whole or in part. In such cases, he gives preference to suprapubic surgery.

As to the details of Dr. Moore's technique, there is little to specifically point out. I will only mention, in addition the Trendelenburg position in which he places his patients, that instead of the Y-shaped or crescent-shaped incisions generally used in France, he prefers a long antero-posterior incision going from the scrotum to the anus. Only in exceptional cases does he find it useful to enlarge the incision by completing it with an inverted V, giving rise to the classic Y.

Most surgeons in the Northwest share Dr. Moore's ideas. I will cite in particular Dr. Archibald MacLaren in Saint Paul, the sister city of Minneapolis, whom I saw perform a prostatectomy following the same technique.

In Rochester, Minnesota, Dr. Charles H. Mayo also prefers the perineal operation. However, he recognizes much more extensive indications for intervention by the suprapubic route than does Dr. Moore. Thus, for example, in obese subjects he always performs suprapubic prostatectomy, sometimes with a perineal incision to facilitate drainage. He also uses the anterior approach if the bladder is very distended. It is the same when the urinary bladder contains stones, or when it is a reoperation after a previous exploration of the bladder for stones or any other cause.

Contrary to Dr. Moore, Dr. C. H. Mayo prefers a transverse curvilinear incision for perineal prostatectomy, because he thinks that by thus creating a vast cavity comparable to that of the vagina, one obtains better access to the deeper parts of the prostatic region.

In Chicago, Dr. Albert J. Ochsner has long been a strong proponent of the suprapubic approach for radical prostatectomy. Currently, he has almost completely abandoned this procedure for the perineal route, except in the case where there is a lobe protruding prominently inside the bladder cavity. One of the main advantages that Dr. Ochsner recognizes in the perineal approach is that it makes it possible to establish satisfactory postoperative drainage of the bladder, which is generally infected in subjects suffering from prostatic hypertrophy. This surgeon has also adopted a horseshoe incision to open the prostatic compartment.

In short, if the treatment of enlarged prostate by removal of the organ cannot yet be considered as a definitively settled question among American surgeons, agreement has nevertheless been established on a certain number of essential points. The question remains on the agenda and they continue to take a keen interest in it, as evidenced by the discussions I have witnessed in various conferences and professional societies. It is likely that prostatectomy will become a settled question in the near future, just like appendectomy.

[p. 312]
Iowa state anti-alcoholism law

At a time when hygienists everywhere are trying to combat the principal causes that threaten society with degeneration and destruction, I thought it would be interesting, during my investigation of medical America, to describe their struggle against one of the most important of these degenerative factors: alcoholism.

By all accounts, alcoholism is very prevalent in the United States. It would be tedious to try to specify the degree of it by using the figures provided by statistics. With the homogeneous and more or less constant population of France, one could conceive of an approximate numerical proportion and say, for example, that in fifty years the consumption of alcohol has quadrupled in our country, but it is quite different in the United States. There, the population has increased considerably during the last half-century; moreover, its components have been so variable over time – I would almost say each year – that the figures would be misleading and would lose all value. Since it is therefore hardly possible to establish a parallel between the two countries, it is nonetheless obvious, for anyone who has stayed in the United States for a sufficient time, that alcoholism is much more widespread there than in France. This explains why, in certain states at least, there has been no opposition to the adoption of almost draconian measures to combat alcoholism.

Having learned that of all the states of the Union it was Iowa that currently had the strictest anti-alcoholic legislation, I went specially to that state to gather precise information on current conditions. It is of this visit, and of the information that I was able to obtain there, that I am going to give an account in the present letter.

We know that from the legislative point of view the various states [20] whose federation constitutes the United States enjoy a certain autonomy, by virtue of which each of them enacts its own laws as it sees fit. Consequently, on many questions, we find different laws from one state to another. Thus, there is no reason to be surprised that the state of Iowa was able to adopt, on 12 April 1902, a law on alcoholism that is not found in any of the other states.

By virtue of the law in question, there has been created in each of the insane asylums belonging to the State of Iowa a division specially intended, according to the law, for the detention and treatment of *dipsomaniacs, drunkards, and individuals addicted to the abuse of morphine or other narcotics.* Obviously, this amounts to putting alcoholics – it is them above all that the legislator is aiming at – on the same footing as the insane or juvenile delinquents.

This assimilation is the fundamental principle of the new law; it shows very clearly in what spirit the measures in question must be considered. It explains, among other things, the provisions regulating the placement of the drinker in an asylum and guaranteeing him against arbitrary confinement. In both cases, the district court or the judge of the county where the drunkard lives is entrusted with the task of having experts examine the person denounced or reported, and deciding whether there is a need for placement in an asylum. The length of stay in this establishment varies according to the number of recurrences. During the first placement, it cannot be less than one year nor more than three years. In case of recidivism, the minimum is two years, the maximum five. The duration of the internment is fixed by the judicial authorities which order the placement: District court or county judge. Alongside these compulsory placements, voluntary placements or placements requested by the family are also accepted.

After a month's stay in the asylum, the director of this establishment, with the assent of the attending physician, may propose to the governor of the state the conditional release of the subject whom he considers cured. To be able to benefit from this favorable provision of the law, the patient must first undertake in writing to abstain from all alcoholic beverages and all narcotics for the duration of the time for which the internment had been ordered when he is not in the asylum; he must also promise to avoid associates who would cause him to resume his old habits of drunkenness.

Such a commitment may seem platonic at first sight: We understand that, to recover his freedom, an alcoholic interned in an asylum would like nothing better than to sign anything that is asked of him, even if it means forgetting his commitments as soon as he is freed. Even among those who sign in good faith, some will not be able to resist the temptation and will fall back into their old mistakes. But this case was anticipated by the law. It orders that any individual given a provisional release by virtue of a voluntary provision be required to provide a report on the first of each month to the director of the asylum in which he had been placed, establishing that he has honored his commitments. The accuracy of this report must be certified, after investigation, by the clerk of the court of the district where the patient resides. If he neglects to send his monthly report, or the clerk refuses his *exequatur*, this is enough for the "released" person to be automatically sent back to the asylum where he will remain until the term prescribed by the judgment, without the opportunity for parole. The preferential provision is also suspended in its effect when three "respectable" citizens make a reasoned request.

At the time when I was in Iowa, the law whose principal provisions I have described had been in force for a year. During this time, several hundred alcoholics were cared for in asylums at *Cherokee, Mount Pleasant,* and *Independence,* where special sections had been created for the new class of patients [21]. Thanks to the kindness of Dr. M. N. Voldeng, I have been able to obtain detailed information on the 150 drinkers treated until then at the Mount Pleasant Asylum, under the direction of Dr. Ch. F. Applegate, information from which it seems possible to draw certain conclusions on the prospects for the new law [22].

The average age of alcoholics sent to Mount Pleasant was forty, three-fifths of them being between the ages of twenty-six and fifty-five. The youngest was only eighteen, but they had also admitted an old man of eighty-four. It is curious to note that 10 patients had not started to drink until after the age of fifty, while in nearly half of the cases the onset of alcoholic habits was prior to the twenty-fifth year.

Of the 150 subjects treated at Mount Pleasant, 137 were born in the United States, including 104 whose parents were also of American origin. This proportion is very high if one considers that, in the State of Iowa, the foreign element is very numerous. It is therefore the native who, in this state, pays the heaviest price for alcoholism.

Alcohol is usually taken in the form of whiskey: This liquor was reported

85 times as the main "corpus delicti"; there is nothing surprising in this when we know how widespread its use is in the United States. Pure alcohol was incriminated for 29 drinkers. It is interesting to note that in 124 cases it was in a pharmacy that the patient stocked up on whiskey and alcohol, a peculiarity which throws a rather singular light on the pharmacies of Iowa.

Quite often, the subjects abused not only alcohol, but also tobacco (61 times), morphine (11 times), etc.

As a general rule, the rest which the patients find in the asylum, the regularity of life which they lead there, and the abstinence from all alcoholic beverages which is imposed on them do not fail to produce in a few weeks a notable change in their state of health. Therefore, aware of this improvement, they soon ask for their conditional release. And what at first is only a request, even a prayer, soon becomes the subject of complaints and demands presented every day in a more imperious tone.

It must not be denied: However attractive the new Iowa legislation may seem at first sight, at least from the theoretical point of view – that is to say with regard to the effectiveness of the cure and the economic advantages – it nevertheless remains, in practice, one of the most difficult and trickiest to implement. How can we get what appears to be real penal repression with deprivation of liberty to be accepted when it comes to an individual whose only crime was to spend too much time with the bottle? As long as these legal provisions have not become part of the culture – and for this time is an indispensable factor – the asylum for drinkers will seem too much like a prison for it to be accepted by public opinion as the best mode of treatment for what is in fact a disease. Furthermore, combining the asylum for drinkers with the asylum for the insane, a precarious alliance dictated by financial reasons, will certainly not make the system popular: We know how a person's reputation – rightly or wrongly – is damaged by having spent time in an insane asylum; how can we hope that the public will understand the distinction between the asylum for drinkers and the asylum for the insane, united under the same roof? This was quickly realized in Iowa, and efforts are now being made to separate the two categories of establishments as quickly as possible.

Excellent in principle, but delicate in practice, conditional release is also one of the weak points of the legislation. Because of the penal nature of the measure ordering internment in an asylum, the judge, in order to make his sentence less cruel, willingly offers the prospect of conditional release after thirty days; the patient then considers it a promise made to him, a commitment made to him, and when the moment approaches, he cries out for a release that may not be justified and perhaps is contra-indicated. Moreover, we must not forget the voluntary placements, for which an extension of the stay in the asylum is even more difficult to impose. Thus, there are many reasons which explain why, without having been very frequent, escapes were not exactly rare.

Finally, it is also important to consider relapses, which are so common in the treatment of alcoholism that some people even deny the possibility of a cure. It must be recognized that from this point of view, the law of Iowa is completely insufficient. It only applies to individuals residing in the state itself; elements foreign to the state are therefore beyond its reach. On the other hand, it suffices for subjects living in Iowa to move to a neighboring state to be absolutely safe. Even supposing the law of Iowa were adopted by all of the American states, we would find ourselves in the presence of a bizarre situation where any state would certainly be rid of its own alcoholics, but on the other hand would harbor those of its neighbors.

We see therefore that if the new legislation of Iowa marks a certain progress in the struggle against alcoholism, it is still far from having taken a final form. With the rapidity of progress in the United States, it is legitimate to think that the improvements for which the first experiments have proved indispensable will not be long in coming.

[p. 330]
On surgical disinfection in the United States

A few months ago, I devoted a letter to describing the way in which operative asepsis is practiced in the United States (see *Semaine Médicale*, 1903, p. 90). I had then only visited the major American cities along the Atlantic coast. Today I need to return to this question to complete my previous observations with the information that I have gathered during my subsequent journey. I will emphasize a few facts which did not find a place in my previous letter.

I previously did not have much to say about the preparation of the patient and the asepsis of the surgeon and his assistants in the United States, because they were mainly using procedures of European origin. This is true of the American East; but as one advances towards the West and the Northwest, one finds opinions and practices a little different.

Throughout the American East, for the preparation of the operating field, major importance is attributed to conscientious brushing – in duration and in force – of the surface to be disinfected; just as in Europe, we rely essentially on the mechanical action of the brush to remove the epithelial layers of the epidermis and, with them, the microbial germs they may contain. In the West, however – in Chicago, for example, on Dr. A. J.

Ochsner's service – brushing has been completely abandoned. Dr. Ochsner attaches the greatest importance and effectiveness to soaping. For him, once the epidermal fats have been saponified by the soap, a simple trickle of water is enough to wash away all the epidermal particles, disaggregated as a result of the saponification. As for the antiseptic liquid with which the operating field is commonly washed after the action of the brush and the soap, Dr. Ochsner finds it completely superfluous, and if he still sometimes follows the preparation of the field with washing with sublimate,[49] it is more because of tradition than with the conviction of doing something useful.

As regards the hands of the surgeon and his assistants, Dr. Ochsner proceeds in a manner analogous to that which he employs for the disinfection of the operative field; only, in order to make the soap penetrate well everywhere around the fingernails, he uses a piece of gauze soaked in sterile water. This surgeon attributes the greatest importance to having smooth and soft hands that are not chapped or cracked. This is why he recommends avoiding rubbing them with a rough object like a brush. What he wants is not to strip his epidermis, but to give it a surface that is easy to disinfect using "gentle procedures." I may add that Drs. W. J. and C. H. Mayo, at Rochester, share Dr. Ochsner's ideas in this respect; they are even so convinced of the merits of this opinion that brushes are entirely banned from their service: One would look in vain for a hand brush at Saint Mary's Hospital in Rochester. As one of them told me, they fear that cracks and crevasses in the hands will become a veritable "garden of microbes," certainly very unsuitable for good antisepsis.

These ideas are also beginning to make their way in the East. In order to keep his hands very smooth and soft, a Philadelphia surgeon, Dr. Allis, rubs them regularly once a week with sand of an extremely fine grain, such as is found on the beaches by the sea.

It is probably also largely due to its softening effect on the skin that the procedure recommended by Dr. Robert F. Weir, Professor of Surgery at the College of Physicians and Surgeons of New York and Chief Surgeon of the *Roosevelt Hospital*, owes the vogue it currently enjoys in the United States. It consists in using a mixture, which is prepared at the time of use, of chlorinated lime and sodium carbonate; this mixture forms with the water a sort of whitish paste which is coated on the hands for a few minutes.[50] The reaction of the two salts on each other gives rise to a release of free chlorine: This gas is the disinfectant. Dr. W. W. Keen, Professor of Surgery at *Jefferson College* in Philadelphia and surgeon in the hospital associated with this school, also uses this means, having first used black soap. Frequently I have seen maize flour (Indian wheat) added to this preparation to increase its softening properties. Any other starch would play the same role; if Americans give preference to cornstarch, it is only because in the United States it is the standard cheap flour.

Dr. R. H. Harte, surgeon at the *Episcopal Hospital*[51] and the *Pennsylvania Hospital* in Philadelphia, combines the use of soap and that of cornstarch: He rubs his hands with a mixture, in equal parts, mustard flour, cornstarch, and soap powder.

Chloroformization and etherization in the United States

I have already described some special procedures of anesthesia which I have seen in use or under trial with various American surgeons. I have waited to give an overview of current American anesthetic methods until having finished my travels. I was particularly curious to ascertain *firsthand* the status of the old quarrel over ether and chloroform in this new country, which is so progressive and so dismissive of former traditions and customs. I must say that my observations have been rather surprising.

In Boston, where my medical investigation began, ether reigns supreme: In the five weeks that I spent in that city, I did not see chloroform administered a single time. As I expressed my astonishment and asked the reasons for this exclusivity, I was rather surprised to hear the reason invoked … tradition. Indeed, it was at the *Massachusetts General Hospital* in Boston that ether was used for the first time by Morton during an operation carried out by Warren, grandfather of the surgeon whose name I have mentioned several times; since then, out of local pride, Boston has remained faithful to ether. Furthermore, this anesthetic is almost as exclusively employed in the three other great medical centers of the East: New York, Philadelphia, and Baltimore; only in this last city is chloroform not so severely blacklisted.

But the more one goes towards the South, the more chloroform gains partisans, and in New Orleans, which is in the extreme South, it is almost the only surgical anesthetic in use: Exactly the opposite of what is observed in Boston.

The Americans explain this state of things by invoking the climate: They say it is the climate that makes ether succeed better in the North, and not be tolerated in New Orleans. It must be said that in the United States, the climate is used to explain everything; it is invoked for everything and for nothing, apropos and irrelevant. In this case, I must confess that it seemed to me to be wrongly blamed, because ether did not seem to me, even in the North, as harmless as I have heard it maintained. It is certain that this anesthetic is responsible, over there, for a considerable number of post-operative pneumonias; the American surgeons do not deny the fact itself, but they contest its interpretation. For them, the patients succumbing to a complication of this kind would have had pneumonia even if they had not undergone operation. It must be recognized that this is passing very quickly onto an argument which is not without value. New England may well be a country with pneumonia, but that will never explain why postoperative pneumonia is as frequent there as it is. Moreover, there are surgeons also practicing in regions with pneumonia, such as the Drs. Mayo in the Northwest, who do not have the same mortality from postoperative pulmonary complications.

Personally, after having traveled all over the country, I have come to attribute a certain value to the historical factor, which I think best explains why the North uses ether, while the South uses chloroform. We all know the influence Harvard University has had on the intellectual development of the United States; its School of Medicine has long – along with that of the University of Pennsylvania – constituted one of the two greatest medical centers in the United States. There is therefore nothing extraordinary in the fact that, in the North, the influence of Boston has radiated far and spread the use of ether. The South, on the other hand, pivots around New Orleans. However, until the last ten years, any doctor wishing to practice in this city had to have done or completed his studies in Paris, and we remember that ten years ago, ether had hardly any followers in the Parisian surgical world; naturally these physicians brought back to their country the habits acquired in Paris, just as their colleagues in the North remained faithful to those which they had obtained in Boston. It seems that this explanation has more plausibility than the argument drawn from the climate, however strange it is to see historical tradition invoked for a country which prides itself on not following traditions.

[p. 338]
The Negro of the United States from the medico-surgical point of view[52]

The United States presents to the observer who wishes to learn about the comparative pathology of the various human races a field of study as vast as it is fertile. There we find together the representatives of the White, Black, Yellow, and Red races. But, in consequence of the war of extermination waged by the White conquerors against the native tribes, the latter have become an almost negligible quantity in the total of the American population, and as for the Asians, their immigration to the United States was becoming so invasive that the flow had to be stopped by laws, restrictive in appearance, prohibitive in fact. It is primarily the White and Black races that need to be considered in the United States: Both are numerically well enough represented for there to be racial antagonism between them; they are also numerous enough for the comparative study of pathology in one and the other to provide useful lessons.

Scattered over the entire territory of the United States, the majority of Negroes are however found in the Southern States, whose warm temperate climate, even subtropical in the extreme south, is better suited to the need for heat experienced by this race of people of equatorial origin. In some states, Blacks even constitute the majority of the population: Louisiana, for example, has fewer White inhabitants than Colored inhabitants.

This is not the place to dwell on the consequences – of such far-reaching economic and political significance in the public and private life of the American people – which result from this situation. It is important, however, to emphasize the facts, in order to show the interest that the special pathology of the Negro presents for doctors practicing in the southern United States. It is through the courtesy of one of them, Dr. Rudolph Matas, surgeon of the Charity Hospital of New Orleans and Professor of Surgery at Tulane University in that city, that I owe most of the documentation on which this letter is based.

When, three centuries ago, the ancestors of the Negroes who now inhabit the United States were imported from Africa – particularly from Guinea – they possessed certain morbid conditions and certain immunities that are still found today in the people of Africa. Since then, the American Negro has preserved almost all the morbid predispositions which his ancestors brought from his native country, but he has also lost most of the immunities which they enjoyed in Africa.

We know, for example, that cancer is a rather rare condition among the populations of Africa. It was the same for the Negroes of America until about fifty years ago: Among them, as among their fellow Africans, cancer was only observed in exceptional cases. At the present time, this is no longer the case, and the immunity of former times has given way to a morbid predisposition which is more pronounced every day. It is fair to add that an increase in the frequency of malignant tumors has also been reported in the White race, where it is moreover considered by some to be more apparent than real; I will not dwell on this point, which was studied at length in this journal last year (see *Semaine Médicale*, 1902, p. 297-302). But among Negroes, this frequency would have increased in much greater proportions than among whites, since at the present time the percentage is almost identical for the two races: For half a century, carcinoma has doubled in frequency every ten years among the Negroes of America, and although the Black population there is very prolific, it is still far from true that the increase in the population follows the same progression as that of cancer.

This is therefore a real and not apparent increase in frequency.

It is also important to make a distinction between the different locations of cancer. Carcinoma of the breast and uterus, for example, affects a quite remarkable proportion, almost double that observed in the White race. On the contrary, cancers of the penis, larynx, tongue, etc., are completely unknown in Negro pathology.

Benign tumors have historically been considered remarkably common among Blacks. This is an epidemiologic particularity that the American Negro also offers. In this respect, it is appropriate to point out in the first line the predisposition that Blacks present to fibrous tumors, a predisposition so marked that one could rightly speak of a true "fibrous diathesis." This diathesis is so widespread that it must be regarded as one of the pathological characteristics of the Black race. The fibrous bodies of the uterus constitute the most frequent manifestation of it: According to the records he has kept in the registers of the Charity Hospital of New Orleans, Dr. Matas thinks he can assign to the fibroids of the uterus a frequency *five* times greater in the Negro than in the white; and this estimate is certainly far below the truth, if we consider the indolence which characterizes the Blacks and keeps them away from the hospital to the last extremity. Be that as it may, this figure suggests what the number of cases of fibroids submitted to the observation of *Black Belt* doctors must be, if one considers that it is a question in this case of an affliction which in itself is already far from rare in the Caucasian race.

Besides the fibrous bodies of the uterus, keloids and elephantiasis complete the series of the most frequent manifestations of fibrous diathesis in the Black race: Keloids are extremely common; elephantiasis is rarer, but observed exclusively in the Negro.

The frequency of benign tumors in the same race is an indication of a formative hyperactivity of the connective tissue. However, it would be premature to attribute an exaggerated functioning to the generality of the elements of the mesodermal layer, of which the connective tissues represent the main derivative. It should not be forgotten, in fact, that certain tumors, such as osteomas, enchondromas, myxomas, lipomas, and a few others which fall into the same oncological group, are remarkably rare in Blacks.

Tuberculosis, in all its medical and surgical forms, is the Negro's most formidable enemy. This is the primary cause of the enormous mortality of the Black population of the United States. From the point of view of the comparative pathology of races, this observation is all the more interesting because three centuries ago, when the Negroes were first brought to America, tuberculosis was entirely unknown among them. Its appearance is therefore correlated with their transplantation to the United States. It is reasonable to think that it was through their contact with the Whites that the Blacks contracted the first germs of this formidable infection, which developed on a ground that had become favorable either because of the new conditions which it found, or as a result of poor hygienic conditions to which the habits of the Negro generally confine him.

There are also certain other afflictions from which the Black man seems exempt in Africa and against which he loses all immunity in the United States: Dysentery, abscesses of the liver, rheumatism, gout. As for malaria, it will suffice to point out that in the United States the Negro seems as subject to it as the White, neither more nor less.

Without dwelling on tetanus infection, since the statements of Dr. Matas simply confirm the greater frequency and seriousness of tetanus in the Black race, we must consider the evolution of syphilis in the Negro. It is generally agreed that this disease, which is much more widespread in the Black race than in the Caucasian race, evolves there with infinitely greater benignity. Now, if on the question of morbidity Dr. Matas finds himself in agreement with the generality of the other observers – whose research, however, is mostly related to the African Negro – it is no longer the same for the question of mortality caused by syphilis. It follows, in fact, from the data he collected in Louisiana that syphilis would give rise there in the Negro to a lethality *three times* greater than in the White.

This is also the proportion that we find for pneumonia, which kills three times as many Blacks as Whites in the United States

In short, the American Negro presents in several diseases a morbidity and a mortality much higher than those of the White. Some of these afflictions are those which plague the Black race in Africa, its continent of origin. A series of others, on the other hand, probably come from proximity to the Whites; these include tuberculosis, cancer, syphilis, etc. Among the immunities enjoyed by the Negro race in Africa with regard to certain diseases, very few have survived in the new habitat of the "African-American"; we can only cite in this order of ideas varicose veins, including under this heading hemorrhoids and varicocele. Very few are the affections which are rife among the Blacks of Africa and which have almost completely disappeared among their relatives in America – affections presenting a distinctly tropical character, such as sleeping sickness – and it seems that the climate suffices to explain the disappearance of these affections among the Negroes of America.

Moreover, if we consider things in a general way, we must not forget that, since the abolition of slavery in the United States (1864), morbidity and mortality have increased in considerable proportions among the freed population. Before emancipation, in fact, the Negro represented for his owner a value which the master took care of with all the respect due to a precious commodity. Since emancipation, the natural indolence and invincible carelessness of the Negro have caused him to concern himself with his health only when he feels driven by necessity, the latter resulting either from the pain he experiences or the inconvenience it creates for his neighbors.

As for the mulatto, one should expect, by virtue of the general principles which govern the crossing of races, that the introduction of the white element would have created more favorable conditions for him. According to the observations that have been collected in the *Black Belt* of the United States, it seems that this is not the case. I found absolute unanimity there on this point: The offspring resulting from the crossing of the White and Black races appears, it is true, to have a superior intelligence to that of the Negro; but from the physical point of view, he is distinctly inferior both to White and to Black, acquiring the weaknesses of the two races without possessing any of their advantages. Certain observations would even tend to suggest that the mulatto is a degenerate product, destined to disappear after a few generations, if new infusions of Caucasian blood do not compensate for the effects of the original crossing.

[p. 347]
On the climate of the United States of America

It is beyond the scope of an article such as this to deal extensively with a subject as vast as that of the climate of the United States. My intention is therefore simply to furnish some general indications and to make some remarks which have occurred to me during the course of my trip to America, either from personal observations, or from conversations with American colleagues. Moreover, one could not hope to collect in such a journey – even when one has devoted nearly a year to it – sufficient data to discuss such a subject in a definitive and complete way. I cannot, however, dispense entirely from dealing here with the climate. I have already had occasion previously to indicate in passing the important role which this factor plays in American life. Without going as far as those who, in all places, at all times and in all things, only know how to invoke the climate as an explanation, we must nevertheless agree that the American climate explains many characteristics that in Europe we generally regard as outside its immediate sphere of influence.

In addition, it must be remembered that the territory of the United States is nearly eighteen times larger than that of France. It is therefore important to also consider the greater distances, and the more pronounced differences that result from them more that we do in Europe. Also the various subdivisions that can be accepted for the territory of the United States, from the point of view of medical climatology, present much more marked contrasts than those, for example, of the natural regions established in France. We will therefore successively review a certain number of zones, namely the East, the South, the region of the Rocky Mountains, the North-West, and California.

The Eastern region is essentially distinguished by the four major cities of Boston, New York, Philadelphia, and Baltimore. Despite their proximity to the coast, these cities have a distinctly continental climate with extreme contrasts between summer and winter that such a qualification entails. What often makes it difficult to live in these cities, especially in New York and Philadelphia, is the great humidity. The fact is explained for the first of these cities by its situation on the marshy island of Manhattan. In summer, the water vapor content of the atmosphere often makes the heat intolerable. It even sometimes becomes so inconvenient that the authorities often allow the inhabitants of poor neighborhoods to go and sleep with their families under the stars in Central Park, hoping in this way to alleviate, especially among young children, the inconveniences that can result from the excessive heat combined with the high humidity. In winter, this same humidity produces the well-known fogs in New York.

Philadelphia is located a hundred miles from the coast. This distance from the sea and the resulting absence of breeze results in the stifling heat that sometimes occurs in the city of the Quakers, which can be more uncomfortable than in New York.

Boston's climate is influenced by its northern location, just as Baltimore's is influenced by its southern location. In the first of these towns, the winter is early and severe; in the second, the summer is long and hot. But because of the greater dryness of the atmosphere, compared to New York or Philadelphia, the climate in both is more tolerable.

The evolution of diseases in the American East presents, except for a few details, the same characteristics as in Europe, in particular as in France. I have already mentioned occasionally the greater severity of pneumonia, the greater frequency of typhoid fever, etc. There is no need to repeat these details here.

As far as the southern United States is concerned, it is important to consider separately, from the point of view of the climate, the Florida peninsula and the Southwest. I will refrain from talking about Florida, which I have not visited. As for the Southwest, which extends along the Gulf of Mexico as far as Galveston via New Orleans, it presents, from the point of view of medical climatology, very specific characteristics which clearly differentiate it from the American East, and also from Europe. The dominant feature of this climate is that it takes on a tropical character, which becomes more pronounced as one advances further towards the South and West. However, the humidity is much lower there than in New York, for example; so that the heat, although torrid, is nevertheless much more bearable in New Orleans than in New York, especially since the breeze blowing from the Gulf of Mexico helps to temper the excessive heat in the atmosphere.

The pattern of evolution of infectious diseases in the American Southwest is noteworthy. Most of the serious infections in this region, if not completely ignored, are at least remarkably benign. It is especially worth mentioning the diseases of children, scarlet fever, measles, etc. I had inquired about the status of anti-diphtheria serotherapy in New Orleans, counting in this way to supplement the information which I had gathered in other US cities. However, it appears from the interviews that I had with the health officers that diphtheria has never been very serious in New Orleans and that, consequently, the documents that could be collected on the question of serotherapy would be of little value.

Unlike the infectious diseases mentioned above, tropical diseases are as formidable as they are feared in the southern United States. I refer on this subject to what I have said of the defense of the coast of the Gulf of Mexico against yellow fever, and, in this case, it is the same for the generality of other tropical (or rather subtropical) diseases.

The region of the Rocky Mountains, which mainly includes the states of Colorado, New Mexico, and Arizona, presents a considerable interest from the medical point of view, in particular the non-mountainous part which extends from the foot of the Rocky Mountains to the East and to the South. The continent, which rises imperceptibly and very gently, but constantly and gradually, as one advances towards the West, reaches the *foothills of the range* – where cities like Denver, Colorado Springs, and Pueblo are located – at an average of 1,600 meters and more above sea level. Moisture-laden winds blowing from the Pacific are stopped by the Rocky Mountains; those that come from the East, having swept across the immense plain which stretches from the Rockies to the Atlantic, have lost all the moisture which they had soaked up in the East. As a result, the climate of Colorado and the neighboring States is found to unite two essential qualities, altitude and dryness. This is why facilities for the treatment of consumptives abound in this region. Thanks to the altitude, the atmosphere is relatively rarefied, even on the plain. As for the dryness of the air, it is quite remarkable; in Colorado, the annual rainfall is considered very heavy when it reaches 50 centimeters; there are hardly more than sixty days without sun. The climate is also rather hot, but with very sharp differences in temperature between the places exposed to the sun and those which are sheltered from it. This contrast, together with the great dryness, makes the heat of summer very bearable at the foot of the Rocky Mountains, especially since the nights are always cool there.

From the physiological point of view, the principal effect of such a climate is to considerably increase the evaporation from all the surfaces, exterior and interior, of the organism. Sensitive at the level of the cutaneous surface, which always appears dry and fresh, this action is even more marked for the mucous membranes. It is manifested, especially in the newcomer, by an intense thirst and an often very unpleasant sensation of dryness in the throat. At the same time, hairs break and fall out. It is also to this drying action that much of the benefits of the Colorado climate in pulmonary tuberculosis are attributed. From a surgical point of view, certain peculiarities also should be pointed out. First of all, it seems that postoperative infections are less frequent and less serious here than in a humid climate, such as that of the Eastern states; in consumptive patients, in particular, cures are generally more rapid and often definitive. In addition, complications arising from surgical tuberculosis in a consumptive are relatively rare. On the other hand, there is a category of patients who are an exception to the rule and tolerate operations in the Far West quite badly: These are the newcomers, still insufficiently acclimatized. The rarefaction of the atmosphere requires a greater functional activity by the cardiovascular apparatus as well as the organs of respiration, so anesthesia is usually badly tolerated, and the disorders which it is often accompanied can be alarming, especially when dealing with a heart damaged by a previous attack. Moreover, in these imperfectly acclimatized subjects, it is generally observed that the suppuration, by its intensity and profusion, contrasts sharply with the rapid and aseptic healing of the wounds which is ordinarily observed in subjects living in the country for some time. Finally, it should be pointed out as one of the peculiarities attributed to the climate of Colorado, the difficulty with which the ether is usually supported. Bronchorrhea following etherization is, in fact, much more frequent than in the East, probably because ether vapors are more irritating due to the dryness of the air. Also, although the surgeons practicing in the Rocky Mountain region have almost all come from the East for health reasons (pulmonary bacillosis) – their origin therefore clearly explains their preference for ether – chloroform, without having yet dethroned ether, nevertheless wins more supporters in Colorado every day.

The Northwest, which one reaches by heading from Colorado towards the North and of which Minnesota with the twin cities of Saint Paul and

Minneapolis serves as a good example, shares many characters with the region of the Rockies. But there, the contrasts are still exaggerated: Very hot summer and very harsh winter, with essentially no spring or fall. Nevertheless, it is a remarkably salubrious climate. From this point of view, it is especially appropriate to emphasize the low frequency of surgical infections.

The different regions we have considered so far are located east of the Rocky Mountains. It remains for us to speak of that which extends between this chain of mountains and the Pacific Ocean, namely California. Two contrary influences act on the climate of California: On the one hand, in the West, the sea tends constantly to load the atmosphere with humidity; on the other hand, the mass of Rocky Mountains forms a sort of barrier to the east, preventing this humidity from being carried away. The strip of land which stretches along the coast and which contains the greater part of the population is remarkable for its extreme constancy of temperature. In places as far south as Santa Barbara – the "Cannes" of the United States – the hottest and sunniest month of the year is January. Epidemiologically, California also differs from the rest of the United States. A compatriot, Dr. de Chantreau, who practices in San Francisco, told me that he had not seen two cases of pneumonia there in ten years. Typhoid fever is also much less prevalent there, and the same can be said of other major infectious diseases, such as scarlet fever, diphtheria, etc.

In short, according to what we have just seen, the United States deserves its bad reputation, from the climatic point of view, only for the zones situated to the East and Northeast of the country. There, one can say that there exists a tiring climate, putting the individuals in a condition of less resistance with regard to disease, without counting that to the action of the climate comes to be added that, equally debilitating, which results from the general overwork in this part of the United States. The South is gradually bringing us closer to tropical regions; the climate, painful to bear on account of the heat which reigns there, nevertheless presents characters quite different from those met with in the East. In the region of the Rocky Mountains (Colorado, etc.) and in the Northwest, we find the dry and invigorating climate to which the aspect of good health exuded by the *Westerner* is attributed. Finally, California, at least in its most inhabited part, enjoys a wonderful climate that cannot be better compared to that of the Côte d'Azur - a Côte d'Azur as large as all of France.

[p. 379]
The practice of medicine in the United States

The practice of medicine has long been unrestricted in the United States, and it is only in the past ten years that they have begun to impose certain obstacles to this freedom of practice by requiring a special license.

These restrictions do not apply generally to the entire territory. As we know, the different states of the federation enjoy a certain legislative autonomy, an autonomy of which they are very jealous, but which sometimes creates a regrettable state of disorder and confusion, as we shall see.

By virtue of their autonomy, each state has retained, among other things, the right to enact special laws on the practice of medicine. As a consequence of this state of affairs, the provisions regulating the practice of our art often vary greatly from state to state. Moreover, their equivalence is not recognized, so the license granted in one state does not give the right to practice in the neighboring state. In short, we find ourselves in the presence of provisions which are not dissimilar to those which until recently governed the situation of health officers in France: We know that before the promulgation of the law of 1892, a health officer could practice only in the department which he had chosen. It suffices to draw this parallel between these two analogous situations to show what is both backward and arbitrary in the present condition of the United States regarding the right to practice.

Even now the practice of medicine enjoys, in some states, the absolute freedom which was formerly the rule in all of the states. But the dominant tendency today is to subject access to a medical career to official control. Where the old arrangements still exist, there is always a special reason. In some cases, it is due to the difficulty presented by the recruitment of medical professionals because the region is still poorly inhabited. Other times, as for Colorado, for example, the best elements come from the states of the East, and health reasons have motivated their immigration; it is conceivable that under these conditions the country has every interest in leaving the door wide open to immigration, and it lends itself to this all the more willingly since, in the primitive Far West, the medical schools still lack the resources necessary to give a satisfactory education and consequently cannot measure up to the universities of the East.

The license to practice in a state is granted following examinations passed before commissions appointed by the state concerned, hence their name of State Boards [23]. These commissions are composed of physicians practicing in the state in question, and who must not belong either directly or indirectly to any school whatsoever. This provision is wise if one remembers the implacable competition between the different schools, and it is only on this condition that it is possible to avoid acts of regrettable partiality on the part of the judges. However, when we know how numerous the schools of medicine are in the United States, we cannot help wondering where the state can find competent examiners, when we see almost everyone belonging to the faculty of one or other of these schools. It must be believed, however, that the educated and honest examiner exists, since each year quite a number of candidates are rejected.

The special examinations required to obtain a license are generally taken by the candidate as soon as he has received a doctorate from the school where he studied. The State Board, which as a rule meets several times a year, holds its main session a few days after the end of the school examinations. The tests to be undergone essentially consist of a questionnaire to be answered in writing and, after passing this, an oral examination. The program includes the following subjects: Anatomy, diagnosis, chemistry, *materia medica*, physiology, obstetrics, surgery, gynecology, diseases of children, medicine, and pathological anatomy.

Such an examination, consisting exclusively of written compositions and oral questions, without any practical test, is clearly too rudimentary. Its insufficiency is even more striking when one considers that the judges have before them candidates whom they are seeing for the first time and on whom previous information is entirely lacking. The examination which the candidate had just taken in his school and which had led him to the doctoral degree was also certainly insufficient; at least the examiners generally know very well the value of their pupils, because of the reputation of the school; in addition, they have school files in which are recorded detailed and daily notes on the work carried out by the student during the course of the education.

To be able to appear before a determined *State Board*, it is not enough to have a doctoral degree issued by any one of the 154 schools of medicine in the United States. As I showed in a previous article, these schools cannot be compared to each other and the diplomas they issue are of very unequal value. The *State Boards* only accept as valid the diplomas conferred by certain specific schools that follow a minimum program of studies. The State of Illinois, which was the first to establish examination commissions, immediately rejected a certain number of schools for the inadequacy of their teaching. Since then, the other states have followed this example, and the most insufficient schools have gradually been eliminated throughout the territory.

Moreover, the *State Boards*, by imposing more and more severe conditions on candidates, gave a new impetus to medical education and thus contributed not a little to raising its level. The doctoral degree itself loses all value if it does not confer admissibility before the *State Boards,* since only the latter can give access to a medical career. The institution of these state examinations has therefore had an extremely beneficial effect on the development of medical studies in the United States. Isn't it interesting to see the assertion of public authority on medical education, in this free America where everything is supposed to emanate only from private initiative?

In some states, a doctoral degree is not required for registration for *State Board* examinations. This is for the sole purpose of leaving everyone the freedom to go and acquire their medical knowledge wherever they want. This unfortunately introduces questions of individual freedom where they have no place, because under the pretext of not infringing on this sacrosanct freedom, one loses sight of simple common sense.

The discussion that took place on this subject in New Orleans, during the meeting of the members of the *State Boards* – or *National Confederation of State Medical Examining and Licensing Boards* – a discussion which I had the opportunity to observe, leaves no doubt in this regard. This is what really happens in the few states, for example Missouri, that admit candidates to the licensing examinations without requiring any prior justification from them: Since medical knowledge can only be obtained in a medical school, all candidates have actually attended one of these schools to acquire their medical background. But those of them who, for one reason or another, are in a hurry to settle down and earn a living, appear at the end of the *second* year before the State Board. One can imagine what the examination of such candidates must be, and one can imagine the proportion of failures they provide. It is more difficult to understand the services that might be rendered by those to whom luck or chance has allowed to pass the examinations.

We see therefore that, under the pretext of respecting freedom, we have simply ended up favoring abuses which the institution of the *State Boards* is intended to prevent. Sooner or later, it will be the case in all states that eligibility is strictly limited to applicants who already hold the title of doctor, as is the practice in most states today. It is also interesting to note that the majority of *State Boards* are no longer satisfied with a doctor's degree. It imposes on the candidate a series of additional and more stringent conditions from year to year. The latest provisions in this regard were enacted at New Orleans by the Congress of *State Boards*.

They prescribe four years of schooling, each of which must represent at least 30 weeks of 30 hours or 900 hours of actual work [24]. In all, the minimum requirement is therefore 3,600 hours – namely, in order of importance of the subjects taught, 560 of medicine, 540 of surgery, 500 of anatomy, 340 of chemistry, 260 of pathological anatomy, 250 of physiology, 200 in histology and embryology, 150 in obstetrics, 130 in gynecology, 115 in bacteriology, 110 in pharmacology, 95 in ophthalmology, 75 in neurology, 60 in children's diseases, 55 in medical diagnosis, 55 in oto-rhino-laryngology,

50 of dermatology, 30 of hygiene and 25 of mental diseases and forensic medicine – a quarter of this time to be devoted to clinical studies.

We see that in this enumeration all the specialties are included; they are indeed all compulsory. The figures which we have just quoted express, moreover, the relative value attributed in the United States to the different branches of medical science.

The establishment of *State Boards* is certainly a great step forward in the regulation of medical practice. Moreover, this institution has not yet borne all the fruits that we are entitled to expect. From certain points of view, it even calls for urgent improvements. Here is an example: for fear of seeing themselves invaded by practitioners from the West, the eastern states have determined that the license issued in a given state is only valid in that state. As a result, a doctor from Boston cannot move to New York – or *vice versa* – without having to pass again the examinations he has already undergone in Massachusetts. This is why it is a question of establishing between certain states a kind of reciprocity by virtue of which the value of the diplomas delivered by some would be recognized by the others.

There is also talk of establishing a *national* commission having its central headquarters in Washington, traveling successively from one state to another to administer the examinations, and issuing, following these tests, a diploma valid throughout the entire United States. This solution, which would present many advantages, has against it the very pronounced particularist tendencies of the various states. Be that as it may, moreover, the question is still only under study, and, in spite of its many inconveniences, it is probable that the present situation is destined to continue for a certain time.

[p. 387]
The medical profession in the United States

I propose to devote my weekly correspondence today to the medical profession in the United States. It would perhaps be more accurate to speak of the medical professions of the United States. This is because, in fact, alongside the followers of what was once called allopathy, there exists a whole series of different medical sects which deny the doctrines professed by the allopaths or *regular* doctors and intend to treat their patients according to certain principles very different from those taught by classical medicine. These include the homeopaths, the osteopaths, the eclectics, the Eddyists,[53] the Dowieists,[54] etc. In short, these are what in Europe are called faith healers rather than doctors: They are, to call things by their name, the charlatans of the medical profession. In the United States, moreover, the so-called regular doctors have no problem using this term with regard to the dissidents.

It must be taken into account, however, that in the great American republic, all these categories of dissidents are officially recognized and have their legal existence. They have their societies, their congresses, their schools, their own *State Boards*, and so on. We can therefore very well speak of each of them as a special medical body. Naturally, I paid very little attention to these different groups in the course of my journey. But the importance of these healers, their number, and their influence on the practice of medicine are such that I have heard of them often enough. I must admit, moreover, that the discussions I have had on this subject have not always sufficed to fully enlighten my religion. For example, I have never been able to get an explanation of how homeopathic surgery or obstetrics differs from conventional surgery or obstetrics. I have been told of a "homeopathic surgeon" practicing his art with great distinction in one of the largest cities on the Atlantic coast, without being able to detect the slightest difference between his procedures and those of his so-called regular colleagues.

By including dissidents in the number of physicians who practice in the United States and are recognized by American law, we arrive at a global figure currently estimated at more than 130,000 physicians. This represents, for a population of approximately 80 million, approximately one doctor per 600 inhabitants. This proportion is almost twice as high in the United States as in the major countries of Europe, where there is on average one doctor per thousand inhabitants. Moreover, this surplus is tending to grow every day: It has been calculated, in fact, that each year the medical schools of the United States train about twice as many doctors as are lost to death or retirement.

Be that as it may, it seems that – apart from the American mindset, and also certain conditions inherent in a new country – this surplus of doctors contributes a great deal to conferring on the practice of medicine the United States this mercantile character so striking, I would say almost so shocking, for the European doctor who travels through this country. While in Europe medicine is considered and practiced as an academic profession, the same cannot be said for most of the United States. Apart from the region stretching along the Atlantic coast, medicine is, in fact, practiced much more like a trade – *business* – than like an academic profession. I am well aware that a number of American colleagues protest vigorously against such a judgment. I cannot, however, exempt myself from expressing it, and I add that certain American doctors, very well placed to know things by experience, have especially drawn my attention to this point. I can cite in particular the feeling repeatedly affirmed by those who, after having worked for several years in the big cities of the East, have had to emigrate to the West for health reasons.

In this order of ideas, we can point out the practice widespread throughout the United States – except in the cities on the Atlantic coast – which consists in having one's consulting room in town, in the commercial center, and not in his private home. Thus we can see certain *skyscrapers* (houses with fifteen and twenty floors) occupied exclusively, or almost exclusively, by doctors' offices. The *Reliance Building*, located at 100 State Street, Chicago, is a classic example and is well known throughout the United States. Most often, a common waiting room serves a number of doctors at the same time. These quite frequently associate with each other and the resulting arrangement can take on all the characteristics of a real commercial agreement. Assuredly, one cannot speak of *collaboration* in all these cases, although such a state of affairs seems perfectly suited to lead to it.

The use of the sign – I say purposely *sign* and not *plaque* – is absolutely general, even on the part of those who could be called the princes of science. For those who are not accustomed to it, the effect is really bizarre, when one stands in front of a medical *skyscraper*, in whose windows are spread out in gold letters half a foot high the name of doctor such and such, with the indication of the days and hours of consultation.

The more one goes towards the West, the more the character of mercantilism is accentuated. Far out on the plains is a town of about 4,000 inhabitants, where two brothers practice, surgeons both very distinguished in their specialty and having provided proof not only of their ability, but also of their science.[55] The way in which they carry out their *business* is quite characteristic; this is why it seems to me interesting to give some of the information that I have collected in this respect, although I have not had absolute proofs in my hands. These two surgeons are located on a ground floor that their *business* occupies entirely. They have eight assistants, all doctors of medicine, who collect the observations and carry out the microscopic, clinical, radiographic, etc. analyses which the circumstances require; these assistants are chosen in such a way that each of them has a special skill in a particular branch of medicine. After having been prepared and evaluated by the assistants, the patient is presented to the masters of the house, who examine him in their turn, and, after having consulted among themselves, decide whether there is reason to intervene or not and if so, what this intervention should be. This is practiced in the morning by one of them in a private hospital, owned and managed by nuns, but of which they are the only department heads. The establishment in question, although it bears the name of hospital, is rather a *maison de santé*,[56] since nothing is free. The surgeon's fees are proportionate to the patient's and family's means. They are calculated, I have been told, in such a way as to represent one month of the patient's income: The data used to evaluate this income are collected by a cashier in charge of accounting and in front of whom the patient passes as soon as his arrival, even before having seen the doctor. The Americans aren't shocked by this at all: It is *businesslike*. In the United States one cannot treat a question without citing figures. I will therefore add that, according to what I have been told, the general expenses of this consulting group are not less than 100,000 francs[57] per year, a figure which will not seem excessive despite everything if one considers that the senior assistant himself receives an annual salary of 40,000 francs.

There is, however, one point by which the practice of medicine in the United States abandons its mercantile character: I mean advertising, which is absolutely prohibited both by customs and by codes of ethics. It is not only a question of the advertisements inserted on the fourth page of the newspapers: The name of one of the most eminent surgeons in America is mentioned, who for a long time was ostracized by his colleagues because he had exposed, in the waiting room of his consulting room, a note of fees handsomely paid by a billionaire client.[58] Advertising by a doctor is considered in the United States as the unmistakable mark of a charlatan. They do not hesitate to use it in political journals, usually without success, I have been told.

From all that we have just said, we can judge the degree of "commercialization" of medicine in the United States, and also the important role that charlatanism plays in the practice of the profession, a double consequence of the oversupply which I mentioned at the beginning of this letter.

[p. 395]
Medical societies and associations in the United States

The spirit of association, which is one of the dominant traits of the Anglo-Saxon character, is also manifested in matters of medicine. In this respect, I will mention the innumerable medical societies, large and small, with which the United States of America is covered as if by a vast network. There is no town, however small, that does not have its medical society organized and functioning according to the rules of parliamentary procedure. In the large cities there are an infinity of these small societies, comprising three, four, six members who meet periodically to work together. Most often, the members of these embryonic societies include a physician, a surgeon, and a representative of the main specialties. In accordance with a program established and distributed in advance, personal observations are read there which generally raise certain difficulties of diagnosis, treatment, etc.; during the discussion which always follows the reading of the communication, the assistants make known in turn their opinion on the question in dispute.

This communication thus leads to a kind of consultation. It is also a true mutual teaching, because of the constituent elements of these societies, and thanks to the existence of the discussions, each member is made aware of questions about which he normally has no dealings, but on which another member of the society is informed because of his special studies.

Undoubtedly, the groups of which we have just spoken exert a beneficial influence on individual education. However, they cannot claim the role of a public utility. This is a function attributed to the great societies whose power and authority are considerable in the United States. To fully understand their importance, these societies should be divided into two distinct categories. On some I will have little to say, because they are groups formed on the same model as the French learned societies. Societies of the second type, on the contrary, play a major role in the professional life of the American doctor, a role whose importance is increasing every day, and these institutions have hardly any analogue in France.

Of the first category, the College of Physicians of Philadelphia, one of the oldest and most powerful medical societies in the United States, furnishes a good example. These are societies whose members, in limited numbers, are recruited from the medical practitioners of the city which is the headquarters of the society. Admission being subject to election, most of these societies confine themselves exclusively to the elite of the medical profession. Scholars not residing in the city itself may be admitted as corresponding members, etc. Sessions are weekly, bi-monthly or monthly. I would add that the great medical libraries of the United States belong for the most part to the most important of these societies.

The other medical societies or associations of the United States have a very particular aim: Their reason for being is indeed not exclusively of a scientific order. All revolve around the *American Medical Association*; it is therefore necessary, in order to make its organization and functioning clearly understood, to first explain how the *A. M. A.* is constituted.

Founded in 1847, originally with views similar to those which accompanied the birth of its elder sister, the *British Medical Association*, the *American Medical Association* owed its creation to the desire of the members of the Society of Medicine of the New York State to institute a regular national *Congress* that would include physicians from all parts of the union. But the aim pursued by the promoters of these meetings was not long in being somewhat set aside, so much so that at the present time the annual meeting from which the A. M. A. had emerged has gradually become secondary to the other concerns of its members. The task pursued today by the *American Medical Association* is more ambitious: It is nothing less than to embody a sort of corporation encompassing and absorbing the whole of the medical profession in the United States, with which the Association would ultimately identify itself even to the point of replacing it.

The reason that is officially legitimizes such a vast project is the need, which is undeniably felt in America, to remove from a profession of honor and dignity the suspect elements, which are widespread in the United States, as I have described in connection with charlatanism in this country. To publicly exclude these doctors from a body recognized for the honorability of its members, by refusing them access, would be to both pillory them and stigmatize their procedures. It is this role that some colleagues would like to reserve for the *American Medical Association*. We see how far we are from the goal proposed by the New York doctors in founding this Association.

To enable the *American Medical Association* to play the role in question, however, it was important to enlist in its ranks all the doctors presenting the guarantees of professional respectability: Only at this price could it be admitted that the excluded deserved their fate and fell into the category of "bad apples." However, at present, out of more than 130,000 physicians practicing in the United States, hardly 12,500 belong to the A. M. A., although the work of reorganizing this society has been going on for several years with the greatest activity. It would certainly insult our American colleagues to suppose that there is not even one reputable physician out of ten in their country. The small proportion of those chosen is probably explained by the inevitable delays inherent in the selection that must be made among such a large number of individuals. This selection obviously constitutes the most arduous and the most delicate part of the purification task that they have set themselves. The difficulties are even such that they involve a whole vast plan of organization, hierarchy, and affiliation. On account of the considerable number of physicians practicing in the United States, and also on account of the immense expanse of the territory, it is impossible for the directing committee of the *American Medical Association*, charged with the preliminary inquiry which takes place in connection with each candidacy, to collect with sincerity and satisfactory guarantees the information concerning the professional integrity of the applicant. Also, the formality of a prior selection is imposed on the latter: In fact, only members of the medical societies of the different states can be part of the A. M. A. Now, these regional societies, affiliated with the *American Medical Association*, or rather placed under its supervision, exact from their members the conditions required for admission to the national association, and within the limited circle of the state, it is relatively easy to establish, with some guarantees of accuracy, the moral record of a man whose slightest acts are, by the very fact of his profession, constantly open to public scrutiny.

Finally, for greater certainty, the *American Medical Association* has just decided that the member of a society of a given state must also be admitted to the county or parish medical society. So here the circle of surveillance is even more circumscribed and rigorous observation is made easier.

We see what the aim is: Nothing less than replacing the title of doctor, the origin and value of which we have shown so unequal in the United States, with the diploma of member of the association, thus making this diploma a certificate of honesty, integrity, and professional competence.

One of the means implemented for this purpose by the A. M. A. consists, as we have just seen, in the hierarchy and the good organization of the regional and local societies. Another resides in the adoption of a code of professional ethics, to which all members of the Association are required to submit on pain of exclusion. I do not have to emphasize the various points raised or settled by this code. In the United States, its adoption is seen as considerable progress. I will only add that in France it would certainly be considered a bare minimum.

From what we have just said, it may be concluded that the *American Medical Association* seems at present to exercise a generally beneficial influence on the development of medical life in the United States. I say *at present*, because what is happening currently in certain European countries warns us against too exaggerated optimism and obliges us to reserve the future.

Suppose for a moment, in fact, that the goal pursued by the *American Medical Association* is achieved, which is not impossible to conceive. Then if this Association occupies the place to which it claims, it will have centralized everything and that it will have monopolized the right to distribute certificates of honesty to those who are willing to allow themselves to be regimented under its banner. What will then become of freedom, this freedom of which they speak so much in the United States, of which they are so proud, of which they so willingly believe they have a monopoly? In France, a country of 38 million inhabitants and eighteen times smaller than the United States, we suffer from centralization. But what will it be then in a country with a population double and an area infinitely greater than that of France, where the contrasts are consequently violent and clashing? Can it be maintained that what suits Maine is good for Louisiana, that New York and Denver, California and the Great Lakes should renounce the individuality which these regions owe to their so dissimilar natural conditions? Once centralization has taken place, everything will take place under the control of the *American Medical Association*, and yet this impersonal label will, in fact, hide only the very real personality of the few members who are the directors of the Association. Under their yoke all American doctors will have to bend: Outside the Association, there is no salvation, and they are the Association. It would really misunderstand the natural course of things to doubt that once the Association is well in hand, the few influential people who direct it – whatever their supposed disinterestedness – do not take advantage of an instrument made powerful and docile only for the purpose of public interest.

There is more. The A. M. A. has an official organ called the *Journal of the American Medical Association*. However, this periodical, instead of being a simple bulletin of the society, is a true journal of medicine in every meaning of the term, with this particularity that the subscription to it is obligatory for any member of the association, since the membership fee includes a subscription. Now, we know that the importance of a journal is often measured by the extent of its circulation, and doesn't this create an absolutely artificial circulation by imposing a subscription on any doctor who doesn't care to be publicly stigmatized as a charlatan? For it is indeed this conclusion that the program of the *American Medical Association* logically entails: Any doctor worthy of the name is a member of the association and as such is necessarily a subscriber to the journal. It is therefore easy to understand what competition the organ of the Association is likely to make for the independent medical press as soon as it leaves its role of "bulletin and report." And what will become of the freedom of speech if, in order to express an opinion, one must first pass under the Caudine Forks[59] of three censors imposed by the rules of the *American Medical Association*?

However gloomy such a picture may appear, it is by no means so black. It suffices, to be convinced of this, to see what is happening in England. There exists, for nearly three quarters of a century, a Medical Association created, originally, with the aim of bringing together the doctors who belong to it, of collecting and publishing the interesting cases which they have observed, of studying the medical topography of the country, epidemics, etc. From provincial as it was at the beginning, the Association later became national, and it was then that itis boxused its program by taking care of everything related to the medical profession: Ethics, teaching, legal reforms medical or sanitary, etc. This work of reorganization completed, and almost all of the doctors once incorporated, we found ourselves in the presence of a powerful, docile organization well in the hands of a few skillful or influential people. Now, such an organism, which owes the cohesion of its elements to the common goal pursued, is obliged to change the day when this common goal is attained. This is what actually threatens to happen in the British Medical Association, where there currently seem to be serious inclinations towards transformation into a Mutual Provident Society; we can already predict that, in the more or less near future, there will be a dislocation of the two opposing camps, unless the only raison d'être of the association is henceforth to sponsor the newspaper which, modest at first, gradually competed fiercely and fatally with other medical journals by taking on a real commercial character and by this very fact became a source of large income, although it had as artificial a circulation as that of the American periodical.

Is a similar fate in store for our colleagues in America? Only the future will show it. However, if it is true that history is only a perpetual restarting, it is good to establish comparisons imposed by the comparison of two organizations which have reached different stages of their evolution, but of origin and of similar aspirations, separated only by their difference of ority.

[p. 411]
Medical meetings in the United States

Having come to America to study its scientific and professional medicine, it seemed to me necessary to attend the most important of the medical meetings during the time that I stayed in the country. In addition to the interesting communications that I might hope to receive there – such as Dr. Councilman's report on the smallpox parasite at the Washington Congress (see Semaine Médicale, 1903, p. 192) – I planned to learn about the organization and operation of these meetings, as well as the amount of actual work accomplished by each of them. Certain information collected from the beginning of my stay in America had made me think that there might be some interest in establishing comparisons between American meetings and European meetings.

One of the first things that strike you when you study the organization of the American meetings are the restrictions imposed on the admission of members. Contrary to what generally happens in Europe, where those in attendance are only required to hold the title of Doctor of Medicine – and even this is not always required, as we rea... the last International Congress in Madrid – this title is not enough to be part of an American meeting; it is also necessary to be invited to participate in the work of the organization. Moreover, the simple fact that some of these assemblies – indeed the majority – only represent the annual meeting of an association with somewhat extended ramifications, shows that it is not a question here of assemblies open to all comers, but many sessions held by closed societies. Other meetings bring together civil servants of the same order – such as the *Congress of Licensing Boards* of which I have already spoken – and these are then more committee sessions than congresses in the sense that we attribute to this term.

The restrictions are not limited to the conditions imposed for admissibility; they often also extend to the presentations themselves. Thus, for example, at the annual meeting of the *American Medical Association*, presenters are only given the privilege of the floor after approval by a committee of three competent members, appointed in advance by the association's Steering Committee. The veto of this committee is absolute and without recourse, and I understand that this is not merely a formality; it is applied, I have been told, as often as the need arises. Such a measure is obviously possible only by requiring the submission of presentations several weeks before the time fixed for the Congress. Thanks to this precaution, it is also possible to prepare programs of meetings that fill in the number of hours available, which is even easier because the time granted to each speaker is strictly limited and that extra time is granted only exceptionally.

The distinction between *report* and *communication* is rarely made in the United States. I hardly heard any actual reports except at the Congress in Washington. I should explain here this triennial Congress, called the "Congress of American Physicians and Surgeons," is the most important of all those that exist in the United States, from the point of view of scientific work, and *Semaine Médicale* has reported on it several times. In fact, only the colleagues belonging to certain societies take part in it, which include, in addition to the Association of American Physicians and the American Surgical Association, similar associations for 14 different specialties of the medical sciences.

These various societies have a method of recruitment analogous to that of the Royal Society of London, namely that one can enter it only if elected by the votes of the present members after an application has been made. The honor of belonging to one of these societies is naturally esteemed, considering how difficult it is to be admitted. The members, whose number is limited, are recruited throughout the country and they are required not only to have a high scientific reputation, but also perfect professional integrity. I cited in a previous letter the case of a well-known surgeon who was ostracized for many years by his colleagues because of a certain strain he had once placed on the professional code.

Each of the societies of which I have just spoken meets once a year, generally in May or June, in a location of its choice. Every three years, they meet together in Washington, where they combine to form the Congress of American Physicians and Surgeons, each society constituting for this occasion only a section of this Congress.

We can see what is special about this meeting: It bears no resemblance to the assemblies of the various associations recruited by the *American Medical Association*. It is not enough, to belong to it, to be a doctor honorably known in his state or his province. Nor is it the triennial session of an association – and that is why I did not have to talk about societies and associations – since there is no corresponding association. Finally, the goal it pursues is exclusively scientific, and this is a quite exceptional case.

One is indeed strongly struck, when one attends the sessions of the various American medical meetings, to see what a subordinate role is attributed to questions of a scientific nature in the work of the sessions. One would be almost tempted to say that scientific communications are only the *pretext* for the meeting. In the state societies, I have seen session after session devoted to questions of admission of members, modifications of statutes, adoption of budgets, etc., all things foreign to the scientific goal which it seems logical to assign to these "scientific sessions." The rare times when medicine is discussed, I hardly hear more than a few lessons in elementary pathology, made, it was explained to me, for the benefit of the colleagues practicing in the rural areas, whose remoteness prevents them from keeping abreast of advances in medicine!

I have to admit that I had the same impression when I attended the sessions at the meeting held in New Orleans by the *American Medical Association*. There was, however, the difference that, by a kind of division of labor, the administrative side which had absorbed a good part of the time of the society referred to above was entirely reserved for special committees holding meetings in the offices. But the work of the scientific sessions hardly seemed to me to represent much more than a "Post-Graduate School" conference.

I can therefore say that if the organization of the medical meetings in America seemed to me on more than one point understood in a more rational way than on the other side of the Atlantic, the net result of their work seems to me to be reduced to very few things.

I would add that the New Orleans meeting caused me another disappointment. It was in the month of May; Since the month of September I had been traveling the United States, busily studying the medical situation, and among the many delegates, I barely recognized a few: The meeting included almost no luminaries, professors, or hospital doctors, there were mostly practitioners who came to New Orleans to take advantage of the benefits granted to members of Congress! It was on this impression that I left Louisiana to go to the Congress in Washington. There I had the satisfaction of finding myself on familiar ground, for the proportion of well-known personalities was the opposite of that which I had observed in New Orleans.

[p. 420]
Conclusions from a medical trip to the United States

Having come to the end of the articles that I was responsible for writing to inform the readers of this journal about medical America, both from a scientific and professional point of view, I have to cast a retrospective glance, considering in a general and analytic way the questions that I have studied: After dealing with these questions, day by day, so to speak, following an itinerary whose layout was subordinated to the need to see as many things as possible during the course of a year, it seems useful to merge everything into a table in which the details, necessary in a faithful and meticulous analysis, do not prevent the general impression from emerging; this attempt at a synthesis is all the more legitimate in that, despite their heterogeneity, the subjects dealt with are nonetheless closely related by virtue of the unity of the idea which guided our investigation in the United States, namely to make known on this side of the Atlantic what doctors and medicine are doing in America.

From the point of view of medical science, Americans are particularly interested in surgery. Undoubtedly, the progress made in this area in recent years has a lot to do with this preference. This factor is not sufficient, however, to explain such a predilection, since the progress of surgery has been similar in the different civilized countries. We must also take into account another element: Contemporary surgery is admirably suited to the national character of the American. Like him, it is active, enterprising, often daring. This explains why in America the best minds turn to surgery: Certainly, one meets distinguished, even eminent, physicians there. But how many are there, compared to the surgeons who in recent years have become a solid group?

Moreover, even in surgery, attention is primarily focused on issues of more immediate practical interest, notably on questions of technique and operative procedure. The fact is striking for anyone who follows an important surgical service in the United States for some time. It is even more obvious when one consults the program of an American surgical meeting or observes the work of its sessions. For my part, I twice had the opportunity to experience this: First at the meeting of *the American Medical Association* in New Orleans, then at the *Congress of American Physicians and Surgeons* which was held in Washington. In both of these meetings, almost all the important discussions revolved around questions of operative technique.

The Americans have not actually innovated much in this area. In reality, in the United States, they are in too much of a hurry to do their own investigations. They prefer to borrow from others; this is partly why the American is constantly traveling: Not for vacation, but to see what others are doing and learn from it. As he is subservient to no school and is born with a fairly well-balanced practical character, he knows how to "pick and choose" along the way, and it is here that the particular merit of the American lies: He discerns remarkably well what to retain, and how to modify a process or combine it with another.

For laboratory questions, it is the same. I have pointed out the enthusiasm which for some time has manifested itself in America for this kind of work. Still, it must be recognized that there are very few laboratories where truly original research is carried out. More often than not, they take on a work done abroad – and it seemed to me that they often take it on with very little critical thinking – they generalize it and go into battle just as if the ideas supported in this work – ideas that have sometimes been put forward only hypothetically or are still very subject to caution – were perfectly proven and definitively acquired by science.

Fifteen years ago, we could have truly said that there was no specifically American medicine; we can no longer say that today. This undoubtedly exists, with its own characteristics that derive from the native qualities of the American. However, this American medicine does not have an autonomous, independent life. It is a graft whose vitality depends on the tree to which it has been attached. American medicine has scarcely created any methods which belong to it alone, but it has sometimes brought important improvements to methods or processes which the genius of other nations had discovered. These nations are those of the old world, notably England – because of the language – France, and Germany. It is on these countries above all that medical America depends; so far, she has not been able to become independent of them.

This explains why each year our American colleagues invade the hospitals of Europe *en masse*. It is a pilgrimage which is essential for them to undertake. It is also unlikely that there will be a current in the opposite direction anytime soon. Assuredly, one would find some conditions in America, at least as far as certain branches are concerned – such as surgery – which bear comparison to what is best in our country. But it is doubtful whether these are sufficient reasons for creating, in medicine, the "thrust towards the West" of which the augurs speak.

Many important advances have been made in recent years in the field of medicine in the United States. More remains to be done. I have pointed out on several occasions how neglected the clinic was there. This is the essential foundation of the practice of our art. It is an education that our American colleagues know they still need to seek in Europe and particularly in France. This situation therefore assures our establishments of medical instruction of a numerous and studious clientele, just as other countries attract those who are eager for this or that special education or laboratory work, for example.

Thus, the current between the new and the old world that has been established can for the moment only be unilateral, going from America to Europe: The hour has not yet come for an exchange based on strict reciprocity. But some day this hour will come, for the impression which dominates among the memories left by a voyage of exploration in medical America is of incessant work, of tireless energy, of steady and rapid progress. These are the factors that have ensured the development made by the United States in the world from the economic point of view. They are also what make it possible to predict what American medicine will be some day, perhaps soon.

Original Notes

1. This school, which enjoys an excellent reputation in America, was originally intended to train civil engineers.
2. To vary the intensity of the light at will, Dr. Williams uses the following method: A series of small brass balls are mounted on a vulcanized rubber rod, at a short distance from each other. This rod is held in front of one of the conductors of the machine by means of a rope which passes over a pulley fixed to the ceiling and carries a counterweight at its other end. This is within reach of the doctor, who can increase or decrease the number of balls through which the current passes by lowering or raising the rod carrying the balls in a brass gutter, and thus regulate the intensity of the cathodic stream.
3. It is not within the scope of these articles to discuss hospital construction. However, I would like to point out that this annex of the Boston City Hospital is considered a model of its kind in America. It includes a pavilion for diphtheria and a pavilion for scarlet fever patients around which are grouped a series of pavilions intended for administration, etc. The basic idea behind the construction of this hospital is to isolate each of the patient wards as completely as possible. I was also rather surprised to find, during my visit to the South Department, that the pavilions actually all communicate by a system of underground galleries.
4. Dr. McCollom considers the place of choice for the injection of the antitoxic serum to be the level of the interior angle of the scapula in the

back. He recognizes in this region the advantage of a great laxity of the tissues with absence of veins. Moreover, this point not being accessible to the child's hand, infection of the place of inoculation by scratching is rendered almost impossible.

5. I will not dwell on the radiotherapeutic technique put into use by Dr. Coley, any more than I will emphasize that of Dr. Turnure, whose work I will mention later in this letter. I find, in fact, among these radiologists as well as most radiographic laboratories in the American East, devices and a technique more or less completely modeled on those adopted by Dr. Williams (of Boston). I therefore limit myself with referring to the description I gave earlier. – FM

6. It is often difficult to determine the exact location of the stone before operation. According to Dr. Beck (from New York), a good X-ray should clearly identify the location of the calculus. – FM

7. Remarkably, despite the cavalier way in which asepsis is treated there, the operative results are as satisfactory in London as anywhere else, judging by the information provided to me by the same colleague. I do not know if this is due, as is sometimes said, to the fact that the peritoneum of the English is particularly resistant. – FM

8. City hospitals in America are more asylums for beggars than anything else (almost the only exception being *Boston City Hospital*). Most hospitals are founded and maintained with the help of legacies and donations, as well as the income they derive from their paying rooms. These replace, to a certain extent, the *maisons de santé* that we have in France. To show the importance of these rooms from the budgetary point of view in American hospitals, I will cite as an example the *French Hospital* of New York, which pays *half* of its expenses solely with the resources provided by its paying rooms.

9. In the laparotomies which he performs in obese subjects, Dr. Deaver, the brilliant surgeon of Philadelphia of whom I have already spoken several times in my former correspondence, places a rubber drain longitudinally in the abdominal wall wound, above the superficial aponeurosis and below the adipose panniculus. This drain is long enough for its ends to extend beyond the ends of the wound: Having closed the skin over it, an aseptic solution is injected through one of the ends until it comes out clear through the other end. This drain is removed during the first dressing. This process would have the advantage of giving a better scar by preventing the suppuration of the cutaneous stitches, to which the abundance of the adipose panniculus predisposes. For the same purpose, Dr. Laplace does not exceed the level

of the dermis by placing his cutaneous stitches, so as not to include the adipose panniculus there. Since adopting this method, this surgeon says he has almost completely eliminated stitch abscesses.

10. In the United States, as in Paris, the curve which reflects the frequency of typhoid fever reaches its maximum in the fall, in September and October.
11. Potable water works similar to those carried out for Paris would not be practicable in America, owing to the geographical conditions of the country.
12. Theoretically, the protective lead shield should be 1.5 millimeters thick to be completely impermeable to Roentgen rays. In practice, a shield half as thick suffices with the exposure time that is usually used in radiology. – FM
13. In France, cocainization of the large nerve trunks as a method of surgical anesthesia was employed two and a half years ago by Professor Jaboulay (see *Semaine Médicale*, 1900, p. 398). –FM
14. In connection with what I wrote a few months ago on the subject of temporary carotid ligation (see *Semaine Médicale*, 1903, p. 16), I can add this: In the operation where I saw Dr. Crile perform this maneuver — an operation to which I allude in the course of this letter — there was, from the moment of the ligature of the carotid artery, a rather abundant venous hemorrhage. Dr. Crile also admitted that there is a possibility of an epileptic attack following the simultaneous ligation of the two carotids in a conversation I had with this surgeon. – FM
15. This process recalls up to a certain point that which was formerly advocated by Malgaigne, but it is distinguished by its greater simplicity.
16. We believe that a European doctor would hesitate to inject such a quantity of strychnine. According to Vulpian (quoted by Dr. Manquat, *Traité elémentaire de therapeutique*, Volume II, p. 622, 4th Edition, Paris, 1900), a dose of 10 milligrams of a soluble salt of strychnine by subcutaneous injection, "would certainly be very dangerous." – Ed.
17. The personal observations collected by Dr. Crile give him an average of 135 millimeters of mercury for the blood pressure measured with the Riva-Rocci device. In the case where I saw the pneumatic trousers applied by Dr. Crile, the arterial pressure, ascertained before the start of the operation, was 160 millimeters. This figure was considered excessive and attributed to the arteriosclerosis from which the patient, a sixty-year-old man, was suffering. These figures, which are quite significantly lower than those generally considered normal (180 millimeters), are probably related to the device used to record them. –FM

18. Of course, we are talking about *abdominal* hysteropexy. *Vaginal* hysteropexy has long since become a historical memory.
19. I do not dwell on the Atlantic ports, which also grant free passage, because, as I said above, yellow fever does not find favorable ground in this part of the United States and it is consequently a much less formidable disease there. – FM
20. The administrative divisions of the United States can be compared to similar divisions of France, although in the United States, because of the greater extent of the territory, the different regional divisions had to be given autonomy much more than in France, a country whose territory is 17 or 18 times smaller. We can therefore say that the American state corresponds to the French *départment*, the governor to the *préfect*, the county to the *arrondissement*, the district to the *canton*.
21. In Clarinda, where the fourth insane asylum in the state of Iowa is located, the alcoholic division had not yet been created at the time of my visit.
22. It should be noted that, about a year ago, the English Chambers passed a law, called the *Licensing Act*, which contains provisions aimed at alcoholics. This law is therefore contemporaneous with the law of Iowa.
23. It is important to add that each state has several examination boards. This is because, besides the so-called *regular doctors*, a series of dissident sects have been officially recognized, each of which possesses its special schools and also a special *State Board*, exclusively composed of practitioners of that doctrine.
24. It is important to specify this clause, since in some schools the duration of the academic year may be only four or five months of study!

Biographical Sources

Münch FE, *Ueber die Entwicklung des Knorpels des äusseren Ohres, Dissertation Kaiser-Wilhelms-Universität Strassburg*, Jena: Gustav Fischer, 1897.

"Nécrologie," *Le Monde*, 12 February 1974, p. 19.

Archives Nationales, Base de données Léonore. Accessed at leonore.archives-nationales.culture.gouv.fr., "Munch, Francis."

Publication Source

La Semaine Médicale (Medical Week) ceased publication in 1914. Historical issues can be obtained through the Hathi Trust or the Internet Archive.

Translation Notes

1) Dr. Williams also published a textbook, *The Roentgen Rays in Medicine and Surgery*, 2nd Edition, New York: MacMillan, 1902. Pages 8-19 describe the Holtz static influence machine.
2) Today the Lankenau Medical Center.
3) Subsequently known as the Philadelphia General Hospital, it closed in 1977.
4) Gluge corpuscles were probably what we would today call eosinophils. See Kay AB, "The early history of the eosinophil," *Clinical & Experimental Allergy* 2015; 45:575-582.
5) The author refers to typhoid fever as *dothiénentérie*, a term proposed by French physician Pierre Bretonneau (1778-1862), but rarely used outside France.
6) See Trivedi S, Chakravarty A, "Neurological complications of malaria," *Current Neurology and Neuroscience Reports* 2022; 22:499-513.
7) Mithridates, King of Pontus (135-63 B.C.) protected himself from poisoners by chronically ingesting sublethal doses of several common poisons.
8) See Adams H, *et al.*, "Harvey Cushing's case series of trigeminal neuralgia at the Johns Hopkins Hospital: a surgeon's quest to advance the treatment of the 'suicide disease'," *Acta Neurochir (Wien)* 2011; 153:1043-1050.
9) See Cushing H, "On routine determinations of arterial tension in operating room and clinic," *Boston Medical and Surgical Journal* 1903; 148:250-256.
10) *Corynebacterium diphtheriae*.
11) The Municipal Hospital for Infectious Diseases was later absorbed into the Philadelphia General Hospital, which closed in 1977.
12) This was a French concept about the effect of climate and weather on diseases. See Godonnèche J, "A propos du génie épidémique," *Toulouse Médical* 1946; 47:594-601.

13) Literally "cold," a term usually applied to a normal appendix in America, but "à froid" is apparently used in Europe to describe a previously inflamed appendix that has "cooled off." See Engkvist O, "Appendectomy à froid a superfluous routine operation?," *Acta Chirurgica Scandinavica* 1971; 137:797-800.
14) Acute or chronic nephritis.
15) Paramedian incision with medial retraction of the rectus abdominus muscle.
16) Now the Memorial Sloan Kettering Cancer Center.
17) Now called *Serratia marcescens*.
18) The Roosevelt Hospital in New York, founded by a distant cousin of the presidents with that name, is now the Mount Sinai West Hospital.
19) In his Note [6], the author actually writes "Dr. Seebeck," but there was no doctor by that name in New York, and he is probably referring to publications by Carl Beck, including "The representation of biliary calculi by the Rontgen rays," *New York Medical Journal* 1901; 73:446-448.
20) Both of these hospitals were later absorbed into the University Hospitals of Cleveland.
21) Now part of the University of Pennsylvania Hospitals.
22) A fiber made from silkworm gut.
23) New York's City Hospital closed in 1957 and its building was demolished in 1994. Blackwell Island is now called Roosevelt Island.
24) The Bièvre River flows through Paris, collects much of the rainwater drainage, and empties into the Seine.
25) *Salmonella enterica*.
26) Pusey WA, Caldwell EW. *The Practical Application of the Röntgen Rays in Therapeutics and Diagnosis*. Philadelphia: W. B. Saunders, 1903.
27) Augustana Hospital was later called the Lutheran General Hospital, and closed in 1989. The name Augustana refers to the Augsburg Confession (*Confessio Augustana*), the fundamental document of the Lutheran Church.
28) Today part of Rush University Medical Center.
29) Today part of Rush University Medical Center.
30) Hypodermic syringe, invented by French surgeon Charles Pravaz (1791-1853).
31) See Mudry A, Righini CA, "Friedrich Trendelenburg's tracheal

tampon-cannula," *European Annals of Otorhinolaryngology, Head and Neck Diseases* 2023; 140:135-138.

32) See Grant WW, "New operation for epithelioma of the lip," *Medical Record* 1899; 55:744-746.

33) See Grant WW, "Bridge for treatment of nasal fractures and deformities," *Annals of Surgery* 1903; 38:441-443.

34) See Halsted WS, "The results of operations for the cure of cancer of the breast performed at the Johns Hopkins Hospital from June, 1889, to January, 1894," *Annals of Surgery* 1894; 20:497-555.

35) The scalene tubercle, where the anterior scalene muscle attaches to the first rib, named for Jacques Lisfranc (1787-1847).

36) The *angulus venosus*, named for Nikolai Ivanovich Pirogoff (1810-1881).

37) Split-thickness skin grafts, named for Karl Thiersch (1822-1895).

38) Now the Mount Sinai Morningside Hospital.

39) Now the Hospital for Special Surgery.

40) See Cushing H, "The employment of local anaesthesia in the radical cure of certain cases of hernia, with a note upon the nervous anatomy of the inguinal region," *Annals of Surgery* 1900; 31:1-34.

41) See Turck FB, "Shock produced by general anesthesia," *Journal of the American Medical Association* 1903; 40:1206-1212.

42) See Crile GW, *An Experimental Research into Surgical Shock*, Philadelphia: J. B. Lippincott, 1899; Crile GW, *Blood Pressure in Surgery*, Philadelphia: J. B. Lippincott, 1903.

43) The pneumatic trousers were repopularized as the Medical Anti-Shock Trousers in the 1970's. See Clark DE, Demers ML, "Lower body positive pressure," *Surgery, Gynecology & Obstetrics* 1989; 168:81-97.

44) The original Alquie-Alexander procedure shortened the round ligaments extraperitoneally via the inguinal canals. See Goldspohn A, "The extended indications and modified technique of the Alquie-Alexander-Adams operation, with important adjuncts," *American Gynaecological and Obstetrical Journal* 1898; 12:155-161.

45) This statement was specifically quoted by the *Clinical Review* (of Chicago), 1904; 19:309-310, which praised the author's letters in "the famous French medical journal" *Semaine Médicale* as "written attractively and truthfully."

46) See "Demonstration of McGraw Ligature," discussed by A. J. Ochsner and others in the Transactions of the Chicago Surgical

Society, *Annals of Surgery* 1904; 39:144-147.
47) Finney JMT, "A new method of pyloroplasty," *Bulletin of the Johns Hopkins Hospital* 1902; 13:155-161.
48) Now called *Aedes aegypti*.
49) Mercuric chloride, no longer used.
50) See Weir RF, "On the disinfection of the hands," *Medical Record* 1897; 51:469-473.
51) Now the Episcopal Campus of Temple University Hospital.
52) Of course, most of the diseases mentioned in this section are now known to be microbial infections, having nothing to do with supposed racial or other genetic factors.
53) Christian Scientists.
54) Followers of faith healer John Alexander Dowie, whose "Christian Catholic Church" was based in Zion, Illinois.
55) The author is obviously describing the Mayo brothers in Rochester, Minnesota.
56) French authors make a distinction between the *hôpital*, a charitable institution, and the *maison de santé*, which we might call a "private hospital" for paying patients.
57) The *franc* was the monetary unit for France, Belgium, and Switzerland, and was equivalent to about $0.19.
58) Probably referring to J. B. Murphy, who was initially denied membership in the American Surgical Association, although he was eventually elected in 1902. See Davis L, *J. B. Murphy: Stormy Petrel of Surgery*, New York: G. P. Putnam's Sons, 1938.
59) In 321 B.C., a Roman Army was trapped at a narrow mountain pass called the Caudine Forks, forced to surrender, and humiliated by being made to bow as they passed two-by-two under an ox-yoke.

7
Roman Barącz (1902-1904)

Roman Barącz was born in 1856 in Lemberg, in a predominantly Polish part of the Austro-Hungarian Empire, a city that also had large minority populations of Ukrainians, Jews, and Armenians (the last group including the Barącz family). He studied medicine at the Jagiellonian University in Kraków. He trained in surgery in Kraków, Lemberg, London, and Vienna, and practiced in Lemberg starting in 1885. He visited numerous surgical centers and participated in scientific meetings all over Europe, and spoke twelve languages.

In 1902, at the age of 46, he traveled to the United States to observe surgical methods, and stayed until 1904. Later that year, he reported on his experiences in both German and Polish journals.

In 1906, he was named *Privat-Dozent* at the University of Lemberg. He published 99 articles in general surgery and was particularly interested in fungal infections. After the First World War, the city became part of Poland, and was known as Lwów (today it is Lviv, Ukraine). Roman Barącz' son Zygmunt also became a surgeon, but was killed during the war with the Bolsheviks in 1920.

Shortly after completing an operation in 1930, Roman Barącz had a sudden fatal heart attack.

Beobachtungen über die chirurgische Technik in den Vereinigten Staaten Americas
Wiener Medizinische Wochenschrift 1904; 54: 530-533, 579-582, 630-633, 667-670, 729-733

Krótki pogląd na obecny stan techniki chirurgicznej w Stanach Zjednoczonych Ameryki na podstawie własnych spostrzeżeń
Przegląd Lekarski 1904; 43:127-129, 145-147, 160-163, 177-180

Observations on surgical technique in the United States of America[*]
Dr. Roman von Barącz
Privat-Dozent[1] for Surgery at the University of Lemberg[2]

One of the most important factors in the progress of modern surgery is the improved surgical technique. If in Europe during the past ten years it has reached a high level of development, nevertheless it has improved at an even more rapid pace in America, advancing by giant steps. I would like to report here on my observations from two centers of medical science in America, namely New York and Chicago.

First of all, I must emphasize that their hospital facilities are not comparable to those in Europe, but are vastly superior. Wealthy industrialists have generally founded the hospitals and bear half of their maintenance costs, while the other half is covered by paying patients. In America, operations are not performed in private homes, but instead even the wealthiest follow medical advice and are admitted to the hospital where their chosen surgeon operates. The larger hospitals have 4 to 6 surgeons, and a similar number of gynecologists and internists. Surgeons operate on their private patients in operating rooms built and equipped for this purpose. Larger hospitals are usually affiliated with a medical school or university, in which case the hospital is then an annex of the university. Hospital surgeons are usually professors at the associated university. For example, the Roosevelt Hospital[3] in New York, furnished according to all modern requirements, is also part of a medical school known as Columbia University, where surgeons of such stature as Robert Weir and L. Stimson lecture. Mercy Hospital[4] in Chicago is part of the medical school of Northwestern University, where the famous surgeon J. B. Murphy is Professor of Surgery.

Asepsis: Asepsis is better managed in America than in Europe, thanks to the superior hospital facilities, which use almost exclusively glass, iron, and even white marble for walls and doors, thanks to the better educated nurses [1], who are only hired and allowed to take care of patients after three years of schooling and passing an examination, and finally thanks to the abundance of sterile hot and cold water.

Hand disinfection is carried out very meticulously. Here I must mention the method of hand sanitization introduced by Robert F. Weir [2] and adopted not only by New York surgeons but also in almost all of the eastern states of America. It uses the emerging antiseptic properties of chlorine. Kümmel's experiments with chlorine water in 1885 had already demonstrated the strong antiseptic properties of chlorine. P. Rauschenberger, pharmacist of the Roosevelt Hospital, first recommended using a mixture of commercially available lime chloride ($CaCl_2O$) with ordinary sodium carbonate (Na_2CO_3), which with a small addition of water releases free chlorine. This mixture saponifies and dissolves skin oils and epidermis. The exact chemical action is not yet explained, but it is established that it results in sodium hypochlorite, which is known by the name of Labarraque's Solution. The method of use is very simple. A handful of plain lime chloride is placed in one dish, and in another a few crystals of common soda (about an inch thick and half an inch wide). After careful mechanical cleansing of the hands with soap, water, and a brush, one puts about a teaspoon of the lime chloride and a soda crystal in the hands and rubs them together with a little water. Rubbing first the piece of soda and then the resulting paste takes 3-5 minutes. The hands are then rinsed with sterile water, and become extremely smooth and smell of chlorine. The chlorine smell can be removed by washing the hands with a 1-5% sterile solution of ammonium water (*aqua ammoniae*). Hands can be sanitized this way 3-4 times a day without seeing or feeling any harm to the skin.

This method of hand disinfection has proven not only better clinically, but also bacteriologically compared to other methods of hand disinfection (Fürbringer method,[5] sublimate[6] disinfection). Out of 42 experiments, the hands were completely sterile in 40; so it may be concluded that 95% of cases will achieve complete sterility.

Despite very thorough hand sanitization, Americans almost always operate wearing the steam-sterilized rubber gloves introduced by McBurney. The number of unexpected postoperative abscesses after clean operations is thought to be greatly decreased since the introduction of rubber gloves. Sterilization of dressings, suture material, and instruments is done the same way as we do. Catgut is mostly sterilized using the Elsberg method (boiling in a saturated solution of ammonium sulfate for ½ hour, hardening in absolute alcohol, and storage in juniper oil).

More recently, N. Senn (Chicago) has had excellent results with iodized catgut, which however he does not prepare with the method of Bloch, recently described by Claudius [3]. Senn first sterilizes the catgut using the method of Hofmeister, then stores it not in sublimate-alcohol but in the following solution: Absolute alcohol 950, glycerine 50, iodoform 100. The alcohol dissolves the iodine, which impregnates the catgut, making it similar to Bloch's iodized catgut, and similarly strong and totally aseptic.

A very widely used suture material for superficial sutures after laparotomy or plastic operations is silkworm gut (*crin de Florence*). It is a very strong suture material, although somewhat too stiff. It can be sterilized in the same way as catgut.

Absorbent gauze is used as a dressing material without the addition of antiseptics, only sterilized.

As a substitute for iodoform, Murphy recommends bismuth subiodide (oxyiodide Merck) (BiOI).[7] It is a very fine powder, brick-red and odorless, which has strong antiseptic properties, can be sterilized easily without harm, and promotes drying and granulation. Murphy also uses gauze impregnated with this material. From personal experience, I can also recommend this preparation.

Since it is known that the abdominal cavity is very difficult to sterilize, Murphy has developed a special adhesive rubber dam,[8] an appropriately sized piece of which is sterilized and stuck to the abdominal skin prior to laparotomy. The incision is made through this adhesive drape and the laparotomy carried out, after which the drape is removed. If the laparotomy is being performed because of peritonitis, the adhesive rubber dam can be left in place postoperatively to prevent eczema due to irritating secretions.

So-called "cigarette drains" are used instead of the usual drainage tubes or gauze packs. These are constructed of various lengths of absorbent gauze, wrapped in rubber sheets and steam-sterilized. These are inserted into the wound. They have the following advantages: 1. They can be removed from the wound very easily and painlessly; 2. They combine features of tube drainage and capillary drainage. I found these drains very practical.

American surgeons use formalin as an antiseptic for three purposes: 1. Gynecologists use it for irrigation of female genitalia; 2. Murphy uses it as a 2% admixture with iodoform-glycerin suspension to strengthen the effect when injected into tuberculous joints; 3. Finally, during my stay in America, Barrows in New York used it as a 1:5000 solution intravenously in a few cases of postpartum infection, with supposedly good results [4].

Anesthesia: Chloroform was most often used for general anesthesia, using the drop method on an Esmarch mask. On the other hand, gynecologists use ether anesthesia, either by itself or starting with nitrous oxide and then continuing with ether. The use of ether for short procedures on children seemed very practical. The basic method is to pour a small amount of ether into a bag that will be applied to the child. This bag can be quickly and easily improvised out of a large piece of paper and cloth. A piece of absorbent gauze is stuffed into the bag, 10-15 grams of pure ether are poured onto it, and the bag is placed tightly over the mouth and nose and held firmly. After just a few minutes this leads to complete analgesia and a sleep of short duration, from which the little patients awaken completely without any recollection of the operation that has taken place. It is an anesthesia similar to that of Sudeck, producing complete analgesia and sedation but requiring less narcotic drug by cutting off the supply of air.

As local anesthetics they use cocaine, beta-eucaine in a 6% solution, and nirvanin. After repeated attempts, anesthesia by injection of cocaine or tropacaine into the spinal canal has been almost completely abandoned in America.[9]

On the other hand, there is increasing interest in methods of anesthetizing larger parts of the body, especially the limbs, by injecting weak solutions of cocaine into the nerve trunks (endoneural injections) that supply these parts of the body. This method was recommended almost simultaneously by R. Matas (New Orleans), Crile (Cleveland, Ohio), and Cushing (Baltimore, Maryland). By injecting weak (1%) solutions of cocaine into the nerve trunks, not only is feeling and power in the limb provided by these trunks abolished, but the nervous reflexes are also abolished. According to Crile, the respiratory and vasomotor reflexes are abolished by intraneural injections of cocaine, and thus also surgical shock.[10] By blocking the nerve with cocaine, conduction in it is stopped only for a few hours, after which power and sensation return completely; and there is never any degeneration or inflammation of the nerve. According to Crile, this method of anesthesia is indicated in those cases where there is a contraindication to general anesthesia. In amputations of the lower limbs, 1% cocaine is injected into the three main nerve trunks supplying the limb, namely the lateral femoral cutaneous, femoral, and sciatic nerves; in operations on the forearm, in places supplied by the ulnar nerve, 1% cocaine is injected into this nerve in its course in the groove between the olecranon process and the medial condyle of the humerus; when amputating the arm at the shoulder the individual branches of the brachial plexus are cocainized, at which time the axillary artery is temporarily clamped (Crile), making it possible not only to remove the entire extremity at the shoulder joint without pain or bleeding, but also to perform this major intervention without shock.

Cushing has also used endoneural injection for repair of inguinal hernia.[11] After cocainizing and incising the fascia of the external oblique muscle, he injects cocaine solution into the following nerve trunks: the ileohypogastric, the ilioinguinal, and the genitofemoral; the operative field is thus anesthetized, and any manipulation of the bowel is painless anyway. Cushing makes use of endoneural injections for major amputations only to avoid shock; he always uses ether for general anesthesia.

This method of analgesia must be tried out more extensively before a judgment can be made about its value. In any case, the protection against shock in major operations on the limbs, especially in debilitated persons, encourages further attempts. The dissemination of this method of analgesia will be hindered anyway by the difficulty of the technique. These attempts should also take note of whether endoneural injections might have any unfavorable consequences on the nervous system!

Roentgen rays are used extensively not only for diagnostic but also for therapeutic purposes. Instead of the Ruhmkorff induction apparatus, the large static influence machines of Holtz are used as a source of Roentgen rays in America.[12] They are using Roentgen rays to treat lupus, acne, psoriasis, eczema, and cancer, and indeed with good success. The treatments take place 2-3 times a week, and healthy parts of the body are protected with lead shields. Not only skin cancers, but also deeper and recurrent cancers shrink due to the effect of Roentgen rays, as I was able to see for myself in Chicago at the Augustana Hospital[13] in the department of Dr. A. J. Ochsner. Pain is reduced even with a few treatments; even neuralgias are affected favorably by the Roentgen rays. A. J. Ochsner also uses Roentgen rays after radical mastectomy to prevent recurrences. Dr. N. Senn (Chicago) has had very good success using them for malignant lymphoma. The mechanism of action is probably the partial necrosis of regenerating parts and resorption of the necrotic tissue. The subject is still too new for one to make any judgment. However, it seems to me that the Americans will solve this problem through further research.

Regarding operations on the skin and subcutaneous tissues, I have to report on Wyeth's management of angiomas and the modification of Thiersch skin transplants by Edward H. Ochsner (Chicago).

J. A. Wyeth's method of managing angiomas is based on the injection of boiling water into the growth. A few drops of water or sometimes more is injected, depending on the size of the growth, until the skin over the growth feels hot and blanches. For larger growths these injections are done in multiple sessions. One must inject the water fairly deep under the growth and compromise the surrounding tissues, in order to avoid emboli. These injections create clots, which are then resorbed [5].

[p. 579]

Ochsner's modification of Thiersch skin grafts is based on performing the entire operation in dry conditions. Whereas Thiersch submerges the pieces of skin in a sterile 0.6% saline solution and advises wet dressings, Ochsner does the entire operation dry. Ochsner disinfects the donor skin 12 hours before surgery, covers it with dry sterile gauze, and after 12 hours cuts dry pieces of skin with a dry sterile razor. This dry method enables every motion of the razor to be very carefully controlled, since the donor extremity is not slippery and the pieces of skin can all be equally thin; they also heal better with this method. The recipient site is also kept dry, although it must be hemostatic; the granulating surface must have only healthy granulation tissue: Deep ulcerations with necrotic debris must be cleaned out with a sharp curette down to the muscle fascia, so that a dry healthy wound surface is created. After transplantation, the pieces of skin are first covered with a sterile dry rubber sheet, then with a thick layer of sterile gauze and immobilized with adhesive tape. The grafted pieces of skin have usually implanted by 10 days at the time of the first dressing change, and the donor site has also healed by the dressing change at 12 days. Ochsner's modification also saves a lot of time, as I saw for myself (St. Mary of Nazareth Hospital, Chicago).

Regarding operations on the skeletal system, I have to discuss the methods of managing deformities of the upper and lower leg in children with rickets. This condition is encountered especially often among Negro children. V. P. Gibney and Whitman (New York Hospital for Ruptured and Crippled[14]) treat this problem with subcutaneous linear osteotomies, but Ridlon and W. Blanchard (Chicago, Home for Destitute Crippled Children[15], Wesley Hospital[16]) treat the deformities almost exclusively with rapid osteocampsis or rapid osteoclasis. For this purpose, they have exclusively employed the osteoclast of N. Grattan (from Cork, Ireland) since September 1892, namely the time when Grattan demonstrated his apparatus at the 6th Congress of the American Orthopedic Association in New York.[17] Grattan's apparatus, a strong two-armed lever, is notable for its very great weight of 36½ pounds, and also for its great strength and the precision with which one can direct its breaking or bending strength. Two arms of this apparatus, made of naked steel, surround the extremity to be fractured, while another equally strong arm is inserted on the opposite side between the first two arms; this third arm is then directed toward the previously determined point of the deformed extremity and brought closer by using a large screw. In an anesthetized child, the whole procedure takes 5½ minutes; the actual osteoclasty takes 7-8 seconds, manual correction of the deformity 5-8 seconds, application of a plaster cast 2 minutes, and hardening of the plaster 3 minutes.

Thus, a whole series of deformities can be treated in one session, in the same time as would be needed for a Macewen osteotomy! Whereas a wedged osteotomy shortens the extremity by an inch, the osteoclasis lengthens it by an inch, since it creates a wedge-shaped fracture at the site where force is applied to the bone. In deformities due to rickets, the osteoclasis should be performed before the child has attained 5 years of age, since after this the bones become harder and have more of the consistency of adult bones. Dr. W. Blanchard (Chicago) has performed the rapid osteoclasis with the Grattan apparatus in 262 cases of deformities due to rickets of the lower leg (*genua valga* and *vara*), always with good success. With *genu valgum* the osteoclasis is made over the femoral condyle (*osteoclasis supracondylica*), and with *genu varum* at the upper part of the tibia. For lesser degrees of deformity, it is only necessary to bend the bone, called osteocampsis. The main requirement for success of this procedure is hypercorrection of the extremity with respect to the original deformity. Thus, the knee is placed in valgus for *genu varum* and vice-versa for *genu valgum*, and immobilized in a plaster cast. Neither Ridlon nor Blanchard have seen soft-tissue complications due to osteoclasis. The advantages of Grattan's rapid osteoclasis are as follows: Speed of performing the operation, minimizing postoperative pain, avoiding the time and expense needed for antiseptic bandages, and finally the most important – lengthening the extremity. Based on my own observations, and to some degree my own experience [6], I can strongly recommend this method of osteoclasis. The wider acceptance of this rapid osteoclasis is only hindered by the relatively high price of the apparatus. (The instrument costs 70 dollars in Chicago.)

Among other orthopedic operations, I saw a lot of reductions of congenital hip dislocations, performed either by Lorenz, who was at that time in Chicago, or by other surgeons using his method. I will not describe the Lorenz method of reduction, since it is well known.[18]

Mastectomy for carcinoma is usually performed using the improved method of Halsted.[19] This improvement in technique is based upon routine excision of the pectoralis minor muscle and systematic removal of the lymph nodes and fat in the angle between the jugular and axillary veins. Halsted recommends the systematic removal of these glands, since he has demonstrated metastases histologically in this location even when they feel healthy on palpation.

Now I will proceed to operations on the digestive tract.

Gastroenterostomy: In America, this is mostly done using Hacker's method, namely a posterior retrocolic gastroenterostomy, since American surgeons take the view that connecting the most inferior part of the stomach to the jejunum is necessary for gastric emptying and avoiding stagnation of undigested food in the stomach.

For gastroenterostomy, the Americans especially emphasize gastric drainage. In order to avoid the so-called "vicious circle," almost all of them add an entero-enterostomy to the gastroenterostomy. For the gastrojejunal anastomosis, most of them use a mechanical aid, namely the Murphy button,[20] or Robson's bone bobbin,[21] or the elastic sutures of McGraw; only A. J. Ochsner (Chicago) advocates the usual suturing. Wm. T. Bull in New York uses the improved Murphy button; this improvement consists of two lateral prongs on the male half of the button inserted into the jejunum, which spring out after closure of the button to hold it in the jejunum and prevent it from falling into the stomach. Bull, Kammerer, and other surgeons do not place a purse-string suture to constrict the incisions in the stomach and jejunum, but simply constrict the incisions by suturing their ends together with a few Lembert sutures following the suggestion of Carle and Fantino, thus keeping the neck of the button in the middle of the wound. If the incisions in the stomach and jejunum are made no larger than necessary to insert the pieces of the button, then the ends themselves never cover the region of the button. W. T. Bull performs gastroenterostomy as follows: He first chooses the appropriate loop of jejunum and incises it about 40 cm from the duodenal-jejunal fold. Through this incision he introduces one half of a small Murphy button into each arm of the loop; about 15 cm from the jejunal incision each half-button is pressed against the free bowel wall, the bowel wall is incised, and the two halves of the button are pressed together. Thus, an entero-enterostomy is first created. Then the anterior inferior gastric wall is also opened with a small incision, the female half of a larger button is introduced into the stomach, and the stomach incision constricted as described above. Finally, the male half of the larger Murphy button is introduced into the jejunal incision, this wound is also constricted as described, and the two halves of the button are pressed together. No further sutures are applied. The button used for gastroenterostomy by W. T. Bull is modified in that the male half of the button placed in the jejunum is provided with two lateral springs, which come out when the button is closed and prevent it from falling into the stomach. I do not know who introduced this modification, but it is a great advance in the technique, which should lead to a wider acceptance of the Murphy button method since one no longer needs to fear the button falling into the stomach.

The second method of gastroenterostomy, which is still being tried out, is that proposed by T. A. McGraw (Detroit, Michigan), which consists of using elastic ligatures. I watched Dr. Willy Meyer use this method to perform a gastroenterostomy at the German Hospital[22] in New York. It involved a case of gastric cancer complicated by infiltration of the greater and lesser omentum. After elevation of the omentum and transverse colon the mesocolon was divided bluntly and its walls were sewn to the posterior wall of the stomach. After identifying the first loop of jejunum it was brought up to the stomach and sewn to it with several Lembert sutures. Next the stomach was folded laterally and about a half inch from the suture line the entire thickness of the stomach wall was pierced with a straight needle about 5 cm long, armed with an elastic suture.

The round elastic suture material was about 2-3 mm in diameter. During the puncture of the stomach wall with the Hagedorn needle, the assistant stretches the elastic suture, which decreases its diameter and allows it to pass easily through the stomach wall; immediately after the puncture, the suture regains its original thickness and thus seals the two puncture sites. In the same way, at the same distance from the suture line and parallel to it the jejunum is punctured with the same needle and suture. The elastic suture is now pulled together tightly, its two ends are crossed, and the assistant ties the crossing point of the elastic sutures close to the stomach and intestine with a thick and tight silk suture, after which the ends of the elastic suture are cut off. Finally, a second row of Lembert sutures are placed on the anterior wall of the stomach and bowel that have been thus attached.

[p. 630]

In order to avoid a vicious circle, an entero-enterostomy is constructed 15 cm below the gastroenterostomy. Willy Meyer surrounds the entero-enterostomy site with a running suture. Of course, the anterior antecolic gastroenterostomy used in this method is an easier procedure. McGraw's experiments have shown that the elastic suture begins to create a communication between the two parts of the intestinal tract starting on the third day after the procedure. The gastric and intestinal portions encompassed by the elastic do not become gangrenous but simply resorb. The patients are at first nourished using enemas, and then receive a liquid diet by mouth starting on the third day. According to McGraw, the enteric anastomosis using elastic ligature is the quickest of all known methods; it is very simple, and even the most debilitated patient is not put into shock; it can be performed aseptically, and the peritoneal cavity is not exposed to gastrointestinal contents. McGraw and Willy Meyer invite further attempts using this method [7].

Most American surgeons perform gastrectomy using the method of W. J. Mayo (Rochester, Minnesota) [8]. Mayo advocates as radical an operation as possible. He advises leaving only the fundus of the stomach, since stomach cancer invades the lymphatic channels and nodes not only along the lesser curvature but also along the greater curvature, and even along the gastrocolic and gastrosplenic omentum, and only the fundus has few lymphatics.

Dr. Mayo operates as follows: First the lesser omentum is tied off from the pylorus up to the left gastric artery. The incision is made close to the liver; the entire lesser omentum is divided; thus, the pyloric region of the stomach is mobilized and brought downward. Guided by a finger in the lesser omental sac, the gastrocolic omentum is ligated as peripherally as possible up to the origin of the left gastroepiploic artery. After double clamping of the duodenum and pylorus, the pyloric portion of the stomach is divided using thermocautery, and the duodenal stump is closed with a blind pursestring suture. A heavy crushing clamp is applied to the stomach along a line from the left gastric artery to the left gastroepiploic artery, and the stomach is divided along this line. Not much more than the fundus remains. The gastric incision is closed with a running suture. Then a gastroenterostomy and finally an entero-enterostomy are performed with a Murphy button.

Management of appendicitis: Cases of appendicitis are seen more often in the United States than in Europe. The reasons for the frequent incidence of appendicitis may be attributed to insufficient nutrition, especially in the working class, eating too quickly, and perhaps also the excessive drinking of ice water (common in America). Regarding surgical indications, most American surgeons operate on every case either in the first hours of the attack (before 24 hours have passed) or soon after the first attack. This opinion is shared by the greatest specialists in this area like McBurney, Deaver, and Robert F. Weir.

After 24 hours from the beginning of an attack, an operation is avoided; at this time most administer laxatives (castor oil, calomel), in order to empty the intestinal tract of strongly irritating feces and very toxic bacteria. General practitioners regard waiting for a second attack of appendicitis to be a major error; every internist refers every case of appendicitis to a surgeon. This eagerness to operate in America is rational, in that surgeons only rarely encounter neglected cases complicated by peritonitis and gangrene; thus, there is almost zero mortality after appendectomy.

The operative technique with appendicitis is different, depending on whether it is a fresh case or a case *à froid*,²³ and different when managing a complicated case.

In fresh cases, the incision is either that of McBurney or of F. Kammerer. The most frequently used method is McBurney's. The skin incision is made 1-1½ inches medial to the anterior superior iliac spine inferomedially in the direction of the fibers of the external oblique muscle. The incision only divides the skin; it should not extend to the aponeurosis of the external oblique; it should be about 4 inches long, perpendicular to a line from the anterior superior iliac spine to the umbilicus, and the upper third of this incision should be above this line. The upper part of the external oblique and its fascia are exposed as widely as possible with a finger, then a small incision is made in the direction of its fibers and the skin incision. The edges of the incised external oblique and its aponeurosis are now pulled apart with blunt retractors, thus exposing the deeper internal oblique muscle. The fibers of this muscle run more horizontal, almost at right angles to those of the external oblique. The fibers of this muscle and the transversus abdominis underneath it are separated with a blunt instrument (a blunt Cooper scissors or the scalpel handle) and pulled apart with another pair of blunt retractors. The wound through these muscles runs perpendicular to that in the external oblique. The exposed transversalis fascia and peritoneum are now divided in the same direction as the fibers of the deeper muscles (internal oblique and transversus); this incision is about 2 inches long. Traction on the wound edges gives sufficient exposure for locating the appendix. This is sought by a finger introduced toward the cecum; it lies either on the posterior or medial wall of the cecum. If there is difficulty locating the appendix, the cecum is delivered, and its anterior tenia followed inferiorly to the point where the appendix is attached. If the appendix cannot be identified due to adhesions or other abnormalities, the oblique incision can be extended medially over to the rectus muscle. The anterior rectus sheath can be divided horizontally, the belly of the muscle retracted medially, and the posterior rectus sheath also divided horizontally as an extension of the incision in the transversalis fascia. This gives very good access to the appendix. The McBurney incision has the advantage that it does not injure any nerves, major vessels, or muscles; the muscle fibers return to their natural place after the operation which avoids incisional hernias. After removing the appendix, the deeper muscles and external oblique are separately sutured with fine silk or catgut, requiring only a small number of stitches; the skin is sutured with strong silkworm gut.

The appendix is amputated as follows: After careful, mostly blunt division of adhesions, the mesoappendix is divided separately between ligatures. The base of the appendix (at the cecum) is ligated with fine catgut or silk, clamped above the ligature, and amputated; the mucosa of the stump is burnt with a pointed thermocautery device, then a purse-string suture is placed circumferentially in the cecum to enclose the stump.

McCosh (Presbyterian Hospital, New York) only cauterizes the mucosa of the amputated appendix, without any purse-string suture in the cecum; nevertheless, he has had no complications in more than 1000 operative cases. Some surgeons (Robert F. Weir) use concentrated liquid phenol applied with a glass rod to cauterize the mucosa of the amputated appendix instead of thermocautery.

Dr. Robert Dawbarn (New York) first places a purse-string suture of fine silk in the cecum around the appendix about ½ inch from its base, amputates the appendix ½ inch above its attachment, grasps the tip of the stump with a fine forceps, and inverts the stump into the cecum; finally, he ties the purse-string suture and removes the forceps.

G. M. Edebohls (New York) inverts the entire appendix into the cecum and prevents it from coming back out by several sutures placed in the cecum.

These last two methods for managing the appendix only seem appropriate if it has sufficiently strong walls and is not stenotic at the base.

The second type of incision for appendectomy is that proposed by F. Kammerer (New York); it resembles those proposed by Jalaguier and Lennander. This incision is made along the lateral border of the rectus abdominis muscle; the sheath of this muscle is split longitudinally, the muscle is bluntly retracted medially, then somewhat more medially the posterior sheath, transversalis fascia, and peritoneum are also incised longitudinally. The rest of the procedure is the same as just described. Objections are made to this method because it damages the nerves entering the rectus muscle, which leads to muscle atrophy and weakening the abdominal wall. This incision is less used.

A third method, the lumbar approach to appendectomy proposed by G. M. Edebohls in conjunction with nephropexy, will be considered when the latter procedure is described.

With periappendiceal inflammatory processes the operative approach is not much different from ours; a longer incision is made, and the direction of the muscle fibers is not considered.

Appendectomies are among the most frequent operations in America. One often sees three or four performed one after the other. Often the appendix is removed incidentally in the course of other laparotomies. In two cases at the Presbyterian Hospital in New York, for example, McCosh first performed an appendectomy through a flank incision following the example of Edebohls, then closed the peritoneum and proceded to carry out a nephropexy. During a laparotomy for pyosalpinx, Dr. Clarence Webster (Presbyterian Hospital, Chicago) encountered adhesions of the right tube to the appendix, and after removing the uterine adnexa he also removed the appendix.

[p. 667]

Appendicostomy for chronic colitis: The clever Americans have also made practical use of the vestigial appendix, namely for the purpose of managing chronic colitis. American surgeons have long recommended a cecal colostomy for colitis (Murray in 1891 for amebic colitis, Keith in 1895 for membranous colitis) to divert the irritating feces and to deliver medication directly to the affected bowel. However, because it is harder to manage a colostomy of the cecum and harder to create a loop, this approach was modified so that a fecal fistula is created instead of a mature colostomy. This approach was used by military surgeons in Manila and Africa. Finally, Bolton at the suggestion of Gibson in New York further modified this method similar to the gastrostomy of Kader.[24] Robert F. Weir also used this Kader-Gibson type of fistula with good success in a case of severe dysentery originating in India. After creating a cecal fistula and introduction of a large drainage tube into the rectum, the large intestine can be irrigated with warm physiologic saline solution containing 5% methylene blue or a 1:5000 solution of silver nitrate, or with bismuth in starch water.

The second time Weir had a similar case and planned to create such a fistula, he found a rather long and thick appendix. Without giving it much thought, Weir sewed the appendix to the abdominal wall, cut into it and demonstrated its patency by introducing a thick Nelaton catheter. Then he tied off the end of the appendix and closed the wound. After two days, the ligature was removed from the appendix and through it he began to irrigate the colon with a catheter. With this treatment, the patient's condition improved, the bloody bowel movements diminished, the red blood count increased, and the patient was discharged after two months.

During my stay in New York, Dr. Bull at the Roosevelt Hospital did a similar operation on another patient with very good success. Similarly, Willy Meyer [9] operated on a third patient with good success. It seems to me that such an operation is only suited to patients who have a long and thick appendix. In any case, this approach ought to be considered in cases of persistent colitis, and further attempts are indicated. Perhaps this management could also be extended to difficult cases of syphilitic ulceration and gonorrheal infections in the rectum!

In America, the radical repair of inguinal hernia is performed using either the method of Bassini or that of Halsted (Baltimore). The latter differs from the Bassini method in that Halsted bluntly separates the venous plexus from the spermatic cord and excises it leaving only a single vein, and that he leaves the cord above the aponeurosis of the external oblique muscle, between this aponeurosis and the skin.

For abdominal wall hernias and larger umbilical hernias, Willy Meyer has had best results suturing a silver mesh (Filigrane) over the hernia defect following the method proposed by Witzel and Goepel.[25] He has achieved durable results in this way.

The radical operation for umbilical hernia of Mayo (Rochester, Minnesota): Considering that the rectus muscles are difficult to use for reconstruction of the anterior abdominal wall because they are too thin and their medial borders are too far apart, Mayo advises strengthening the anterior abdominal wall by overlapping the rectus aponeurosis using silver wire. He advises an oval horizontal resection of the hernia defect, separating the peritoneum over a long segment and closing it horizontally with catgut, and then suturing the two leaves of the aponeurosis one over the other. For sewing together the two leaves of the aponeurosis Mayo uses three or four mattress sutures of silver wire such that the loops placed in the lower leaf pull it under the upper leaf. The inferior border of the upper leaf is then sewn to the lower leaf with catgut.

Here I should also mention the method of managing hernias in children used by A. J. Ochsner (Chicago). Ochsner considers increased intra-abdominal pressure to be the primary cause of hernias in children. This increased pressure results from: 1. Gaseous distention of the stomach and intestines due to poor nutrition, 2. Constipation, 3. As a result of phimosis, coughing, or vomiting. Only in the minority of hernias in children is there a congenital weakness of the abdominal wall. Ochsner believes that 95% of hernias in children can be healed by regulation of the diet, preventing cough, and circumcision along with appropriate care of the children for 4-6 weeks. The foot of the bed should be elevated 20-30°; thus the hernia sac is emptied and will become obliterated. Only the cases where this bed rest cannot be carried out are treated with a truss. Even after reduction of an incarcerated hernia, which is always possible in children, the narrow hernia defect will close with the management described. Ochsner only performs a radical operation such as Bassini or Halsted in cases of very large hernias or an enlarging defect or congenital laxity of the abdominal wall. Most American surgeons do not perform a radical operation in the first year of life. In older children they simply tie off the hernia sac and close the skin. This minimal intervention achieves a lasting cure.

For typhoid bowel perforations the right side of the abdomen is opened at the lateral border of the rectus abdominis, since the perforation is usually found in the lower portion of the ileum. The site of perforation is closed in the direction of the bowel with a two-layer Lembert suture; one should not assume there is only one site of perforation since there are usually several. Since typhoid ulcerations can also affect the appendix, it should be examined in every case of typhoid perforation and removed if there is even the slightest doubt about its involvement. After closing the site of perforation, the abdominal cavity is irrigated with a large amount of warm physiologic saline solution or a weak solution of hydrogen peroxide and the abdomen is drained at the site of perforation. With larger perforations a bowel resection should never be performed; such defects can be covered with a flap of omentum in order to terminate the operation quickly and avoid shock. In these perforations, the Americans are opposed to making a midline incision with greater externalization, since these are associated with severe shock.

J. B. Murphy has demonstrated that good results can be obtained with appropriate management even after generalized peritonitis due to perforated gangrenous appendicitis or typhoid in six (!) consecutive cases, of which I observed three at the Mercy Hospital in Chicago. According to Murphy, the course of a generalized peritonitis depends on the following factors:

> 1. The type of infection: If the infection is caused by toxic streptococci, the peritoneum quickly loses its epithelial layer; this is followed by rapid absorption and generalized sepsis. The less toxic staphylococcus or colonic bacilli do not cause such immediate denudation of the bowel epithelium, so that the toxins are absorbed only later (not until the 4th-6th day) and death does not occur until much later with this type of infection.
> 2. The time elapsed from perforation until laparotomy: An early operation, before the purulent secretions have been absorbed, gives much better results than a later operation.
> 3. The degree of pressure of the purulence on the peritoneum: The greater the abdominal pressure while the purulent secretions remain, the quicker they are absorbed; this pressure must be eliminated by an early laparotomy.
> 4. The spread of the infectious material in the abdominal cavity. If the exudate spreads to the upper part of the peritoneum, the danger

is greater, since absorption occurs more quickly in this area than in the lower part. Therefore, the patient should remain in a semi-upright position after operation.

5. The administration of antitoxin and other means to weaken the effect of the toxins absorbed from the peritoneum (antistreptococcal serum, Credé's ointment,[26] intravenous saline infusions).

6. The length of anesthesia and the amount of bowel manipulation.

Murphy proceeds as follows: The laparotomy incision is made on the right side of the abdomen at the lateral border of the rectus abdominis muscle. The site of perforation is located and sutured in the direction of the bowel; with perforated gangrenous appendicitis the appendix is removed. The sutured site of perforation is not left exposed; two thick drainage tubes are placed in this location and the rest of the abdomen is closed up to the location of the drains. The patient is then kept in a semi-upright position at an angle of 35° and the bandage is changed frequently; Credé's ointment is applied.

The six consecutive cases of diffuse peritonitis handled in this way (one from a perforated typhoid ulcer and five from ruptured gangrenous appendicitis) all survived.

Murphy does not not remove the exudate mechanically with wiping and saline irrigation – as is usually done – but only allows for drainage (the thick tubes and semi-upright position), and he attributes great importance to this factor. Every one of these cases healed, despite a penetrating odor of the secretions at the first dressing changes; no irrigation was used. These successes have encouraged further attempts with this approach.

Excision of carcinoma in the upper rectum: Dr. R. F. Weir excises high rectal carcinomas using the modified method of Maunsell (New Zealand). Maunsell's method, which is not as well known to us, deserves great consideration, since it preserves the lower part of the rectum.

Maunsell opens the abdominal cavity through an incision in the lower abdomen, divides the peritoneum transversely over the part of the bowel identified by the tumor and frees the peritoneum bluntly from this part of the bowel. Then an assistant dilates the anus digitally or a posterior exposure of the rectum is performed, and the bowel with the tumor is invaginated and brought out through the anus. Now the bowel is resected in the region of the tumor, the stump of the invaginated bowel is sutured circumferentially, the sutured portion of the bowel is reduced back into the abdominal cavity, and the parietal peritoneum and abdominal wall are closed. The operation is performed in Trendelenburg's position with the use of a special dilator for the abdominal wound and a special bowel retractor.

[p. 729]
Weir's modification is based on the following points: To protect against the possibility of bleeding, the superior hemorrhoidal arteries are ligated. After dividing the peritoneum, it is freed up widely from the piece of bowel involved with the tumor down to the coccyx; the bowel is doubly ligated above and below the tumor and resected through the abdominal cavity. The mucosa of the two resected stumps is cauterized with pure liquid phenol and wiped off with an alcohol swab. Then both the distal and the proximal ligated ends are invaginated and brought out through the dilated anus. After the ends have been sutured together, the anastomotic site is reduced back into the abdominal cavity, and the peritoneum and abdominal wall are closed.

This Maunsell method, as modified by Weir, allows high rectal tumors to be excised without bleeding, maintains control of defecation by preserving the lower rectal segment, and makes the bowel anastomosis easier.

Operations on the urogenital system: Surgical kidney diseases are evaluated in America with all the new methods used to monitor the function of the other kidney: palpation, ureteral catheterization, fluoridzine test,[27] cryoscopy of blood,[28] and even separate collection of the urine from each ureter by separating the bladder. A radiograph is made in every case, especially when there is suspicion of kidney stones. Thanks to this apparatus the localization of stones is very precise, which in turn simplifies the kidney operations.

Among kidney procedures, I have seen several nephropexies and pyelotomies. Nephropexy is mostly performed using the technique proposed by G. M. Edebohls (New York).[29]

The patient is positioned prone with the back elevated by placing a special cylindrical air pillow beneath the upper abdominal region. An incision is made over the lateral border of the erector spinae muscle from the twelfth rib to the iliac crest. The fibers of the latissimus dorsi muscle are bluntly divided along the lateral border of the erector spinae, without opening the fascia of the latter muscle. Then the transversalis fascia is divided with protection of the iliohypogastric nerve. The sheath of the quadratus lumborum muscle is opened from the twelfth rib to the iliac crest. The kidney is freed up bluntly along with its fatty capsule, delivered into the wound, and its fatty capsule cut away. Now the kidney and the upper end of the ureter are palpated to determine where an incision or puncture should be made. If appendicitis is also present, the peritoneum is incised at the outer border of the kidney, which is temporarily replaced into the abdomen, the ascending colon and cecum are identified and the appendix is inverted or amputated. After closure of the peritoneum, the kidney is again brought out and traction sutures are placed. The true capsule of the kidney is incised longitudinally over its convex border, split against a hollow probe, stripped from up to half of the kidney on both sides, and folded back. Now the four retraction sutures on the kidney applied so that two are on the anterior side and two are on the posterior side. Suturing is done with chromic catgut, silkworm, or kangaroo tendon. Every suture pierces through the folded back capsule close to the folding point. The upper sutures are placed in the middle of the upper half of the kidney and the lower sutures in the middle of the lower half of the kidney. Each suture is passed first through the folding point of the capsule from inside to outside, then with a straight Hagedorn needle passed through the non-mobilized part of the capsule and the renal parenchyma parallel to the long axis of the kidney for a distance of about 3 cm, and finally passed through the capsule from outside to inside. The resulting eight suture ends are now passed through the anterior and posterior edges of the abdominal wall muscles. The medial sutures are attached to the fascia of the quadratus lumborum, the quadratus itself, and the erector spinae, the lateral sutures are attached to the transversalis fascia and the latissimus dorsi; all then appear on the external surface of the latissimus. They are not yet tied. First the the muscle and fascia wounds are closed with four to six mattress sutures, such that the cut surface of the quadratus lies next to the kidney. These sutures include laterally the latissimus dorsi and the lumbar fascia, and medially the fascia of the erector spinae and the external border of the quadratus lumborum. Only now the traction sutures are pulled together and tied, so that the no longer encapsulated kidney is fixed next to the quadratus lumborum. The skin wound is closed. The patient must lie in bed for three weeks.

Edebohls has performed 206 nephropexies in 186 patients; in 68 cases he did both kidneys in one session, and in 6 cases he did both kidneys in two sessions; in 46 cases he also inverted the appendix through a lumbar incision and in 6 cases amputated it; in many cases he performed other fairly major procedures at the same time or in separate sessions; he has lost only three patients with this procedure; the mortality is thus only 1.55%. Following these cases for years, he has not seen any loss of attachment of the kidneys or occurrence of a lumbar hernia.

While I was present, Drs. Elliot and McCosh at the Presbyterian Hospital in New York operated on several cases following the method of Edebohls;

McCosh also removed the appendix in two cases; the combination of the two procedures was very easy; the resected appendix contained pus in both cases.

At this point, I should mention that Edebohls first noticed the frequent association of wandering (right) kidney with appendicitis several years ago. Edebohls explains the conjunction of these two diseases by proposing that the wandering kidney puts pressure on the duodenum and pancreatic head and thus compromises blood flow through the superior mesenteric vessels that run between the pancreatic head and the vertebral bodies, resulting in venous congestion of the appendix. This stasis leads to pathologic changes in the appendix. According to Edebohls, 60% of people with wandering kidneys develop pathological changes in the appendix.

Murphy makes use of a different operative technique. He performs an oblique lumbar incision; the fatty capsule is not disturbed; after delivering the kidney into the wound, the capsule is peeled away from both sides of the kidney over almost half of its surface, folded and held in place with sutures of thick catgut or silkworm. Using these sutures through the folded fibrous capsule, the kidney is fixed to the deep flank muscles; then the skin is closed.

As seen from the above, American surgeons have given up all methods of nephropexy that include the kidney parenchyma itself in the suture; they limit themselves to the decortication of the kidney and fixing it to the deep muscles by suturing the peeled-off fibrous capsule to the muscles; thus, stronger and more lasting adhesions are achieved.

For nephrolithiasis, a pyelotomy with immediate closure of the renal pelvis is usually performed in America. Murphy does this operation as follows: Incision as for nephrectomy, blunt mobilization of the kidney with preservation of the perirenal fat capsule, careful displacement of the kidney, exposure of the renal pelvis, precise determination of the stone location, opening the renal pelvis, extraction of the stone, controlling the mobility of the ureter by inserting a ureteral catheter, suture of the renal pelvis with fine silk, repositioning the kidney, and abdominal wall closure without drainage.

For prostatic hypertrophy, a radical operation is usually performed in America. The majority elect perineal prostatectomy, and one could say it is regarded as standard practice and the operation of choice; galvanocaustic prostatectomy or the so-called Bottini operation are seldom used.

Murphy (Chicago) does a total subcapsular prostatectomy. His method is the following: The patient is placed in lithotomy position. With a Ferguson bladder sound in the urethra, he first makes a horseshoe-shaped incision whose branches are at the level of the anus, then a median incision, so that the incision is Y-shaped. Both incisions are carried down to the membranous urethra. A broad Sims speculum is inserted into the rectum. Guided by a finger in the rectum, the soft tissues between the urethra and the rectum are divided; in this way the prostate is exposed and separated from the rectum. Aided by the bladder sound, the tip of which is turned posteriorly and inferiorly, the prostate is retracted downwards. Now the capsule over one of the lateral lobes of the gland is split parallel to the urethra, and the lobe is retracted downwards and bluntly mobilized. The other lateral lobe is similarly mobilized. Finally the middle lobe is shelled out including the posterior wall of the prostatic urethra; the anterior portion of the gland, the so-called isthmus, is left in place, since it is known that this does not undergo anatomic changes and does not cause urinary retention. The bladder should never be injured by this operation. The bladder is drained by a tube through the perineal wound for several days. The wound is partially closed with a few deep sutures of catgut and a few superficial sutures of silkworm, but partially left open with a gauze pack.

In order to get better drainage, the patient is kept in a sitting position for 5-7 days; after 5 days, Murphy allows the patient to stand. After removing the drain, a soft indwelling catheter is inserted for several days. The patient is given much water to drink, and urotropine as a bladder antiseptic. Murphy restricts the use of suprapubic prostatectomy to cases of extremely large hypertrophy. He considers perineal prostatectomy to be the best, simplest, and least bloody, and affords the best protection for the rectum and best drainage of the bladder. He has excellent results in several cases.

Although it cannot be denied that the prostate can be resected as radically as possible using Murphy's method, I consider it significantly more traumatic and less protective than the subcapsular prostatectomy (excochleation) recommended by L. Rydygier at the Ninth Congress of Polish Surgeons in Kraków in 1900 [10]; therefore, I would definitely prefer this to Murphy's method. In Rydygier's resection the anterior portion of the middle lobe and the urethra are preserved and the ejaculatory duct and verumontanum are not injured, which is important especially for younger prostate patients; with the older ones it is important that the latter operation is also significantly less traumatic.

A. J. Ochsner (Chicago), who previously favored suprapubic prostatectomy, has abandoned it and gone over to perineal prostatectomy.

Willy Meyer also performs a perineal prostatectomy in the usual uncomplicated cases. However, in cases complicated by bladder stones he either makes a bladder incision or, more recently, does a lithotripsy followed by a Bottini galvanocaustic prostatotomy.[30] Meyer's experience with the latter method is limited to only three cases; further experience will determine which of the two methods used by W. Meyer will be preferred; it seems to me that such cases must be individualized.

Americans are mostly conservative with respect to uterine myomas; myomectomy is performed only for multiple or large tumors; hysterectomy is normally used only in postmenopausal women. Patients decide to undergo surgery more readily if they are assured that the uterus will be preserved.

McCosh, who did several myomectomies while I was at the Presbyterian Hospital in New York, told me that a patient can still have an uncomplicated pregnancy even after her uterus has been divided into two parts because of a large number of myomas or interstitial location. The broad-based myomas are shelled out through an ovoid incision; the wound is closed with catgut. If the uterine cavity is opened, it is curetted and the uterine wall then closed in layers. If there are numerous myomas extending into the uterine cavity, either the anterior or posterior wall of the uterus is opened, or the entire uterus is split in half, and after enucleation of the tumors the uterus is carefully repaired with deep and superficial sutures of catgut; the uterine cavity is then drained through the vagina.

With retroflexion of the uterus, the Americans perform either the Alexander-Adams operation (shortening of the round ligaments) or an abdominal hysteropexy. Hysteropexy is usually done using Kelly's method. After opening the abdominal cavity, adhesions are divided bluntly or between ligatures; the uterus is displaced into extreme anteflexion; a strong suture is placed through the posterior superior wall of the uterus and it is fixed to the peritoneum of the abdominal wall. Two sutures are generally sufficient; the extreme anteflexion soon returns to normal anteflexion.

In addition to the usual extraperitoneal method of shortening the round ligaments (the Alexander-Adams operation), an intraperitoneal method recommended by H. T. Byford (Chicago) is often performed.[31] After a lower abdominal laparotomy, the round ligaments are identified and brought together to form an anterior sling. Both arms of the sling are sewn together and the point of the sling is fixed to the inguinal ligament. The Byford procedure is actually a modification of the method recommended earlier by W. Gill Wyllie, which consisted of bringing the ligaments together to form a posterior sling.

In my opinion, the Byford method may be rational but should be performed only as an adjunct to a laparotomy performed for other indications.

My report only partially illuminates the present situation of American surgical technique, since it considers only methods of management or operations for which I myself was present during my short stay in America. Thus I have not addressed many important operations, for example those on the vascular system, the brain, the liver, or the bile ducts, since I did not personally witness any of these. I also omit many methods of well known operators such as B. F. Kammerer, Arpad Gerster, B. Farquhar Curtis, Lewis Stimson, and others, since they had only less interesting cases at that time or I could not be present for their operations.

Original Notes

* As presented to the 13th Congress of Polish Surgeons in Kraków on 15 July 1903 and at the Lemberg Medical Society on 13 November 1903.
1. Affiliated with every large hospital there is a training school for nurses. They accept young women age 25-35 who can give evidence of the necessary education. In addition to bedside teaching at the hospital, didactic courses are held for them by the hospital doctors. After graduation from the three-year program of study they undergo an examination and receive diplomas as certified nurses.
2. See the *New York Medical Record* from 3 April 1897.
3. See the *Deutsche Zeitschrift für Chirurgie* 1902, Volume 64.
4. Barrows' experiments with intravenous formalin should be taken with great caution, firstly because of the highly irritating effect of formalin, and secondly because Barrows did not use a physiological solution of common salt to dilute the formalin, but pure distilled water. We know that pure water for intravenous injection causes hemolysis and therefore has a deadly effect on the animal organism. These experiments were later repeated by W. Bauer (*New York Med. Journal*, 21 March 1903) who noted the adverse effects of similar injections. One case of streptococcal infection resulted in the death of the patient; in another case, cyanosis immediately occurred so the injection was stopped and only a saline infusion was administered; Bauer thinks only the latter was responsible for the patient's recovery. Experiments undertaken by Bauer on rats showed that those treated with intravenous formalin died sooner than control animals. I can add that since my return from America I have not seen the slightest harm from injection of tuberculous joint infections with a 2% formalin solution in iodoform-glycerine, although the period of observation is too short for me to issue a report on the potential success or benefit of this method. I have also tried intravenous formalin in a physiologic saline solution in a severe case of tuberculous meningitis and in a case of abdominal typhus along with Dr. V. Arnold (in his Department of Infectious Diseases in the Lemberg General

Hospital) without any effect on the course of illness; the patient with meningitis died.
5. I have very successfully treated two angiomas in small children with this method.
6. These two Chicago surgeons generously supervised my performing a few osteoclasties with Grattan's instrument.
7. Up to November 1903, A. J. Ochsner has already performed 40 gastroenterostomies using the McGraw ligature without a single fatality. Since beginning to use this method, he performs it in those cases where he could formerly only do a non-therapeutic laparotomy. Theoretically, he considers intestinal suture with needle and silk to be the ideal, but the latter technique has many drawbacks. See Transactions of the Chicago Surgical Society, 2 November 1903, *Annals of Surgery*, January 1904.) (*Added in proof.*)
8. In America, W. J. Mayo enjoys the reputation of one of the greatest specialists in the area of gastrointestinal surgery.
9. In the 28 October 1903 session of the New York Surgical Society (see *Annals of Surgery*, February 1904, pp. 208ff.) Willy Meyer and Howard Lilienthal report five more appendicostomies for chronic ulcerative colitis and colonic polyps. They had particularly good success with the first type of disease and W. Meyer considers this new management of colitis to be the method of the future.
10. See *Zentralblatt für Chirurgie* Nr. 41, 1902, and *Przegląd Lekarski* Nr. 52, 1903.

Biographical Source

Donigiewicz S, "Prof. Dr. Roman Barącz," *Posłaniec św. Grzegorza* 1931; 5(44):3-10. Accessed through wiki.ormianie.pl.

Publication Sources

The *Wiener Medizinsche Wochenschrift* (Vienna Medical Weekly) is still published (today in English as well as German). Historical issues can be obtained through the Hathi Trust.

Przegląd Lekarski (Medical Report) is still published. Historical issues can be obtained through the *Jagiellońska Biblioteka Cyfrowa*, jbc.bj.uj.edu.pl.

Translation Notes

1) *Privat-Dozent* is a European academic title approximately equivalent to Associate Professor.
2) Lemberg at this time was part of the Austro-Hungarian Empire. After the First World War it was part of Poland, and known by its Polish name, Lwów. After the Second World War it became part of the Soviet Union, and today it is the city of Lviv in the western Ukraine.
3) The Roosevelt Hospital in New York, founded by a distant cousin of the presidents with that name, is now the Mount Sinai West Hospital.
4) Mercy Hospital in Chicago just closed in 2021.
5) Fürbringer's method was standard in Europe, and involved washing with soap, then alcohol, then another disinfectant.
6) Mercuric chloride, no longer used.
7) Murphy mentions bismuth subiodide in "Arthroplasty," *Annals of Surgery* 1913; 57:593-647.
8) See Murphy JB, *Journal of the American Medical Association* 1901; 36:1246. The drape was manufactured to his specifications by Johnson & Johnson, who still make a similar product today.
9) The drugs mentioned in addition to cocaine were semi-synthetic derivatives of it.
10) Crile was a tireless investigator of surgical shock (see his *Blood-Pressure in Surgery* published in 1903), but decades would pass before our current (still imperfect) understanding of shock evolved. The idea that nerve blocks would prevent shock persisted for some time, and has been partially revived by the current notion of pre-emptive analgesia (see Katz J, "George Washington Crile, anoci-association, and pre-emptive analgesia," *Pain* 1993; 53:243-245.
11) See Cushing H, "The employment of local anaesthesia in the radical cure of certain cases of hernia, with a note upon the nervous anatomy of the inguinal region," *Annals of Surgery* 1900; 31:1-34.
12) See Williams FH, *The Roentgen Rays in Medicine and Surgery*, New York: MacMillan, 1902. Pages 8-19 describe the Holtz static influence machine.
13) Augustana Hospital was later called the Lutheran General Hospital, and closed in 1989. The name Augustana refers to the Augsburg

Confession (*Confessio Augustana*), the fundamental document of the Lutheran Church.

14) Now the Hospital for Special Surgery.
15) Now the University of Chicago Comer Children's Hospital.
16) Now part of Northwestern Memorial Hospital in Chicago.
17) See Grattan N, "Osteoclasia," *Transactions of the American Orthopedic Association* 1892; 5:128-132.
18) See Mueller F, "Bloodless reposition of the congenitally dislocated hip joint versus arthrotomy, with statistics of 34 cases operated on by Dr. Lorenz during his visit to the United States in 1902," *Journal of the American Medical Association* 1905; 44:1915-1919.
19) See Halsted WS, "The results of operations for the cure of cancer of the breast performed at the Johns Hopkins Hospital from June, 1889, to January, 1894," *Annals of Surgery* 1894; 20:497-555.
20) See Murphy JB, "Cholecysto-intestinal, gastro-intestinal, entero-intestinal anastomosis, and approximation without sutures," *Medical Record* 1892; 42:665-676.
21) See Mayo Robson AW, "A method of performing intestinal anastomosis by means of decalcified bone bobbins," *British Medical Journal* 1893; 1:688-689.
22) Today the Lenox Hill Hospital.
23) Literally "cold," a term usually applied to a normal appendix in America, but "à froid" is apparently used in Europe to describe a previously inflamed appendix that has "cooled off." See Engkvist O, "Appendectomy à froid a superfluous routine operation?," *Acta Chir Scand* 1971; 137:797-800.
24) See Magowska A, "Surgery, fame, and misfortune: The life of Bronisław Kader," *World Journal of Surgery* 2012; 36:1998-2002.
25) Witzel O, "Über den Verschluss von Bauchwunden und Bruchpforten durch versenkte Silberdrahtnetze (Einheilung von Filigranpelotten)," *Centralblatt für Chirurgie* 1900; 27:257-260. Goepel R, "Über die Verschliessung von Bruchpforten durch Einheilung geflochtener fertiger Silberdrahtnetze (Silberdrahtpeloten)," *Centralblatt für Chirurgie* 1900; 27:458-461. Today, mesh repair is generally preferred for large umbilical hernias.
26) "Unguentum Credé," containing metallic silver.
27) Phloridzine was a substance given to induce glycosuria, used as a test of renal function. See Krotoszyner M, Willard WP, "Experience with the methods of determining physiological kidney-function for operative procedure," *American Journal of Urology* 1905; 2:35-40.

28) A method to estimate specific gravity by freezing point depression. See "Cryoscopy of the urine," *Journal of the American Medical Association* 1901; 36:1254-1255.
29) For historical perspective, see Moss SW, "Floating kidneys: A century of nephroptosis and nephropexy," *Journal of Urology* 1997; 158:699-702.
30) The Bottini procedure cauterized a transurethral passage through the prostate. See Meyer W, "The treatment of prostatic hypertrophy associated with stone in the bladder by means of litholapaxy and Bottini's operation at one sitting," *Annals of Surgery* 1902; 36:17-28.
31) The original Alquie-Alexander procedure shortened the round ligaments extraperitoneally via the inguinal canals. See Goldspohn A, "The extended indications and modified technique of the Alquie-Alexander-Adams operation, with important adjuncts," *American Gynaecological and Obstetrical Journal* 1898; 12:155-161.

8
Jean-Louis Faure (1904)

Jean-Louis Faure was born in 1863 in Gironde, France. He studied medicine at the Faculty of Medicine in Paris, and practiced general surgery at its various affiliated hospitals for the rest of his career, with a special interest in gynecology. He performed the first successful radical hysterectomy for cancer in France in 1896.

In 1904, at the age of 40, he traveled extensively through North America, and reported on his experiences in July of 1904.

He returned many times to the Americas, including Greenland and South America. He was a consultant to the French Army in the First World War and treated many war casualties. He was also known as a philosopher and poet: His *L'Âme du Chirurgien* [*The Soul of the Surgeon*] was widely quoted, and his *Hymne à la Paix* [*Hymn to Peace*] was set to music by Camille Saint-Saëns (Opus 159).

He was appointed Professor of Gynecology in 1919, after the death of Samuel Pozzi. He was named Emeritus Professor in 1934, and died in 1944.

Impressions d'Amérique
La Presse Médicale 1904; 12(*Articles originaux*):476-478

Impressions of America
by J.-L. Faure

We should be careful not to rush into hasty conclusions or premature judgments. America is so large and I have traveled through it so quickly that I would not presume to present anything other than some impressions. When it comes to the natural world, first impressions can actually be more vivid and more profound than those brought forth after long contemplation, and we do not need a prolonged visit to feast our eyes on all the spectacles offered to us in this great land that nature is constantly renewing.

I can see, as if they were still before my eyes, the rivers of Florida creeping through the virgin forests with their waters inhabited by alligators, the deep and verdant woods of Louisiana, the formidable Mississippi – a river of mud carrying tree trunks as if they were a few wisps of straw in one of our French rivers, the desolate plateaus of the Mexican sierras, lush California with her greenery and flowers, the dark forests and giant trees of the Rocky Mountains, the bleak expanses of the Great Plains, the wide and majestic St. Lawrence, and, above all, that miracle of nature, the Grand Canyon of the Colorado with its incomparable splendor and superhuman beauty!

But institutions and men are more difficult to judge; in my quick study, I may have been able to learn something about American surgery and the surgeons who practice it, but it was impossible for me to go into anything in depth! Therefore, I repeat that I cannot give here anything other than impressions.

To begin with, from a purely technical point of view, and for all the material aspects of our practice, there are no great differences between what is happening in France and what goes on in America. Countless journals, books and their translations, international congresses, constant travels, increasingly numerous and cordial personal relationships have tended to unify the great modern surgical ideas all over the world. These have spread throughout the world, surgeons from all nations have contributed to their formulation and development, and thus there cannot be very serious differences between them. The general doctrines are the same, with some individual variation, which is generally no greater between the surgeons of France and America than among individual surgeons within each of these two countries.

The structure in which American surgeons work is essentially the same as that in which we work ourselves. The most beautiful operating room I have ever seen is in New York, at the Mount Sinai Hospital. The entire walls, and even the ceiling, are covered with huge slabs of white marble. The doors are also of white marble – and in one piece! But this splendor, instead of commanding our admiration, seems rather to be uselessly overdone. It is indeed an extraordinary room, but I cannot say the same for every one I saw. I saw good, bad, and in between, some being built and some being rebuilt. In this respect, things are pretty much the same as in Paris, and the older hospitals, which are very uncommon in this new country, would be better suited for demolition than the always imperfect restorations. The hospitals I saw in Mexico City are probably the oldest in America and these are in lamentable condition, even compared to our old Hôtel-Dieu. I hasten to add that this situation is about to change and that, thanks to the activity of Professor Liceaga, Dean of the Faculty of Medicine, a new hospital[1] is under construction and today almost finished at the gates of Mexico City, which will be comparable to the finest hospitals in the world. And when its 21 individual pavilions, its lecture halls, and its operating rooms are covered with the greenery and flowers that always flourish in the perpetual spring of this admirable climate, we will have in Paris no great hospital to match it.

The washbasins, with their sometimes pedal-operated faucets, do not differ significantly from ours, and they have the same problem mixing the water as we do, so it is sometimes boiling hot and sometimes ice cold. It seemed to me that the sterilization apparatus and especially the autoclaves, which are almost always large and arranged horizontally, are perhaps on average superior to those we possess, although it is naturally impossible for me to comment on their functional performance.

For the actual operations, surgeons and their assistants are usually covered from head to toe in sterile clothing. Nearby observers have the luxury of gowns, such as are unknown to us; the nurses even forgo the usual vanity of their sex and cover their hair completely under sterile caps. Almost all operators and their assistants wear rubber gloves. Alongside these unobjectionable but perhaps exaggerated precautions, on the other hand, it seemed to me that skin preparation on anesthetized patients was done with less care and asepsis than it is here, and I especially found that the number of assistants is usually excessive. Two, three, or four assistants who touch the patient or the instruments, plus two or three nurses who take care of the bandages and pass them from hand to hand, seem like too many for those of us who have been trying, and for some of us succeeding, to limit ourselves to one assistant.

As far as I could tell, the operating tables are no match for ours. None of those I saw can bear comparison to Mathieu's admirable table. The most common table, made of thick glass plates that can be easily dismantled, was fairly good but cannot be tilted enough to comfortably perform all the maneuvers for pelvic surgery, which I think is a serious defect.

One point on which we have an undeniable superiority is the instrumentation. At least for general and gynecological surgery, American instruments are heavy, primitive, and sometimes almost crude.

At first, this is surprising for a people who have such a great sense of practicality and excel in the production of industrial tools.

It is because they have not developed workers capable of building a delicate instrument. To make these elegant, flexible, and solid instruments, it takes real artists working with their hands and their brains and not with machines; it requires long education, tradition, and direction which are still found only in old Europe and particularly, I would like to say, in our old France.

The general organization of services only remotely resembles what we see here. The free hospital - the hospital for the indigent - hardly exists in America, partly because there are not many poor people; partly because everyone, from the richest to the poorest, finds it natural and appropriate to pay for the care they receive and the time devoted to them, just as they pay for anything else; and also no doubt because public welfare agencies have not had time to become organized in many towns, some of which have not even existed for fifty years.

City, county, or state hospitals are therefore relatively rare. On the other hand, private hospitals abound. Some, comparable to our surgical *maisons de santé*, are private enterprises which may either belong to a surgeon or live off his exclusive clientele or that of a few others. Others, less modest in appearance, may be due to the generosity of some billionaire. We have seen the competition, sometimes ostentatious but in any case beneficial, among the "kings" of industry in America, to donate certain great works of public interest, especially universities and hospitals. The results are often beautiful and long lasting.

In these hospitals, there are almost always rooms where the sick belonging either to certain nationalities, or to certain associations, or quite simply to the immense army of the unfortunate are treated free of charge. But next to them are also almost always either rooms or pavilions for the private patients of the surgeons of the hospital. No one in America thinks it strange to see the rich cared for under the same roof as the poor; and it would be desirable that this were the same elsewhere, and specifically in Paris. In this respect, we should model ourselves on the Americans, and nothing would be simpler and more profitable for everyone than to establish in the hospitals of Paris "wealthy districts" where, for example, we could care for patients suffering from surgical conditions or acute and contagious diseases, such as eruptive fevers, which are so difficult to monitor and impossible to isolate in the patient's home. From the surgical point of view, in particular, the surgeon would gain precious time from which the patients on his service would benefit; he would gain the security afforded by an operating room he supervises himself and a staff whose education he supervises himself. The patients would be more likely to find a cure, and their appropriate fees could be returned to the charitable operations of the hospital, a considerable sum which now only makes a fortune for the numerous surgical *maisons de santé*. This would furthermore be an admirable example for the secondary staff, who would find many advantages in the transition to "wealthy districts" and would work accordingly to achieve it!

All this would be excellent and very simple to organize, but I am afraid we will never witness such a revolution.

The nurses and other auxiliary personnel are constantly increasing their education and value. They are mostly women who have excellent intelligence for their important functions and who often add to this first quality an admirable devotion to duty. I do not believe that most of our hospital staff match the value of an average American nurse. They are often of a fairly high social status and their general education and instruction are almost always far superior to those of the great majority of our staff. On this basis, it is difficult for us to oppose having young girls with a good education and sound instruction enlist as nurses in our hospitals and, although there is today some movement in this direction, it is only exceptionally, whereas it happens all the time in America. Also, American nurses perform certain functions that ours do not. In particular, they are the ones who write the daily progress notes of patients including those who have undergone surgery. Once the vital signs have been recorded by one of the students on the service, the nurse updates the record on a special sheet each day noting diet, mealtimes, temperature, pulse, and any specific incidents. They do so in a precise, correct, and conscientious way, which allows them to make observations that could serve as a model for most of our external students, who too often make them in a rather superficial way. In any case, it seemed to me that the observations are generally recorded in a more complete and more methodical way than with us. For example, in several departments I saw a page devoted exclusively to anesthesia, with graphs making it possible to see how long the patient was asleep, the state of the pulse and respiration at every moment, any reactions to the anesthesia, and the required amount of ether—which is incidentally the only anesthetic I saw used.

The only objection I might have to these records is how extensive and voluminous they are. Even one page a day leads in the end to a frightfully cumbersome stack of paper, which can take a certain amount of courage to attack.

In sum, the recruitment of auxiliary staff is superior to what we see here.

Is this true for the selection of the surgeons themselves? This is a very serious question and I do not think I have sufficient information to make a firm judgment.

There are many surgeons in America, and most of them continue to practice general medicine. It is an absolute right, just as in France, and it is even sometimes a duty, especially for the rural doctor who often has the difficult responsibility for emergency surgery. But the surgeons in charge of a public service are relatively few in number, as with us, because these services themselves are few in number. They are not chosen competitively, but are appointed either by the board of directors of the hospital, or by the founders of the hospital or those who represent them. When the hospital belongs to a university, as often happens, it is naturally the professors of this university who are responsible for the services of the hospital. But when the hospital is owned either by private associations or by political or municipal organizations, such as a city or county, the surgeon is appointed at the discretion of the directors of the association and at the mercy of political currents. This is basically what happens in France in private hospitals and in many small towns where public assistance is not organized as in Paris.

It is thus that two or three years ago the surgeon of the French Hospital[2] of San Francisco, Dr. Dudley Tait, a man whom I hold in high esteem, was summarily dismissed after a disagreement with the hospital administrators and was replaced by another doctor of the same establishment! We know that in America thousands of civil servants have their situation linked to that of the President of the Republic. And so quite often the ownership of a surgery department will change at the time of the presidential election!

Undoubtedly, there are eminent surgeons who are sheltered from these fluctuations by their reputation, but it is obvious that a hospital surgical practice may be under regrettable conditions of arbitrariness and instability. And we complain here about the institution of competition!

Be that as it may, there is great surgical activity in the United States. Americans favor quick fixes, and in this respect the education of the American people is more advanced than ours. I can offer no better proof of this than the rapidity with which President McKinley was operated on during the attack which cost his life.³ An hour after his injury, he underwent an operation in a private hospital, by the nearest surgeon. It was not considered desirable to wait for this serious determination until the leading surgeons of America were assembled at his bedside, during which time the disease would be allowed to worsen hour by hour. On the contrary, it is understood there that any penetrating wound of the abdomen requires an immediate laparotomy; so the belly of the president was opened without delay, as one would have opened the belly of a common citizen. Although things certainly happened with comparable rapidity in France after the assassination of President Carnot,⁴ in even more tragic circumstances and in an environment not conducive to success of the operation, this was only because the signs of internal bleeding were sufficient to remove any hesitation and because surgeons were present at the scene of the tragedy who were able to take on such a formidable responsibility.

Thus, we see that surgical interventions are more deliberately offered and accepted there. And to show how this state of mind common to surgeons, doctors, and patients can sometimes lead to extraordinary results, the story of the Mayo brothers is a striking example.

In the fertile and pleasant regions of Minnesota, 500 kilometers west of Chicago, not far from the Mississippi, which here is still a beautiful and peaceful river, there is a small town of 6,000 inhabitants, almost a village for this country of huge cities. This village is called Rochester. The two Mayo brothers, young surgeons without titles or academic appointments, live here simply, modestly, and peacefully. They have at their disposal a small hospital, with a little more than a hundred beds, now rather cramped, and two small operating rooms where both operate together. And there, every morning except Sunday, they do an average of ten operations – about three thousand a year. The day I arrived there, I was able to see the following with my own eyes: Extraction of a polyp from the uterus, excision of tuberculous nodes from the neck, two prostatectomies, an abdominal hysterectomy for fibroids, a gastroduodenostomy for pyloric stenosis, a gastroenterostomy for cancer, and finally a cholecystostomy and a cholecystectomy for cholelithiasis. Such is, more or less, the program for each day.

In the afternoon, a crowd arrives at their "office," which is what they call a medical practice in America, a hundred patients, who are first examined by assistant doctors, eleven in number, responsible for simplifying the task. One examines the eyes; another the throat and the ears; another the heart and the lungs; another analyzes the urine; others, if necessary, perform radiography, examination of sputum, or laboratory investigations. And the two surgeons, on whom all the information converges, and who can barely keep up with this overwhelming load, finally make their decisions.

Patients come from everywhere, from Mexico and Canada, from the distant shores of the Pacific and Atlantic. And the crowd is not drawn to this extraordinary center by the usual methods of quacks and miracle workers or by the attraction that supernatural practices exert on childish and credulous imaginations, but rather by the legitimate reputations of these two fine surgeons who practice their art in all conscientiousness and who heal their patients.

American hospitality is admirable, and that which I encountered among my colleagues touched me deeply. They opened their practices to me, they opened their homes to me. Futhermore, some of them have even done me the honor of entrusting me with their patients on whom I have endeavored to show our American colleagues what may be interesting in certain operating procedures which are still, I believe, special to French surgery.

Therefore, I do not want to end these few notes without thanking all those who welcomed me so well: Cullen and Sampson in Baltimore; Albert and Hurtado in Mexico; Ward and Stapler in San Francisco; the Mayo brothers in Rochester; Professors Ochsner, Murphy, and Senn in Chicago; Boldt, Beck, Edebohls, and Pryor in New York; Bristow in Brooklyn.

And how can I begin to thank Professor Clark for his charming hospitality, and the illustrious Keen, who did me the honor of personally assisting me in an operation, and who combines an already long experience with the brain and hands of incredible youth! And my old friend Baumgarten, with whom I found a piece of France in Mexico, and Valentine of New York, who for me exceeded the limits of the most extreme kindness, and Dudley Tait in San Francisco, who works with admirable energy to spread the ideas of the French School, which he often knows better than we do and represents France over there more and better than many French people, and above all Howard A. Kelly, who showed me how one can combine the qualities of a perfect clinician with those of an excellent operator on his fine service at the Johns Hopkins Hospital, and who received me like a brother.

As for my old comrade Merlin,[5] who followed me without a murmur in this race around a continent, what do I not owe him for having been my support in this battle against space, the slowness of trains, the dust of the deserts, and the monotony of the ocean, a daily battle, which continued for more than eight thousand leagues!

And now, where is Surgery most beautiful and most powerful? Is it in this New World, among this effervescent people who carry on their backs a whole future of greatness? Is it in our old France, whose past alone may be greater than this unknown future? I do not know. On both sides of the ocean, we are all walking parallel paths, working our best.

But what I do know is that Surgery is great and recognizes its greatness, and that we have the duty to know what we are worth, and the right to say so.

No, the old land of France is not exhausted. She is still alive, maternal and fruitful! And from her soil, where so many vanished generations lie for eternity, new generations are still constantly arising. As of old, her children labor and expend their treasures of intelligence and energy in all manifestations of human activity. Surgery is neither the least elevated nor the least exciting. And to see men who serve it with all the ardor of their enthusiasm and all the depth of their faith, it is not necessary to go around the world – it is enough to travel around France – or even to travel around Paris.

Let us therefore deplore the decadence of those who do not feel their chests are large enough to breathe freely, nor their backs strong enough to walk straight ahead. Let us travel, let us voyage around the world. Let us learn from others what they can teach us, and teach them in turn, giving them perhaps more than we receive. Let us strive that from this generous example may be born fruitful works which will live after us for the greatness and for the glory of immortal Surgery.

Biographical Sources

Faure J-L. *L'Âme du Chirurgien*. Paris, 1921.

Menegaux G. "Jean-Louis Faure (1863-1944)," *Mémoires de l'Académie de Chirurgie* 1952; 78:103-117.

Karamanou M, Saridaki Z, Piagkou M, Laios K, Androutsos G. "The great surgeon Jean-Louis Faure (1863-1944) and his contribution to the treatment of uterine cancer," *J BUON* 2013; 18:296-298.

Publication Source

La Presse Médicale is still published. Historical issues are obtainable through the Internet Archive.

Translation Notes

1) The Hospital General de México.

2) Now the "French Campus" of the Kaiser San Francisco Medical Center.
3) See Trunkey D, Farjah F, "Medical and surgical care of our four assassinated presidents," *Journal of the American College of Surgeons* 2005; 201:976-989.
4) Carnot bled to death from a stab wound to the portal vein, despite immediate laparotomy by a prominent surgeon in Lyon. See Régnier C, "L'assassinat du président Sadi Carnot," *La Revue du Practicien* 1994; 44:2008-2012. Alexis Carrel was a medical student in Lyon at this time, and his biographers have speculated that this event may have led to his interest in vascular suture.
5) A brief note in the *Journal of the American Medical Association* (1904; 42:1029) identifies this person as "Dr. Stephen Merlin," visiting Howard Kelly in Baltimore with Jean-Louis Faure and departing 8 April 1904 for Florida and a "tour of the country."

9
Albert Hoffa (1904)

Albert Hoffa was born to German parents in South Africa in 1859 and was educated in Germany, graduating with a medical degree from the University of Freiburg in 1883. He became an assistant in the surgical department of Hermann Maas, followed his professor to the University of Würzburg, and was appointed a *Privat-Dozent* there, practicing and teaching general surgery. He became interested in the relatively neglected area of orthopedic surgery, published a textbook on fractures and dislocations in 1888, and opened a private clinic in Würzburg that attracted many patients and students. In 1902 he was called to be Professor of Orthopedic Surgery in Berlin.

During his transition from general to orthopedic surgery, he had visited numerous centers in Europe, and had also traveled to America in 1891 and 1893, especially to learn about the nonoperative management of hip tuberculosis. His American colleagues invited him to return in 1904, at the age of 45, among other things to receive an honorary degree from the Jefferson Medical College in Philadelphia. He wrote the following report of his experiences.

Back in Berlin, he pursued an active program of clinical surgery, monitoring childhood deformities in the population, and developing pediatric hospitals. However, he developed signs of heart disease and died suddenly on New Year's Day 1907.

Reisebriefe aus Amerika
Deutsche Medizinische Wochenschrift 1904; 30:996-998,1141-1143

Letters from a trip to America
by A. Hoffa

Atlantic City, 5 June 1904

Dear Dr. Schwalbe:[1]

As promised, I am sending you these lines to describe the impressions that the land of "unlimited possibilities"[2] has made upon us.

As you know, I came to Atlantic City in response to an invitation from my American specialty colleagues to attend their meeting here at the beginning of June,[3] and I also have the assignment from our Ministry to study the conditions and circumstances related to my area.

I started my journey on May 12 upon the steamer *Blücher* of the Hamburg-America Line, accompanied by my former assistant Dr. Hans Spitzy, who is now at the Pediatric Clinic in Graz, and my brother-in-law Bang. After a relatively pleasant crossing, we arrived in good condition at New York on May 22. I had been to New York before, and was amazed at how greatly the city had grown during the 12 years since I last saw it. The growth of the city is even faster than that of Berlin, but I have to say that the skyscrapers of 20-30 stories did not make a favorable impression on me.

We were most cordially welcomed by our colleagues, and I was greeted by my friend Dr. R. H. Sayre, the son of the well-known founder of American orthopedics.[4] As soon as we arrived, a detailed campaign plan was presented, which was indeed followed and hardly allowed us a quiet moment during our time here. The time was spent partly with visiting hospitals and partly with performing operations that my colleagues here asked me to demonstrate at different hospitals.

These colleagues wanted to learn about our German surgical methods, especially our operative techniques, since last year Professor Lorenz from Vienna had limited himself to closed manipulations.[5] I performed a variety of open hip joint reductions, a large series of tenoplasties, subtrochanteric osteotomies, club foot corrections, etc. and very much enjoyed the approval that was paid to our methods by the usually numerous assembled colleagues.

American orthopedics is at a relatively high stage of development, and we can learn quite a lot from the Americans especially in technical-mechanical aspects; our visit was therefore very fruitful in this respect. The Hospital for Ruptured and Crippled[6] is excellently equipped, with more than 200 beds devoted exclusively to orthopedic patients. Professor Gibney[7] leads this hospital; his principal assistants are Dr. Townsend, Dr. Whitman, and Dr. H. L. Taylor, also well known to us for their excellent contributions. They have a clinic every day from 1:00 to 3:00, where they see more than 100 patients. Most of these are cases of spondylitis, tubercular joint disorders, and palsies, with relatively few congenital deformities. The cases are carefully examined and appropriately managed. Those cases that require operative intervention are admitted to the hospital. The wards are extremely bright, airy, and well ventilated. It is a pleasure to see the extreme cleanliness here; all the children are bandaged so that they can be out of bed, every child has his own little wheelchair so he can move about by himself. In addition, there is a large common room in which the children have an hour of school every morning; they say a prayer and sing together, and learn some elementary subjects. The building has five stories, with the operating room and kitchen on the top floor. The roof is flat and is used as a garden in the summer, so that the children can be outside in the fresh air all day. In the basement is a large workroom, where all the necessary splints and orthopedic apparatus are made. The entire enterprise is exemplary, and I only wish that we had a similar orthopedic hospital in Berlin. As a special annex there is also a department for hernia patients; every day they see a large number of hernia cases with trusses, and they perform a radical operation on every patient willing to undergo surgery. The method of Bassini is performed with American efficiency by Dr. Bull and Dr. Coley.[8] The results are excellent, with only five recurrences out of the last 1300 children who were operated upon.

After thorough and repeated observation of the orthopedic hospital, we also visited the other large hospitals. Our pavilion system is not possible in New York, since there is generally limited space due to the fantastically high cost of real estate. In order to accommodate a large number of patients, the hospitals are therefore built much higher. In general, the arrangement of these hospitals made a good impression on me. We visited St. Luke's Hospital,[9] the Mount Sinai Hospital, the Presbyterian Hospital, the German Hospital,[10] and Bellevue Hospital. The first two of these, and especially the Mount Sinai Hospital just completed six weeks ago, provide almost excessive luxury for doctors and patients.

At the Mount Sinai Hospital we saw the Chief Surgeon Dr. Gerster operating, and at the German Hospital we witnessed several very nicely performed procedures by Dr. Kammerer. We were welcomed everywhere in a most friendly way, and all the details were kindly explained to us. The

German Hospital has been renovated since the last time I saw it, with a new pavilion for private patients; the facilities are not as luxurious as in the more richly endowed hospitals, but quite adequate in every respect and consistent with all the modern requirements. For suture material, they mostly use catgut, which is provided by the pharmacies reliably sterile. The sterilization is so complete that stitch abscesses are hardly ever seen.

The greatest impression we had during our visits to the hospitals was the excellent quality of the nursing staff. Their pleasing appearance and their extraordinary competence mean that any comparison with our nurses would favor the American colleagues. The reasons for this are probably that the American nurses come from the educated classes and furthermore that every large hospital has an associated nursing school, in which they undergo three years of instruction. After this course they undergo an examination, and if successful they are permitted to work as public nurses. It would be very desirable if more of our young educated ladies in Germany would devote themselves to this profession, which is indeed demanding but very rewarding, honorable, and so appropriate for the female sex.

I was very interested in how they managed the emergency services here. The larger hospitals have an associated "Ambulance Service." Each hospital has its district; if there is an accident within this district, the police will call the responsible hospital. The hospital has its own building for the Ambulance Service, where 4-12 ambulance wagons and horses are kept, depending on the size of the hospital. A horse and wagon are always ready for immediate dispatch. I was repeatedly able to see the wagon driving out of the gate within a minute of the telephone call, carrying the doctor assigned to the Ambulance Service. The patient is then retrieved from the scene of the accident and brought to the hospital. Here he is evaluated and managed, and if he cannot be discharged is admitted or perhaps observed further. Special arrangements are made everywhere for heat stroke, which is very common here in the summer. The daily number of emergency cases is very large; one morning at the New York Hospital[11] House of Relief, which is led by the well-known surgeon Professor Stimson, we saw 22 acute fractures along with a large quantity of other injuries, large and small. The management is generally very appropriate. If possible, the patients are discharged home with their bandages. Among the accidents requiring the Ambulance Service, there are also many who are severely intoxicated, and there are extra rooms for their management.

Following an invitation from the German Medical Society of New York, I attended one of its meetings[12] and, as desired by its chairman Dr. Boldt, gave an introductory talk about congenital hip dislocation. In addition, cases were presented and one colleague, Dr. Weber, shared his experiences and impressions from a trip to the St. Louis World's Fair. He could not say enough good things about the educational exhibits of the German universities [1],[13] and spoke enthusiastically about the German accomplishments in this area, which overshadow all the others.

After ten days in New York, we traveled to Philadelphia, and were once again cordially welcomed by our American colleagues. Here I had the honor to receive an honorary degree from the famous Jefferson Medical College, one of the oldest universities of North America. With great ceremony, on the stage of the Academy of Music in front of 3000 people, including the active participation of the leading women which is customary for such occasions here, I was awarded a doctoral diploma and actually had a doctoral hood placed on me. As far as I know, the only other German colleague to share this high distinction was *Geheimrat*[14] Dr. von Mikulicz from Breslau.

The hospitals in Philadelphia are older and therefore not as efficient and up-to-date as those in New York. However, they are building new hospitals. That of the Jefferson Medical College should be ready about a year from now and will have all the modern facilities. I also held many "clinics" and performed a series of operations in Philadelphia, and was greatly pleased by the interest shown by the medical community on these occasions.

Among the colleagues who were especially helpful to us, I would especially mention Professor Wilson and of course Professor Keen, who is well known to us as an Honorary Member of the German Surgical Society.

One of the unpleasant things here is the plague of reporters.[15] It is absolutely impossible to avoid them. Wherever you go, they snap your photograph with their Kodaks, and you find your picture displayed in the newspapers, sometimes during the operation and sometimes while departing in the automobile. One clever reporter even managed provide his readers with a photograph of the "arm and hand of the famous German surgeon." They especially wanted to interview me about my relationship to Lorenz; the visit by Lorenz here last year had created quite a stir. The newspapers talked a lot about his closed methods of managing congenital hip dislocation, especially the complications that inevitably occur among older patients.[16] Now these people thought I was coming to "kill Lorenz," and were quite astounded to realize that I agree with Lorenz in many areas, and that along with every other specialist in this area I believe that closed reduction is the best method of management for appropriate patients with this condition.

From Philadelphia, we proceeded to Baltimore, where we visited the new orthopedic hospital under the excellent leadership of Dr. Tundstall Taylor. From there we went on to the majestically beautiful garden city of

Washington, with its Capitol and the wonderful library.

Now we are in Atlantic City, one of the most fashionable seaside resorts of North America, where about 3000 doctors will be attending the meeting of American physicians and surgeons. Once we have gotten through this, we will travel on through Buffalo and Chicago to St. Louis, and I will report from there about our experiences.

With cordial greetings,
Sincerely,
Hoffa

[p. 1141]
En route from Chicago to Boston.

Dear Colleague:

The Exhibition in St. Louis is behind us. Now we are on our way home again. Yesterday we traveled eight hours from St. Louis to Chicago, and now there are 31 hours of travel ahead of us from Chicago to Boston. However, the facilities on the train are so comfortable that you can make such a long journey quite nicely. Our train has a smoking lounge and a reading room in addition to the dining car, you can get a shave and take a bath, so there is everything your heart could desire.

A trip such as we have made is socially educational. You get to know the land and people, and develop a new opinion about many things from what you had before. Thus, the general impression is that things are nicer back in Germany than they are in America; at least the educated classes of the population at home have a much more interesting life. Our old culture surrounds us with advantages that are completely absent in America. The pleasure we have in the arts and sciences, theater, and music, are chiefly replaced there by sports, which are pursued in every possible variation. We should find the good where we can, so it is this enjoyment of sports and healthy exercise that I would gladly see introduced at home. When our American colleagues are done with their day's work, they dedicate themselves to outdoor activities. One might enjoy horse and wagon, another sails, another goes out and plays a game of golf that refreshes the lungs and nerves.

We should also do this, and our schoolboys at the *Gymnasium*,[17] our older daughters, and especially our university students should be out in God's open air instead of wasting their time in the taverns, and should build up their physical strength in the peaceful competition of sports. Germany has always been recognized as a nation of thinkers, and the St. Louis Fair demonstrates again that Germany leads all other countries in the intellectual area. However, the others are making strenuous efforts to catch up. If we are to remain on top, we will need to use all our potential strengths, and we can do this if our young people take care of their bodies as well as their minds so that we are strong enough to combine the necessary physical efforts with mental efforts without fatiguing through nervous exhaustion.

We made the acquaintance of quite a few doctors during our journey and tried to get a clear picture of the present status of medical practice through our conversations. The general impression was that, despite all the well-known internal and external social conditions, the status of a doctor in Germany is greatly superior to that in America. The German doctor, even in a rural area or small town, carries with him the solid foundation of his *Gymnasium* and university education.

Here in America, on the other hand, you very often meet doctors who have chosen this profession after failing to make a living in some other way. We met a whole series of doctors who were previously pharmacists, dentists, journalists, secretaries, etc., and then obtained a doctoral degree at some college, usually in the West. These colleges are not connected with the government but are purely private enterprises that compete with each other.

In every large city there are several such colleges; apparently there are seven in St. Louis, which are soon supposed to be merged into three. Clearly, with this system there can be no thought of a fundamental standardized education for physicians; the larger colleges of the eastern states consider themselves, with justification, to be far superior to many of their sister institutions in the West. The education that a medical student receives in New York, Boston, Baltimore, and Philadelphia, for example, is similar to that in our German universities; in the western colleges, the doctor is generally only trained as a practitioner. Related to this difference in education, the doctoral degree necessary for a medical license is only valid for the state where it was awarded. The German doctor graduating from any of the German universities achieves the right to practice anywhere in the entire Empire; whereas the American doctor, who graduates for example in St. Louis, can only practice in New York if he passes an additional state examination.

The "postgraduate school" is an excellent institution that makes an effort to remedy the deficit in undergraduate medical education. The same idea, which we are now attempting to provide in Germany by introducing the practical year and the academies on our larger cities, has been realized in the postgraduate schools of America for many years. These schools are extended hospitals where the leading doctors teach all the theoretical and practical branches of medicine that are important for the practitioner. They are well attended and fulfil their purpose of truly preparing the practitioner for his profession.

One consequence of the profusion of colleges is that the number of doctors is excessive, even more than with us. The ill effects caused by this overproduction of doctors are fortunately minimized for us by our medical organization — but here there is no such organization: everyone works for himself, often without any consideration of his colleagues. The German doctors who have immigrated here especially regret the lack of collegiality, and the inability to appeal to any authority in a given case.

Because of the excess number of doctors, the prospects for young German doctors who want to settle here are hardly favorable. The cost of living is generally greater than in Germany, and the rents for office space are high, especially in the large cities. The young doctor therefore has more of a struggle here than at home before he earns enough to make a living. His chances only improve if he succeeds in joining the staff of one of the larger hospitals. Such a hospital appointment is the best advertisement to the public. In the larger hospitals here, there is not one surgeon or internist or gynecologist etc. who is the chief and runs everything, but instead a number of doctors share the work, so that the same hospital will have four or five surgeons, for example, each of whom only operates on a certain day; consequently these surgeons are often active at 3-4 different hospitals, and might operate today at one hospital and tomorrow at another. The hospital doctors are also involved with teaching the students. Even at the university hospitals there is the same division of labor; each professor supervises his service only for a few months and then is replaced by another. Therefore, the student does not receive a consistent education; the personal training that a student receives at our German institutions, and is passed on from generation to generation, is almost completely absent here; only a few universities, for example the Johns Hopkins University[18] in Baltimore, are based on the German model. The young doctors graduating from this university have approximately the same preparation as our German students.

The earnest striving for improvement certainly exists here; there is an extraordinary amount of scientific work, often with more lavish support than we have. However, there is not always a correct evaluation of the results; Germany is recognized everywhere as the leader in the field of medicine, and many colleagues here gratefully acknowledge their indebtedness to German universities for the advancement of their knowledge.

At a big dinner given in our honor by the surgical and orthopedic society in Chicago, with about 80 colleagues present, this devotion to German science was expressed most touchingly. All of those present had at least briefly studied in Germany; all were enthusiastic about what they had learned in Germany. One after another stood to raise his glass to the health of his German teacher, and in a sparkling address, Chicago's famous surgeon Murphy celebrated Germany's leading role in all areas of medicine.

The World's Fair in St. Louis also gave a shining example of how Germany truly serves the whole world as an educational model. The German educational exhibit was clearly the best thing that the fair had to offer. This was not only our opinion, but that of everyone who visited the fair. Our educational methods were presented in exemplary fashion down to the smallest detail, as they are used in the universities and technical schools, in secondary schools, or in the institutions for the blind or deaf. The medical department was especially distinguished. An overview was presented for the instruction in surgery, the individual specialties of internal medicine, normal and pathologic anatomy, ophthalmology, and otology using exhibits, wax models, x-rays, posters, instruments, etc. There was a special presentation of bacteriology, including serum therapy and immunology. The presentation by the imperial health office also made a memorable impression. In addition, the German precision optical instruments were incomparably beautiful; in particular, the Zeiss ultramicroscope and epidiascope created a justifiable excitement. The latter was set up in a small auditorium, where there were lectures every Wednesday and Saturday. At the request of the German exhibit directors, I myself gave a talk about *coxa vara*[19] with x-rays and demonstrations, which was eagerly attended by the doctors of St. Louis.

Extraordinarily beautiful color photographs, produced by the apparatus of Prof. Miethe,[20] were also projected in this auditorium. – Germany also came off well in other areas of the World's Fair. The German building was praised not only because of its prominent location right next to the Festival Hall, but also because of its internal and external appearance.

The abundant anthropologic material at the fair was very interesting. Almost all nations were represented. We were particularly interested in the "wild" people, of whom we were able to see the various tribes of Filipinos thanks to the kind guidance of the responsible American military doctor. For the amateur there will probably never again be such an opportunity to study comparative anthropology.

The fair had many more interesting things for the doctor; there was especially a lot of nice things to see in the area of electricity.

German surgical instruments were only represented by the well-known Berlin company of Louis Löwenstein. The representative of the firm said he had done good business over there.

The well-known New York company Marx had some very nice artificial legs and arms.

I will close with a few words about the American medical congress in Atlantic City. The meeting had the same character as our *Naturforscher*[21] congresses; lectures were generally given in separate sections. The chairmen of the individual sections performed their offices with exemplary punctuality. If the time allotted for a presentation or discussion had expired, the chairman rapped on the table with a large hammer (called a gavel), and the speaker had to stop in the middle of a sentence; permission would not be granted to speak further, and every speaker abided willingly by the rules.

If you travel from the large cities of the East more into the interior, the "provinces," the older hospitals leave much to be desired; however, new hospitals are being built everywhere. Everything here gives the impression of development, of becoming. When comparing Germany and America we must not forget that the entire American culture is still young, scarcely a century old; but the people have an abundance of surplus energy, which will not be completely matured for many decades. We had the impression that German thoroughness and American ingenuity make a good combination, as the Americans can learn much from us; similarly, we found that there is an extraordinary amount that is exciting and worth knowing, and so I recommend that more colleagues should cross the great ocean and get a picture of this great country. Their American colleagues will receive them with open arms.

Looking forward to seeing you again soon, yours
Hoffa

Original Notes

1. See the article by Wassermann in this journal, No. 17. (Editor)

Biographical Sources

Hoffa A, *Lehrbuch der Fracturen und Luxationen für Ärzte und Studierende*, Würzburg, 1888.
Osgood RB, "Albert Hoffa," *American Journal of Orthopedic Surgery* 1908; 6:7-12.
Baudach E, *Eine Studie über Albert Hoffa und seine Resonanz in Amerika*

unter Berücksichtigung der Zeitumstände, Dissertation, Julius Maximilians-Universität Würzburg, 1977.

Hernigou P, "Authorities and foundation of the orthopaedic school in Germany in the 19th century: Part II: Richard von Volkmann, Julius Wolff, Albert Hoffa, Friedrich Trendelenburg and other German authors," *International Orthopedics* 2016; 40:843-853.

Publication Source

The *Deutsche Medizinsche Wochenschrift* [German Medical Weekly] is still published. Historical issues can be obtained through the Hathi Trust.

Translation Notes

1) Julius Schwalbe, editor of the *Deutsche Medizinische Wochenschrift*.
2) *Das Land der unbegrenzten Möglichkeiten* (*The Land of Unlimited Possibilities*) was the name of a popular book by economist Ludwig Max Goldberger, published in 1903.
3) This was the Annual Meeting of the American Medical Association. Dr. Hoffa gave a talk on "The influence of the adipose tissue, with regard to the pathology of the knee joint" in the Section on Surgery and Anatomy. See *Journal of the American Medical Association* 1904; 43:44-60.
4) See Zampini JM, Sherk HH, "Lewis A. Sayre – The first professor of orthopedic surgery in America," *Clinical Orthopedics and Related Research* 2008; 466:2263-2267.
5) See Jackson RW, Pollo FE, "The legacy of Professor Adolf Lorenz, the 'bloodless surgeon of Vienna'," *Baylor University Medical Center Proceedings* 2004; 17:3-7. For a description of the nonoperative methods see Lorenz A, *Ueber die Heilung der angeborenen Hüftgelenks-Verrenkung durch unblutige Einrenkung und functionelle Belastung*, Leipzig: Franz Deuticke, 1900.
6) Now called the Hospital for Special Surgery.
7) See Brand RA, "Biographical sketch: Virgil Pendleton Gibney MD, 1847-1927," *Clinical Orthopedics and Related Research* 2010; 468:308-311.

8) See Coley WB and Hoguet JP, "Operative treatment of hernia," *Annals of Surgery* 1918; 68:255-268.
9) Now the Mount Sinai Morningside Hospital.
10) Now the Lenox Hill Hospital.
11) Now the Weill Cornell Medical Center.
12) The German Medical Society of New York meeting on 3 June 1904, as recorded in the *New Yorker Medizinische Monatsschrift* 1905; 16:385.
13) Wassermann A, "Die medizinische Abteilung der deutschen Unterrichts-Ausstellung in St. Louis," *Deutsche Medizinische Wochenschrift* 1904; 30:638-639.
14) *"Geheimrat"* was a title bestowed by the emperor on deserving subjects. The British equivalent is "Privy Councillor," and even this sounds rather silly to Americans.
15) On the other hand, the extensive documentation of the author's visit by newspaper reporters as well as professional journals enabled an interesting doctoral dissertation 70 years later (see Biographical Sources).
16) See Mueller F, "Bloodless reposition of the congenitally dislocated hip joint versus arthrotomy, with statistics of 34 cases operated on by Dr. Lorenz during his visit to the United States in 1902," *Journal of the American Medical Association* 1905; 44:1915-1919.
17) The *Gymnasium* in Europe is a secondary school that prepares the student to enter a university. It is generally equivalent to a college preparatory course at an American high school plus one or two years of college-level work.
18) The author makes the common mistake of calling it the John Hopkins University.
19) A congenital hip deformity.
20) Adolf Miethe was an early developer of color photography using three images taken through red, green, and blue filters.
21) *Gesellschaft Deutscher Naturforscher und Ärzte*, still active.

10

Julius Hirschberg (1905)

Julius Hirschberg was born in 1843 in Potsdam, Germany. He received a classical education and excelled in school, going on to study medicine at the University of Berlin. He met the great ophthalmologist Albrecht von Graefe at a cholera hospital during the Prussian-Austrian war of 1866, and became his assistant and disciple. He began his own private practice, was among the first to adopt aseptic surgical methods in ophthalmology, and developed a reputation for skill, diligence, and innovation. He pioneered the use of electromagnets for extraction of metallic foreign bodies in the eye. He never became a full professor, but was a prolific author and a demanding and rewarding teacher who attracted many students from Germany and abroad.

Hirschberg traveled extensively, including to North America in 1887 and 1892 (on the latter occasion continuing to Japan and around the world), each time writing an account of his experiences. His third trip to America, at the age of 61, is described in the following pages.

In 1907, he gave up clinical practice and concentrated on completing his magnificent 11-volume history of ophthalmology, for which his research included reading Arabic, Latin, Greek, and Egyptian hieroglyphics. He generally did not draw attention to his Jewish heritage, but in 1914 led a successful protest against a Russian policy limiting the participation of Jewish ophthalmologists at an international congress. He was intensely patriotic and bitterly disappointed at the outcome of the First World War. Impoverished during the postwar period, he sold his extensive library to a Japanese colleague, and it is now a valued possession of Tokyo University. Julius Hirschberg died in 1925.

Meine dritte Amerika-Fahrt
Medizinische Klinik 1905; 1:1056-1061, 1084-1088, 1135-1140,1191-1196

My third trip to America
by J. Hirschberg, Berlin

At the special request of the Editor of this esteemed journal, I have undertaken to record my impressions from my last trip to America. However, I must ask the interested reader to grant me some leniency if my account is more subjective than expected, even compared to the descriptions of my first two voyages in 1887 and 1892 [1]: On the one hand, it is necessary in the following to talk more about myself than I usually prefer;[1] and on the other hand, because of the speed at which I covered the gigantic distances, to be satisfied with the personal impressions that the fleeting experiences made on me. Nowhere did I have the opportunity in any single place to call out in the words of Goethe: "Only linger here, thou art so fair."[2]

After having been the guest of honor at the ophthalmology section of the British Medical Association in Summer 1904, I received a friendly invitation that same fall from the chairman of the ophthalmology section of the American Medical Association, Prof. C. R. Holmes of Cincinnati, to address the section at their 56th Session in Portland (Oregon), to be held July 11-14, 1905. This was in accordance with a new arrangement whereby each section was permitted to invite a guest of honor.

In 1902 Prof. Haab from Zürich and in 1904 Dr. A. Maitland Ramsay from Glasgow had been invited by the ophthalmology section and had attended. The former had spoken about removal of foreign bodies from the eye [2], and the latter about the general management of ocular diseases [3]. The colleague invited for 1903 – I think it was a Frenchman – had cancelled at the last moment. The number of potential candidates from Europe is somewhat limited. Acceptance of this invitation requires someone who enjoys traveling, can afford it, and can speak English adequately.

As much as I adhere to the principle of using only the German language at international meetings [4], it is necessary to speak English at a national conference of American doctors.

I accepted the invitation despite the enormous distance [5] of about 12,500 kilometers, nearly a third of the circumference of the Earth. I have always considered it valuable to maintain good international relationships in science, and I think Germany should be represented on important occasions.

These considerations of duty coincided with my personal desires.

I wanted to make my third (and perhaps last) journey to the United States, which has made such gigantic progress in the last ten years, in order to form a judgment based on direct observation. Therefore I did not follow the most comfortable plan, to return from Portland in the hot summer by taking a ship to the coolness of Alaska and then crossing Canada back to Europe; indeed, I had already seen glaciers falling into the sea in Spitzbergen in 1895: Instead, I decided to travel through the United States, despite the heat and the effort, to the fabulous Queen of the West, San Francisco, continuing on to southern California and then returning through Denver and Chicago to Boston and the Atlantic Coast. Neither the two gentlemen I mentioned nor any of my acquaintances or colleagues from Berlin who had been invited to America had ventured so far to the west and southwest. I must admit that my trip to southern California in the month of July was a risk, but it all went well.

For the subject of my talk, I chose a purely theoretical topic, namely the history of Arabic ophthalmology. On the one hand, I had been continually involved in studying the source material of this area for the last five years and had just finished reviewing the proofs of the final manuscript [6] before my departure; on the other hand, I wanted to demonstrate that such investigations were valued in the United States, even though they could only satisfy the scientific sense of educated men and had nothing at all to do with clinical practice, healing the sick, or making money. Some people who have never been to America nurture and spread false ideas about the "Empire of the Dollar," but let me say from the beginning that I was not disappointed; the lecture captured the undivided attention of the audience.

Of course, I wrote down my talk in English [7], read it aloud to my wife and an English listener, and wrote it out in clear text [8]: The lecture lasted 50 minutes. A speaker who respects his audience should always make careful preparations.

The voyage across the Atlantic Ocean can be easily imagined by anyone who has experienced it, at least if he shares my good fortune in having no tendency toward seasickness [9]. Three months before leaving, I had reserved a well-ventilated single cabin on the promenade deck of the North German Lloyd express-mail steamer *Kaiser Wilhelm der Große*. At 9 P.M. on June 19, I departed from the busy capital of the German Empire on a special train of this company; sleeping in a comfortable single compartment, I reached the shore of the North Sea; early in the morning of June 20 the train stopped at the dock in Bremerhaven, where we could directly board the proud vessel [10].

Captain Cüppers is an especially kindly and reassuring example of a real

German sailor. I immediately got to know the ship's doctor Dr. Katerbau,[3] who is among the oldest and most experienced health officers of the North German Lloyd fleet. Of course, at mealtimes I sat at his table, on his right hand. To his left were an American ophthalmologist and his wife, whom I met through the following special circumstances.

Once an experienced person has boarded the ship, inspected his cabin, and confirmed that his luggage is present, he signs up for a bath time – I chose 6:40 for my daily bath – and rents a chair on the promenade deck that is in a good location near some cover [11], where he alone has the right to sit every day and evening. Once I had attached my card to my chair, I read the name on the one next to it: Mr. Frank Allport. I knew this name well from the specialty literature. I walked up to the chair with the question, "Are you Frank Allport, the oculist of Chicago?" He answered in the affirmative. I introduced myself. He was returning with his wife from Italy; they were enthusiastic about Germany and Berlin, where they had spent several days, and became very pleasant table companions. He is one of the leaders of the ophthalmology section of the American Medical Association [12].

As soon as I set foot in the United States – in the great arrival hall of the North German Lloyd at Hoboken on the Hudson, across from New York – I was enveloped into the tender care of my American colleagues, who arranged to make my excursion as enjoyable as possible, as they had promised in their letter of invitation. My old friend Hermann Knapp, who could not be there in person (since he was preparing for the wedding of his youngest daughter) sent his faithful servant: These do exist in the United States!

Prof. J. C. Weeks, who 20 years ago attended my clinic and at that time completed a microscopic study using my case of an ocular abscess resulting from meningitis [13], came in person as a representative of the New York ophthalmologists to accompany me and my luggage in a carriage [14] to the hotel and invite me to a reception that evening. While he was dealing with my luggage and the customs procedures, and I was looking through some letters that had just been delivered to me from former students with greetings and invitations, a gentleman approached me and asked in German, "Do I have the pleasure of addressing Professor Hirschberg of Berlin? I am on assignment from the *New Yorker Staats-Zeitung*." Well, I knew from both my earlier visits that you cannot avoid the press, and allowed him to interview me for the minute that was available. Anyway, I enjoyed being able to send my wife a newspaper clipping in which, along with other inaccuracies, it literally stated "Professor Hirschberg is a gentleman of medium size, with a short, white beard, against which the lively, sparkling, light-brown eyes are a notable contrast, giving him a youthful appearance."

I will not try to describe New York. It is half Babel and half Bellamy's paradise.[4] The gigantic buildings of 20 stories (skyscrapers) are well-known to everyone – at least from the windows of the North German Lloyd and the Hamburg-America Steamship Line. They result from the high cost of real estate and are safely enabled by the rock-hard ground: But they are not beautiful, at least for the eye trained in classical architecture, which is unwillingly drawn to the roof and then follows the external fire-escapes slowly back down to the first floor. In addition, these buildings block the wind and at night radiate back the solar energy that they have absorbed all day, and so create New York's unbearable warmth, which caused so many to collapse and die from heat stroke during the days after my arrival. Indeed, I found it more tolerable at the equator than during July and August in New York and Washington.

I stayed at the Waldorf Astoria Hotel, 5th Avenue and 34th Street, a huge elegant building with 1500 rooms that takes up a whole city block and reaches up to a roof garden on the 18th floor, where you can sip a glass of beer or another drink and listen to the band in relative coolness. I was on the 12th floor – just as accessible as those below due to the numerous well-attended lifts, which they call elevators here; the higher floors are actually preferable because they are cooler and have less street noise – a spacious, nicely furnished room with an excellent bed, private bathroom, and storage area, for the moderate price of 5 dollars. Everything was provided for health and comfort, hot and cold water for the sink and bath, electric lights, desk, bed, and ventilation. Every day they made up the bed and provided new hand and bath towels. I sadly compared the status of this new culture to the old one that has passed, and remembered from my first trip to Olympia in 1886 how, with the encouragement of my new Hellenic friends, I had to supervise the innkeeper at Pyrgos while he removed the new bed sheets [15] and replaced them with newer ones from the closet.[5]

All the American hotels where I stayed – of course, I always chose the best ones – demonstrated the same high quality. However, when I told my San Francisco friends that their new St. Francis Hotel was the best of all, they responded to my surprise that the Bristol Hotel in Berlin was just as good, which I myself had no way of knowing.

After I had visited my friend Knapp and had breakfasted, I took the streetcar down to the Battery at the south end of the metropolis, and proceeded from there on foot, with Baedeker [16] in hand, to see again the most important downtown buildings up to City Hall and the huge suspension bridge[6] that has always fascinated me. Only a pedestrian can get the right impression. But in downtown New York, it is not a trivial matter to be a pedestrian [17]. Every second it seems that you are about to be run over or crashed into: You just have to pay attention, and the drivers also pay attention [18]; so nothing happened.

In two multiple-hour automobile rides, I again toured downtown and then uptown to the farthest border, so I could see the street scenes and principal buildings, walked through Central Park, visited the Art Museum, which has made great progress since 1887, and observed two eye clinics. This time, I could not devote more than three days to the metropolis.

The first evening, I was brought to the reception by Prof. Weeks and Prof. de Schweinitz, who had come from Philadelphia to New York for the occasion. They took me to the famous Delmonico Restaurant, of which I still had a good memory from my previous visit. Several rooms were set aside for us. After the initial reunions – since I already knew most of these colleagues from their visits to Berlin, my visits to New York, and international congresses – and after a few introductions, we sat down to a nicely appointed Round Table. I myself was seated next to the Toastmaster, Dr. Thomas Pooley, who had been my guest in Berlin 24 years ago and has since won great acclaim for his introduction of the magnetic needle for diagnosis of iron splinters in the posterior chamber of the eye.[7] In front of each person was an artistically rendered menu with the colorful flags of the United States and the German Empire [19] and the inscription in gold letters: Dinner in honour of Professor J. Hirschberg given by American Confrères, Wednesday, June twenty-eighth 1905, Delmonico's New York. I will skip over the menu items including the wines, but I have to share the last page, which contained the toasts. These are spoken after finishing the meal, one after the next. They were as follows: "Our guest. Hands across the Sea. American ophthalmology. Ophthalmology in the universities. Ophthalmological echoes. The toxins in ophthalmology. The ophthalmology of the future. *Auf Wiedersehen*." I was embarrassed at what was said to my face by my old friend H. Knapp, who has brought such honor to German medicine on the other side of the ocean; fortunately, he concluded by praising my wife, my true companion in my long scientific work, which gave me great pleasure to hear from the mouth of an old friend. I answered this toast immediately in English. Prof. Weeks and E. Grüning also spoke very friendly words. The rest of the toasts concerned American issues, sometimes very incisive and earnest, sometimes very humorous. Professor de Schweinitz, one of the best speakers, spoke about university teaching in ophthalmology and his own very practical principles and rich experiences. Since the United States cannot constitutionally do anything for the universities, and the individual states and cities have so far done very little, the medical schools are basically private enterprises, which are partly affiliated with the hospitals supported by religious institutions and charitable organizations; thus there are not insignificant difficulties in the United States, especially for teaching ophthalmology, which requires expensive laboratories and instruments, modern operating rooms, and hospital beds. The question was raised whether there is truly a unique American school of ophthalmology, which was answered in the negative. This is also my own opinion.

The United States has yet to produce a man like A. v. Graefe, Helmholtz, or Donders. There are excellent ophthalmologists, of whom some have immigrated from Europe, and indeed chiefly from Germany; the practical work is basically no different from that in Europe; the scientific work follows the same paths, where of course the younger region has not quite overtaken the older one. Progress is guaranteed by the existence of numerous archives and journals of ophthalmology [20]. Certain innovations of individual American ophthalmologists in the areas of refraction and muscle disorders do not justify distinguishing a separate American school of ophthalmology from the European.

Perhaps it would be appropriate to add a few words here about the history of ophthalmology in the United States and Canada [21], since this information may be relatively unknown back home.

Georg Frick's treatise on *Diseases of the Eyes*, Baltimore 1822, was the first ophthalmologic work published in America. Colleagues from America maintain that in England it was also considered the best book at that time. But it should be mentioned that the full title read "Management of Eye Diseases, including the Teaching and Practice of the Leading Wound Surgeons of the Present and especially of Prof. Beer"; and that the detailed review in the *Philadelphia Journal of Medical and Physical Sciences* added the following: "The author seems to be well acquainted with the German literature, and we are indebted to him for introducing it to us." Then in 1850 there followed the work of Henry Howard in Montreal, *Anatomy, Physiology and Pathology of the Eye* (517 pp.) But the first modern *American Textbook of Diseases of the Eye* was published by H. D. Noyes, Professor of Ophthalmology at Bellevue Hospital Medical College (738 pp.) The author took his own observations and opinions as a basis, but also become familiar with those of others not only through study of their writings but also through repeated observation of European clinics.

The multiple-volume handbook *A System of Diseases of the Eye* by W. F. Norris and Charles O. Oliver may be considered an English counterpart to our Graefe-Saemisch (First Edition); however, it should be mentioned that several excellent chapters were also written by professors and colleagues from Germany [22].

The idea that strabismus surgery was invented in America I consider unproven. There is no documentation before 1841 [23]! Dr. William Ingalls is said to have advised dividing the muscles of the eye in 1812-1813. Dr. Gibson relates (1841) that he divided some muscles in 1818, three times with minimal success and once with a major complication, the greatest possible secondary divergence; and "will not propose myself as the inventor or challenge the priority of that excellent surgeon (Dieffenbach)." The triumphs of the United States lie in other areas.

We are indebted for very fundamental work in refraction and accommodation by Edward Jackson, first in Philadelphia and now in Denver, Thorington in Philadelphia, Wurdemann in Milwaukee, John Green in St. Louis, and Risley in Philadelphia, among others. Intensive studies of disorders in eye motion have been made by George T. Stevens – to whom I am not very grateful for inventing the name heterophoria[8] – G. C. Savage in Nashville, and Duane in New York, among others.

It should be recognized that these investigations in the United States are generally performed very carefully and that the glasses prescribed are well made and well framed [24]. This fact is familiar to any doctor with an international practice. M. Gould in Philadelphia has improved bifocal lenses, de Schweinitz ophthalmometry, Thomas Pooley in New York sideroscopy [25],[9] and Edgar G. Loring ophthalmoscopy.

In the area of bacteriology, the name of John E. Weeks of New York is most prominently associated with that of Robert Koch. In the area of ophthalmic surgery, H. Knapp has made immortal contributions. Karl Koller, the discoverer of topical cocaine anesthesia for the eye, is now an American citizen. Our area of science follows the same law as in economics: Growth can occur through immigration from Europe as well as through natural increase [26].

This may suffice. It is difficult, indeed almost impossible, to write the history of today: History can only judge the past, our present times await the judgment of the future.

On the afternoon of July 1, I left the bustling city on the Hudson on the express train to Cincinnati. (Approximately 1300 km in 20 hours.) I must emphasize one thing. Whoever leaps into the powerful whirlpool of American hospitality has to have a strong constitution, a resilient stomach, and a certain audacity, because he will be dealing with gigantic distances and unusual stresses. During the next 9 days, I never slept in a hotel, only in a sleeping car.

At about noon on July 2, I reached Cincinnati, which has about 400,000 inhabitants, of whom a third are Germans. Indeed, their original settlement was called "Over-the-Rhine," that is, on the north side of the Miami Canal.[10] At the train station, I was met by Dr. C. R. Holmes and Dr. R. Sattler with a comfortable carriage.

Dr. C. R. Holmes is chairman of the ophthalmologic section of the meeting to be held in Portland; he has repeatedly studied for long periods in Europe, including at my institution, but has especially pursued intensive and important investigations with Waldeyer of the paranasal sinuses, which are so important for us [27]; he is a professor at the university, chief of a large modern and well-equipped private clinic for diseases of the eye and ear, which we immediately went to see, and a director of the Cincinnati General Hospital. In the latter capacity, he has to review the plans for renovation and has made extensive hygienic studies of lighting, heating, and ventilation, about which he made an interesting presentation at the opening session of our section. From Cincinnati to Portland, and then from Portland to San Francisco, Dr. Holmes never left my side, and without my noticing he took care of all the little annoyances that are inevitably associated with a journey over such a huge distance. I have to acknowledge him as "my son in science and my father in love."

As we traveled through the city, we had the opportunity to admire its principal work of art at the city center. It is the fountain donated by Tyler Davidson, which was cast using August von Kreling's molds in Munich, and presents the refreshing spray with enchanting motifs of its pleasantness, its use, and its magic.[11] After we had seen the business district, which had the huge buildings and familiar bustle of an American city, and the German Quarter with its smaller buildings and numerous workshops, we drove to the beautiful spacious suburbs with their endless rows of garden houses, the homes of the well-to-do.

At the home of C. R. Holmes I bathed and dressed, and had a nice breakfast with him and his first assistant, as well as Dr. Sattler and two of the leading jurists of the U.S.; then changed clothes for an automobile ride in the area, returned, bathed, dressed, and drove to the Cincinnati Country Club House, where another reception was given. This was indeed the high point of all these arrangements. On the terrace of the clubhouse, 65 gentlemen were seated at 16 small tables, leading doctors and ophthalmologists and other citizens. I will skip over the food and wines and mention only the toasts, which were especially cordial:

To our guest: On behalf of the medical profession of Cincinnati, Dr. Joseph Ransohoff. 2. Welcome to Cincinnati, Robert Ramsey, Esq. 3. The American Medical Association. Dr. Charles A. L. Reed. 4. "Speed the parting guest," *auf Wiedersehen*, Dr. Daniel Milliken.

I repeated twice, first in English and then in German, a well-known saying of Goethe [28],[12] which unleashed a storm of applause. Everyone shook my hand and said it had been a wonderful evening. It is different in America than in England. In Edinburgh, at the welcome ceremony of the international ophthalmology congress in 1894, three people shook my hand; when a friend from London asked me about it, I explained that these were my students – whereupon he said he did not have three students in Scotland. But everywhere in America there are dozens of doctors who have been with us, studied diligently, and enjoy seeing us again.

At eleven we drove home, put on traveling clothes, drove to the train, and went to bed in the sleeping car. The train did not leave until 3 A.M., but we were already asleep.

Here I had the stateroom of the sleeping car to myself (ticket cost 7 dollars), so I slept just as comfortably as in the best sleeping car of my fatherland. Around noon of July 3, we arrived in Chicago and got off at the new Hotel Auditorium-Annex [29].[13] This is extremely luxurious with marble and a Pompeiian picture gallery, although not very tastefully decorated.

After a bath we had another automobile ride through the majestic boulevards and the huge parks of this newest metropolis, in the company of colleagues who filled three vehicles and took turns sitting next to me.

Then bath, dress, reception at the Athletic Club, with a friendly toast to the "magnetic man," which I answered briefly. Then back into traveling clothes for the special train that would take us from Chicago to Portland, leaving at 10 P.M.

This special train had been arranged by Mr. Gates of Chicago, an American Stangen,[14] to transport a flock of more than a hundred doctors and their companions through Canada to the site of the meeting, of which one part would later take a steamer to Alaska and the other part would return to Chicago by way of Yellowstone Park. I baptized the train with the name "Land Steamer," which stuck. We were a fellowship, indeed a very compatible one: It included Dr. Holmes, the chairman; Dr. Bulson, the secretary of our section, with his family; Prof. Risley, my old acquaintance with whom I had lodged the previous year at Keble College in Oxford; my faithful old student Prof. Posey [30] from Philadelphia; Prof. Weeks with his wife and daughter; my own humble self; and others. Thus, we had the opportunity for pleasant and instructive conversations.

I had one section for myself, that is, nobody sleeping above me.

Our train included a dining car, smoking room, and library [31] – however, no bath. It stopped, not exactly wherever it might wish; however, at numerous preselected locations, so that to the naïve observer it seemed as if the railway was being used like a highway. Of course, this is only possible in regions where the daily number of trains is so small, as it is in Canada.

[p. 1084]

We traveled first the Chicago Northwestern, then the Soo-Pacific Line, which runs from Sault-Ste.-Marie, the passage between Lake Superior and Lake Huron, through St. Paul, and finally to the Canadian Pacific Line, which terminates at Vancouver and Seattle on Puget Sound, that is, on the Pacific Ocean.

Our first day of travel was July 4, which is Independence Day, the national holiday of the Declaration of Independence in the United States. Most readers of this report will be as horrified as I was the first time I read the following excerpt from the Portland edition of the *Journal of the American Medical Association* (3 June 1905, p. 1781):

"In 1903, the Fourth of July tribute was 466 dead and 3983 injured; in 1904 it was 183 dead and 3986 injured. The first year the reported cases of tetanus numbered 415, while last year there were but 105. Within one year the deaths from tetanus were reduced by 25 per cent. [32], although the deaths from other causes were increased by over 50 per cent., and the total number of recorded injuries was practically unchanged … the chief reason for the great tetanus mortality lay in a lack of appreciation of the danger that lies in every blank cartridge wound … Just before the last Fourth of July a vigorous 'campaign of education' on this point was carried on throughout the country, by both the medical and the lay press, and to this cause alone can be attributed the great reduction in tetanus mortality. The average parent learned that a blank cartridge wound was a serious injury that needed surgical attention; the average physician learned that simple dressing of such wounds was little better than nothing at all, and that thorough surgical cleansing with prophylactic injections of tetanus antitoxin were required." [33]. I had previously been appalled to learn the terrible number of ocular injuries associated with each "Independence Day," reported in a study by Dr. Robert L. Randolph in the same journal on 10 December 1904.

More pointed popular instruction about this phenomenon was provided by the comic strips in the morning newspaper, which portrayed the lad Buster Brown celebrating the Fourth of July by exploding fireworks under chickens, ducks, calves, and pigs; and the Great Alderman who does not say a word when the street urchin puts a lighted rocket into the coat pocket of a policeman, etc.

So I was quite happy to experience Independence Day in a moving train car; I hoped I could avoid the fireworks. However, I was disappointed. Our train had barely stopped in St. Paul when people began throwing firecrackers right next to our car and setting off rockets. We had a plentiful supply of these celebratory items in the train. The doctors' children, the childlike Negroes from the railroad staff, and several adults were actively taking part. Fortunately, there were no problems for us. And plenty of doctors were available.

We had an hour in St. Paul and drove around in a car. It is amazing how these cities in the west grow and thrive. St. Paul is said to be overshadowed by its sister city Minneapolis. But in 1887 it had 110,000 inhabitants and in 1900 it already had 163,000. It is not satisfied with its old Capitol. We saw the new edifice of white marble with a cupola like the Baptistery in Florence. Plus beautiful school and hospital buildings. Our Goethe, who indeed felt very warmly toward America and prophesied its prosperity, dedicated the following well-known verses to the United States [34]:[15]

> America! You are not vassals
> To Europe's decadence and thrones.
> You have no kings, no crumbling castles,
> No basalt stones.
>
> You do not harbor petty feuds
> Or quarrels from an age before.
> No ancient memory intrudes,
> No pointless war.
>
> Embrace the future that awaits,
> And someday may your children wonder
> How they were spared by kindly fates
> From tales of ghosts and knights and plunder.

Of course, every word in this poem cannot be taken literally. I have seen basalt stones on the Hudson River. But the first line is true. On the entire journey from New York to the Canadian border I did not see a single soldier, and also none at the border.

On July 6 we reached the picturesque portion of the Canadian Pacific Railway [35] and stopped in Banff, the Canadian version of St. Moritz, which is 4500 feet above sea level, 2346 miles from Montreal, and 560 miles from Vancouver. Although a foreigner, I was the only traveler on the entire train who had previously (1892) stayed in the lodge of this resort; I was able to identify improvements in the spa facilities at the warm sulfur spring; the ecstatic testimonials and discarded crutches had disappeared from the stairway to the lodge.

An excellent breakfast at the hotel – at which we eye doctors and our ladies kept together – allowed us to add some refreshing variety to the monotonous menu of the "Land Steamer," and we were able to enjoy a carriage ride into the mountains. In the evening the train continued and we stopped again the next morning in Loggan, to make a very efficient tour on foot into the mountains to see Lake Louise and Mirror Lake. In the evening we drove in a carriage from Field through a long avenue cut through the primeval forest to a chalet beautifully situated on a small island in the Emerald Lake, where we had dinner: Then we drove by moonlight back to the train. Our coachmen were tall, strong, and very educated young men – Canadian medical students, who do this work in the summer to earn money for the winter and their studies.

Some of us might consider this beneath our dignity. But working as a tutor, as some of our less wealthy students do, especially for less educated families, is just something different, not something better. I was impressed by these young people. They did very well on my brief quiz about the anatomy of the larynx [36].

On July 8, we stopped at the Glacier House station, and walked to the foot of the glacier. It is about the same size as the Grindelwald glacier, but not as beautiful.

On Sunday, July 9, we rode in the train along the Fraser River, which empties into Puget Sound at Vancouver. The vegetation is luxurious, with an undergrowth of tall ferns beneath the gigantic trees. Of course, "you cannot avoid the flame."[16] You could see the active fires beside the train. The flames leapt up from inside the broken-off burned-out stumps; the flames lapped eagerly at the feet of lush living trees. However, the smoke was not as bad as it had been 18 years before, shortly before the end of this stretch, when I was completely unable to see the 14,440-foot-high Tacoma Mountain, or I should say Mount Rainier, as the jealous residents of the sister-city Seattle have properly named it [37].

Completely isolated, it rises broad-footed from the plain; its center is obscured with horizontal layers of clouds, and its sharp peak projects into the clear sky, crowned with snow and glaciers. Late in the evening, when the plain is already quite dark, the peak glows alone in the rosy light, a unique sight that we enjoyed until 9:30 P.M. (in the smoking room); the counterpart of Goethe's "Look up and see! The giant mountaintops proclaim the festive golden hour."[17]

Anyway, on this Sunday afternoon we had stopped in Seattle. This city is like a dream. In 1870 it had 1100 inhabitants, but now 100,000. Our train stopped at the great harbor with its large ocean steamers. The main streets have buildings and stores like those in the capitals of Europe. A public library, built of marble in the Greek style, was a gift of the former steel king Carnegie. Large school and hospital buildings catch the eye. We raced through the main streets on an electric train, through the suburban avenues laid out for another 100,000 residents with building lots available for 50-100 dollars according to numerous advertisements, and finally to the beautiful freshwater Lake Washington, which is entirely bordered by an amusement park [38]. Then, back to the city and the new Hotel Washington, not even mentioned in the 1904 Baedeker, which rises from an inviting hill (accessible by a special electric train) like a castle, and in whose great hall our ophthalmological society enjoyed a 6-course dinner, from oysters (which I never touch so far from home) through baked chicken, to sherbet, with a drinkable red wine and music.

During the night our train was carried across the Columbia River on a giant ferryboat, and we arrived as planned on the morning of July 10 in Portland, the location of the meeting. In the majestic hall of The Portland, the city's leading hotel and headquarters for the ophthalmologic section, it was humming like a swarm of bees that does not know whether to fly in or out. I wrote my name in the register [39] and with some difficulty (despite reservations and confirmations) obtained a good room with bath on the first floor that had just become available for the usual price of $7.50 per day; I verified that my luggage had arrived and put the room key safely in my pocket.

The cause of all this chaos was that Portland, which has increased its population from 40,000 to more than 140,000 since my first visit in 1887 [40] and has increased its area tenfold – since all these cities lay out their streets "to grow on" – had just celebrated a "Lewis and Clark Centennial Exposition" to honor the discovery of Oregon and these parts of the Pacific Coast by Lewis and Clark after their overland trek 100 years ago, and had attracted an enormous number of visitors with inexpensive special trains and all kinds of conventions [41], including that of the American Medical Association.

I drove over to this miniature World's Fair on the afternoon of my arrival, found huge wood and plywood buildings and visited a nice lake, where you could ride on motorboats or walk across a long bridge to reach the exhibition hall of the United States, which had an honor guard of soldiers in khaki uniforms and offered instructive materials about botany (of useful and harmful plants), the treasury and internal administration, the navy, and the mineralogical collection of the Smithsonian Institution that could be studied for hours.

On the morning of July 11, I entered the huge hall of the Armory for the opening session of the convention, adorned as requested with the convention badge that had a ribbon on which "Guest" was printed. Up until a half hour before they had still been diligently hammering and pasting, but now everything was ready. The walls were decked with numerous American flags and the names of the individual states in large letters; several thousand new chairs were occupied by gentlemen and ladies in the hall and the galleries. Representatives of the state of Oregon, the city of Portland, and the American Medical Association spoke eloquently and wittily.

Then I, as the only guest, was called to the platform and introduced to the society, which I had not expected; and after the applause that is customary in America, I extracted myself from the situation with a few words, which I will report as they literally appeared in the evening edition of the *Oregon News*.

"Dr. Hirschberg, professor of diseases of the eye in Berlin University, was introduced, and said: 'I claim one honor, of being the only European oculist who has made his third trip to this country; so you see I enjoy America.'"

Then followed the address of the President of the Association, Doctor Lewis S. MacMurtry (from Louisville, Kentucky). Because of the lively and unruly audience, this was only somewhat understandable by those nearby, but it was also available in print [42], so I can relate the main points:

"When the American Medical Association was organized in 1846 it is doubtful if there were more than 25,000 physicians in the entire United States of America. It was organized as a representative body, composed of delegates from affiliated societies, colleges, and hospitals throughout the states. It was a body of delegates from all state, district, county, and other medical societies which adopted the code of ethics of the national association. The apportionment of delegates was on a basis of one for every ten members of the societies represented.... With the rapid increase in population, the admission of new states to the Union, and the settlement of new territories, came a vast increase of physicians, with a corresponding multiplication of state and county societies.... The sections [developed. The Journal was founded and] has leaped into the very front rank of scientific publications, and in all that a great weekly medical journal should be it has no superior in the world.... It has been the most potent instrument in building up this Association to its present proud position as the largest medical organization in the world.

"[Since 1901, we have] a new constitution, which altered the basis of apportionment for delegates, so as to reduce the delegate body to 150, and definitely established a close relationship between the national organization and the state, district, and county societies. [In addition to the scientific work of the Sections, the House of Delegates can now address matters] appertaining to medical education, to the public health, to national legislation, and to the welfare of the profession. [However,] few of the states have over 50 per cent. of the eligible members of the profession enrolled as members of the society.... The disregard of the good work of the medical profession in the public service ... on the part of Congress is notorious.... In acting as the representative and agent of the 120,000 physicians of the United States the Association is assuming great responsibilities...."

The *Journal of the American Medical Association*, published weekly under the direction of the Board of Trustees, has a press run of more than 36,000 copies and has deservedly received the attention of the German reader, since our important journals regularly report about its contents. I will limit myself to a brief description of one issue (No. 4 from Vol. XLV, 22 July 1905). The issue contains 70 pages and has the following articles:

Intravenous injections of ergot, by E. D. Brown, M.D., Cleveland Ohio. Inguinal hernia of the bladder by S. C. Plummer, M.D., Chicago. Fetal death from looping of cord, by Herbert C. Jones, M.D., Decatur, Ill. Chronic acetanilid poisoning, by Alfred Stengel, M.D., Philadelphia. Potassium chlorate poisoning, by Lester W. Day, M.D., Minneapolis. Then follow editorials, medical news, association news, and current medical literature.

After this description of the association and its journals, you might expect me to make a judgment. (I will first say that I am not one of those tiresome fellows that are called "fault finders" in America.) [43] In my opinion, the American Medical Association, in the manner of its organization and effectiveness, is of great importance for everyone, and not only for the medical men of the United States.

For us, the tighter organization of our German Medical Association with its Doctors' Parliament as well as our Doctors' Councils is probably better, so that we do not need to borrow anything from America. They have, for example, generally suppressed unethical advertising, which is also among the earnest desires of the better doctors in the United States and in many European countries such as Italy.

Freedom of movement for physicians, as it has existed for a generation in Germany, has never arisen as an issue in the United States, since several of the individual states have far too few requirements in their medical licensing examinations!

The combination of social and scientific medical societies is also not worth the effort. Our scientific life is so rich and varied that gathering all our local and specialty societies into a single organization does not seem either appropriate or feasible. The same is true for our medical journals.

The general session I described was the only one at the Portland meeting. The remaining 3½ days were used for the sectional meetings. We ophthalmologists had seven of them, so that I was unable to visit any other sections, and furthermore we were located apart from the others since we needed electric light for our projections.

I will therefore briefly report on the activities of the ophthalmology section, which I attended and in which I participated through presentations and discussions [44].

1. The first session was devoted to the chairman of the section, Dr. C. R. Holmes, who talked about ophthalmologic studies of school and hospital hygiene, illustrated with projected slides. The object of school lighting is relatively simple. The builder is obligated to include as much window area in his plans as is compatible with the safety of the building. Among 30,000 schoolchildren tested in Cleveland during 1889-1900, 20% had poor vision, as did 32% of the schoolchildren in Indianapolis. In hospitals, there must be free access to sunlight and daylight. The question of ventilation is more difficult. All schoolchildren should be promptly examined.

2. Dr. Leartus Connor addressed the question of whether keratitis was caused by rheumatism. Rheumatism can appear first in the dermis and later in the cornea, or the other way around. Most eye doctors say that they have never diagnosed a rheumatic keratitis; it is not even mentioned in most textbooks [45]. The presenter had observed three cases of recurrent keratitis associated with rheumatism (rheumatic arthritis); the keratitis appeared with the rheumatic attack and disappeared when it improved: all three had the advantage of antirheumatic management.

3. Dr. W. H. Snyder from Toledo, Ohio, spoke about the physiologic action of dionin. Corneal edema was seen on postmortem sections from white rabbits whose eyes had been exposed to this powder.

4. Correction of exophoria by the development of the interni, by Dr. W. H. Roberts, Pasadena [46], California. Recommends exercises with prisms.

5. Lateral displacement of tendon insertions, by Dr. Edward Jackson, Denver. If one displaces the attachment of the superior or inferior rectus muscle in a lateral direction, it can improve strabismus.

6. Transitory paralysis of the abducens, by Dr. Meyer Wiener, St. Louis. His cases were unilateral, in young women or girls without other signs of

hysteria.

7. A simple method for localizing ocular foreign bodies using x-rays [47], by Dr. Vard H. Hulen, San Francisco.

8. Blast injuries of the eye, by Dr. John A. Donovan, Butte, Montana.

9. Some eye injuries and their lessons, by Dr. F. C. Heath, Indianapolis.

10. Traumatic lesions of the eye, by Dr. Frank W. Miller, Los Angeles. This was followed by a detailed discussion, in which I myself took part. Dr. Smith of Detroit stated that he had been successful with Hirschberg's magnet in many cases where Haab's had failed.

11. An advancement suture, by Dr. Mark D. Stevenson, Akron, Ohio.

12. On the second afternoon I gave my talk about the ophthalmology of the ancient Arabs. The room was packed full. The audience stood to express its thanks "for the eloquent and learned address" and requested that it be printed in the transactions.

13. Ocular symptoms in sinus diseases, by Dr. W. C. Posey, Philadelphia. It is difficult to diagnose these diseases with nasal examination alone. The ophthalmologist can assist by appreciating certain effects on the eye, for example papilledema, alteration in visual function, displacement of the eyeball, and palsy of ocular muscles, which are so often blamed on rheumatism.

14. The extraction of uncomplicated immature cataracts, by Dr. A. E. Bulson, Jr., Fort Wayne, Indiana. The presenter follows the example of A. Graefe, Hirschberg, and Schweigger. He prefers the combined operation with large keratotomy and wide opening of the capsule; and of course rejects artificial ripening.

15. Endothelio-cylindroma of the orbit, by Dr. John E. Weeks, New York. Vision and mobility of the eye were preserved. These are mixed tumors. But the presenter agrees with Verhoeff that the name cylindroma should be retained, because of the remarkable hyalin change in the mesoblastic parts of these tumors.

16. Preservation and cure of advanced axial myopia through appropriate treatment of the medial and lateral rectus muscles, by Dr. F. S. Crocker, Chicago.

17. Rat-tail tendon for sutures in eye operations, by Dr. Kaspar Pischel, San Francisco. An absorbable suture material, aseptically prepared of course.

18. Tuberculous iritis,[18] diagnosed and managed using Koch's tuberculin, by Drs. W. E. Gamble and E. V. L. Brown, Chicago. The presenters follow the elder Hippel and demonstrated a successful outcome (43rd case in the literature).

19. New test types following a geometric progression, by Dr. C. H. Williams, Boston. Green in St. Louis was the first to specify these, then Javal.

20. Subconjunctival salt injections, by Dr. S. D. Risley, Philadelphia. Weak saline solutions are better than solutions of mercury salts.

21. Sympathetic inflammation after panophthalmitis, by Dr. W. Zentmayer, Philadelphia. The sympathetic inflammation followed a cataract operation and resulted in blindness.

22. Non-toxic amblyopia, by Dr. T. W. Moore, Huntington, West Virginia. He considers visual disturbances due to amblyopia from disuse [48], hysteria, and anesthesia of the retina.

23. Amblyopia caused by wood alcohol (methyl alcohol), by Dr. C. S. G. Nagel, San Francisco. Blindness results from ischemia of the retina. (This toxicity from contaminated liquor is sadly not uncommon in America – fortunately it is rare in our country thanks to laws against contamination of food and drinks.)

24. Spastic astigmatism, by Dr. F. B. Eaton, San Francisco.

25. Melanotic sarcoma of the choroid, by Dr. L. H. Taylor, Wilkes-Barre, Pennsylvania.

26. The etiology of pigmented sarcoma of the choroid, by J. Hirschberg, Berlin. Concerning the role played by congenital pigment particles and Cohnheim's theory.

The chairman closed the successful session with a review and finally announced that the House of Delegates had elected me an Honorary Member of the American Medical Association. Everyone gathered around me and shook my hand cordially.

After my return home, I received the following letter:

> American Medical Association,
> Office of General Secretary.
> 103 Dearborn Ave., Chicago
> 24 August 1905
>
> Prof. Dr. J. Hirschberg, Berlin, Germany
> Dear Sir:
>
> It becomes my pleasure and duty to officially notify you that the House of Delegates of the American Medical Association, at the meeting held in Portland, Oregon, July 11-14, 1905, unanimously elected you an honorary member of the American Medical Association.
>
> Permit me to say that the number of honorary members to be elected each year is limited to three. This year you were the only honorary member elected.
>
> Very truly yours,
> George A. Simmons
> General Secretary.

The pleasures offered by this meeting were numerous and various. There are festivals in the Orient and festivals in the Occident! One great advantage was that the temperature here, near the Pacific coast, was quite tolerable – while the newspapers reported every day about the many cases of heat stroke in New York and Chicago.

On the fairgrounds, a huge wooden hotel (American Inn) had been built on the water. We had a reception there on the first evening, with music, fireworks, snacks. On the second evening we were invited to three private homes, but unfortunately could not attend, because we could not get cabs for the ladies in our party; so we took the streetcar again to the fairgrounds, where the President of the American Medical Association did the honors and pleasant young ladies served us an excellent cold punch.

The third day included a breakfast offered by my old student and friend Prof. Posey for me and several other eye doctors at the University Club, and a dinner at the home of the Portland ophthalmologist Dr. Connor, whose lovely wife was further distinguished by her mastery of the German language. Late in the evening we made another coach and motorboat ride to Oaks, one of the electric-lighted fairgrounds that have been built all over the United States (Chicago, New York), with slides, mazes, funhouses, and other silliness. The chief amusement, on the day after the meeting concluded, was a boat ride up the Willamette and Columbia past the salmon fisheries, where giant wheels turn slowly to catch the great fishes and throw them onto dry land, up to a pleasant clearing in the woods, where the ladies of Portland had arranged a picnic for us. Fifteen hundred pounds of cold cooked salmon meat had been prepared for 2500 people. I received my fair share, and thanks to the consideration of my friends a glass of beer to go with it. That was my last day in Portland, Oregon.

[p. 1135]
On the afternoon of Saturday, 15 July 1905, Dr. Holmes and I boarded the train for San Francisco. It was a "Pullman," that is, with curtains for sleeping, not an individual compartment; however, almost as nicely equipped. The train had a smoking car and dining car, where you can dine *à la carte* at specified times [49]. All through Sunday, in southern Oregon and northern California, we did not encounter any place that could be called a city, but only very small settlements. But the grain in the fields was being harvested with machines that looked like a peaceful version of the murderous scythe chariots of ancient times. There is space here for hundreds of thousands if not millions of inhabitants.

On Sunday morning, the 16th of July, my faithful companion Dr.

Holmes got off the train in Oakland, near San Francisco, in order to catch the next train to New York that was leaving two hours later; I myself took the steamer across the bay and checked into the Hotel St. Francis in San Francisco, one of the most brilliant and best managed in the world in my experience.

I was met there by Dr. Kaspar Pischel, President of the San Francisco Association of Eye-, Ear-, Nose-, and Throat-doctors, who was born in Austria, and was formerly an assistant of Prof. Borysikiewicz in Graz. Dr. Pichel invited me in the name of his association to a reception on the following day, and transported me to his summer residence in San Rafael, not far to the north of San Francisco. It took an hour and a half with streetcar, steamship, electric train, and one-horse carriage to reach our destination.

Thus I spent Sunday afternoon in pleasant company [50]. I was especially interested in his four children, boys and girls ages 6-12. They were treated very considerately, but were obedient and well-behaved, each with a definite individuality. They all swam very well in the artificial pool in the garden – to the distress of their neglected Spitz puppy. They could also ride horseback, except for the smallest one.

During the long time until evening and on the way home questions naturally came up about women and servants. In the course of the lively discussion, I made the perhaps subjective remark that our women had everything they wished; but heard in response that they should be wishing for more: I feel obligated to report this opinion to any colleagues who might want to share it with their wives.

In Europe, it is often said and written that the American husband is kept at hard labor by his wife, but this is certainly not based on the facts. There are very fond marriages in the United States, just as with those of us who enjoy them. It is true that the smaller number of children in true American marriages raises questions for the physician as well as the economist. The easy availability of divorce, just like lynching and graft [51], belong to the childhood diseases of this huge young land, and every observer here and there heartily wishes that they will soon be eliminated. It is a completely false view that the middle-class American woman is pampered; she works harder than her European sister in the same situation. The pleasant and elegant young wife of a lawyer told me that she runs a small household with only one maid and does all the cooking herself, since she has never in the 7 years of her marriage been able to keep a maid who knew how to cook: As soon as one began to make progress under the housewife's supervision in this important skill, she would resign. The housewife also has to manage the children herself. Reliable governesses are difficult to find. This is one reason why the exclusion of Chinese from California has been found so difficult; the Chinese are the most dependable and useful servants. There are not many Negroes in California. The number of Japanese is increasing, but they are not considered reliable and do not make good servants. It should be noted that there is a strong immigration of Japanese doctors into San Francisco. In the Chinese quarter and in the poorer sections of town you see their English and Japanese-Chinese placards: they still mostly care for the Asians, but will soon be competing for the care of Caucasians.

On the morning of July 17, I could see from the "Observation Car" that San Francisco has grown significantly in the past 18 years (since my first visit in 1887). The population has risen from 300,000 to 400,000 [52].

The growth and expansion have especially occurred since the war with Spain (1898). The City Hall, whose construction cost so many millions beyond what was necessary, was nevertheless finished 9 years ago and stood before us with its towering dome, next to the great Californian Monument that was given to the city by the German-American James Lick [53]. I will not say much about the new giant buildings; the largest is the Spreckels Building, constructed by the Sugar King Spreckels, who also came from Germany.[19]

The climate of San Francisco may also be of interest to the medical reader. It is wonderfully temperate. The average annual temperature is 14° C; September is the warmest month (16° C), January the coldest (10° C); in mid-summer it may reach 32° C on some days [54]. At this time it was cool and foggy. As soon as we crossed the bay to the northern peninsula, where the summer residences are, we found bright sunshine and pleasant warmth.

At noon, I visited Dr. Pischel at his office. If you asked a European ophthalmologist who had no idea about American conditions what he would think about an eye doctor's office on the 5th floor – or on the 12th, which I saw in Chicago – he would think it was a ridiculous question. But in a bank or insurance company, or some other giant building constructed by some very rich private man with hundreds of offices, if you can ascend quickly and gently with an electric elevator more comfortably than climbing one flight of stairs in an old-fashioned house, you understand that it all depends upon what you are used to. American patients think nothing of it. Nor do I, as long as the doctors limit themselves to the interventions that we undertake on ambulatory patients.

After I had breakfasted with Dr. Pischel – in a French restaurant for a change – I visited the giant department store [55] that belongs to his father-in-law and brother-in-law, and in particular the art department, which is managed by a knowledgeable associate. I was amazed to learn that

80% of these items came from Europe, even though the tariff constituted 60% of their value. I noted the absence of classical reproductions among the bronzes; these are not in much demand here.

In the afternoon I drove to the famous Cliff House [56]. The trip was inexpensive by streetcar; it cost only 5 cents. First, I visited the old Sutro Park [57], established by the German-American Adolf Sutro (mining engineer and mayor) and opened to the public after his death; and in addition the new Sutro-Seabaths,[20] which are accessible for 10 cents and which I discussed extensively with the founder 18 years before. The surf itself provides the water – similar to the seawater mills of Argostoli on Kephalonia, which I saw in 1886. These sea baths are a healthy establishment for the citizens of San Francisco. A giant wooden building has been constructed: First, you come to zoological and ethnographic collections that seem rather special, to panoramas, taverns, and a theater; then finally you reach the baths themselves.

These consist of six pools in a row; the seawater enters the first, is heated, and then flows into the 2nd, 3rd, 4th, 5th, and 6th, each of them 3-4 feet deep. In No. 2-5 are little boys and girls happily together; only No. 6 is labelled "For Ladies Only" and was almost empty when I saw it. Pools 2-5 each had a slide. One after the next, the boys and girls climbed up the ladder to the top and then slid down the chute, which was kept wet with a flow of fresh water, either on their backs or on their bellies, and shouted for joy as they splashed into the seawater. A huge amphitheater, spanning the length of the row of pools, provided space for thousands of onlookers and was occupied by several hundred.

I spoke to an employee of the baths about a few things that caught my attention, in English of course. But my accent betrayed that I was German, at least for a practiced ear. The young man in charge of the panorama (who I soon discovered was born in Berlin) immediately invited me in German to see his work of art for 10 cents. This gives me the opportunity to point out that German is spoken quite a lot in the United States. Several times on the streetcar or railroad cars I received a German answer to an English question – of course, from German-Americans [58]. In my elegant Hotel St. Francis the maître d'hôtel was a German, who immediately came over to me when I sat down for breakfast in the dining room and took my order in German. Several waiters could and did speak German [59].

That evening, my "reception" was at the Hotel St. Francis. Dr. Pischel was the chairman. My old friend Dr. Barkan had returned to San Francisco for this occasion from his summer vacation (at Lake Tahoe, on the border with Nevada, an 8-hour railroad trip with his entire family!) All the eye doctors of San Francisco were there, the English-speaking and as a third German-speaker Dr. Nagel, as well as other specialists and general practitioners.

The food was excellent, as was the California wine.

The first toast to me was given by Dr. Pischel, in very friendly words. In my response, I alluded to the fact that this wonderful metropolis of the Far West was no older than – the ophthalmoscope, namely about half a century; but similarly had introduced a new era. After Dr. Barkan made some kind remarks and the song "He is a very good fellow" had been sung, he took the floor again and requested that I say something about Albrecht von Graefe. Without hesitation, I described for them a typical day of my mentor from the morning rounds, through the outpatient clinic, operations, private office hours, and finally the evening rounds – ending about midnight. They were entranced. None of them had known A. v. Graefe.

The evening concluded in an elegant hall with marble pillars and space for 1500 people, where we enjoyed a glass of good beer with music and a colorful fountain.

On Tuesday, July 18, my friend Barkan picked me up early in the morning for an excursion to Mount Tamalpais [60]. As usual, we traveled from the hotel by streetcar to the Union Ferry Depot, and from there in a steamer across the bay – with spectacular views of the city, the islands, and the Golden Gate – and then on the northern peninsula first with electric train – whose middle third rail must be avoided since it is lethal to touch; – and finally with the mountain train, which gradually climbs with numerous curves to the peak (795 meters). In addition to my friend's family, there was also a professor of pathologic anatomy, who had grown up in Germany and spent two years as assistant to Prof. Orth, along with his lovely wife. The view included San Francisco and its bay, the coastal mountains, and the ocean. For the trip down, my friend Barkan had rented a small private "gravity car" for us, which descends using its own weight. To be sure, there is a brakeman in the car who said "all right" when I explained that I had promised my wife to return home with all four extremities. This trip is exciting for people with no fear of heights, which included all of us. At the foot of the mountain was Dr. Barkan's summer residence, where we had breakfast. Everyone, including the ladies, spoke only German. The children were bright and good-looking, the young women quite pretty. One thing I learned here was that university studies for women are starting to become less common [61].

I spent the afternoon strolling through the main streets of the city on foot.

As I was dining peacefully at the hotel that evening, a group arrived that included some of my new friends from Portland, and they invited me to join them for the usual tour of Chinatown. I went along like a good sport. But I had concluded 18 years before that this whole show is nonsense that only staged for the benefit of the tour guide (and Chinese beggars). Having visited Hong Kong and Canton 13 years ago had only reinforced my opinion. Who is foolish enough to believe an old Chinaman that he smokes 100 opium pipes every day? The fellow is quite hale and hearty.

On Wednesday the 19th of July, I made an excursion by train with the youngest son of Dr. Barkan out to Palo Alto (34 English miles) to visit the famous Leland Stanford Junior University. This was founded by Mr. and Mrs. Leland Stanford in memory of their only son, who died accidentally at a young age. It was provided with a huge endowment, and since Mrs. Stanford died and left almost her entire estate to the university, it is now valued at 50 million dollars. If money were the only requirement, it would be the top university in the world.

Even Professor Münsterberg [62], who typically takes an optimistic view of American conditions and called this university "a dream in stone, that has grown up under the California palms," had to add: "The thirty million dollars did not create much internal value, since the West is dependent upon western students and mostly western teachers, and it has to take what it can get."

The university opened in 1891. When I was traveling through Canada in 1892, I met two newly appointed professors, of whom one, a young mathematician, came from England. Now it has 150 teachers and 1400 students, the latter including 500 women [63]. It has schools of law, philology, natural science, and engineering. The university is like a small walled city; it occupies a nicely situated area of 3360 hectares at the foot of the coastal mountains that was once a stud farm belonging to the founder. To my disappointment it was vacation time, so I had to be satisfied with looking at the buildings.

I regret to say that the library owns the book collection of Hildebrand (1824-1894), the perpetuator of Grimm's dictionary – just as the books of E. duBois-Reymond have migrated to Chicago. [64]

The art museum is unimportant. Two statues adorn the entrance. One statue representing the founder of newer Attic Comedy has letters engraved by the (Italian) sculptor; he calls it Meandro instead of Menandro. The ornate church has a façade like the cathedral in Siena, except that it does not portray any artwork and is thrown together with no particular style.

You see college buildings with large passageways, laboratories, faculty housing, large dormitories for male and female students, and finally smaller houses called fraternities, somewhat like our student corps, which manage their own finances – even renting out the house during the summer holidays. These fraternities have certain secret activities and are named with certain Greek letters, whose explanation is even difficult for members: for example, ΦΧΒ = φιλοσοφια χυβερνητειρα βιου.[21] At least that is how I understood the words that I heard. Of course, there are also sororities for the women.

I will mention in passing that the university does not permit any alcoholic beverages within its walls. Even worse, the entire surrounding town, apparently through covenants in the property deeds, prohibits the enjoyment of beer, wine, etc. It even required a great effort to obtain a bottle of Appolinaris Water for my modest lunch at the university restaurant. So you can see that not everything is free in the Land of Freedom.

Finally, the reader will be more interested to learn that the university in Palo Alto is used as preparation for medical study. The oldest son of Dr. Barkan has just passed the examination there, will attend the medical school in San Francisco, and finally go to Europe for further education.

On Thursday, July 20, I took the coastal train south to Los Angeles in southern California (Southern Pacific Railroad, 476 English miles in 15 hours, from 7:30 A.M. to 10:30 P.M.), through fruitful regions, past the university in Palo Alto, past the famous observatory of the German-American on Mt. Hamilton, which is visible from a considerable distance. I did not stop to see the beautiful gardens and coast road in Del Monte, nor in Santa Barbara, the American Mentone.[22] The new Angelus Hotel in Los Angeles is almost as good as the exemplary one in San Francisco; for 4½ dollars, I received a room with bath and sitting-rooms. That was really wonderful. Until 1880, this city was of minimal importance. It is located on a small river of the same name, 32 km above its mouth and 23 km in a straight line from the coast, was founded by the Spanish in 1781 with the name of La Puebla de Nuestra Señora la Reina de los Angeles (City of our Lady, Queen of the Angels), and was incorporated into the United States in 1846. With the growth of California's fruit agriculture, it increased its population and importance; in 1900 it already had more than 100,000 inhabitants. In 1910, it will have more than 200,000 – at least that is what we read in different places that were selling house lots.

The growth has been especially rapid in the last few years, since the Spanish War. A captured Spanish cannon in the main plaza is a reminder. It is much more ornate than the usual chimney-like monstrosities, tastefully decorated, and adorned with the motto of Frederick the Great "Ultima razon del rey,"[23] but better here as decoration under a pretty group of trees than on a warship – for it bears the date 1750.[24]

The Americans call this the "mushroom city"; it has indeed sprouted up like a giant fungus. It has skyscrapers like New York, although not as many; there are the same streetcars and large stores. The automobile dealers are no smaller and perhaps no less numerous than in many large European cities. The jewelry stores have nice displays of the most expensive goods. One thing that distinguishes Los Angeles from New York is the abundance of palm trees that one can admire in the suburban streets. There are wonderful fruit markets. All the food is inexpensive. A pound of good beef costs 5 cents, which is as if it cost 20 pfennigs at home. On the other hand, everything that requires skilled manufacture is significantly more expensive in the western United States compared to at home in Europe. Thus, a nice house in the suburbs of Los Angeles costs about as much as in the suburbs of Boston, say 8000 dollars; the land and space are cheaper in Los Angeles, while the building costs are greater.

I learned all this as a pedestrian on my first morning (Friday, July 21) – after having been greeted at my hotel early in the morning by Dr. Babcock, the president of the ophthalmologic society of Los Angeles, and after the inevitable reporter had inquired about my impressions of America.

One American city is very much like another. Unless you want to study something specific in industry, business, or teaching in the United States, you are soon finished. One educated lady in Chicago asked me: "What are you looking for in the United States? When I leave our city, I only travel to Europe."

I will also note that Los Angeles has a mild and consistent climate (average temperature in January 11°, in August 21° C.) although it is not generally considered a winter resort. A Negro who had moved there said to one of my colleagues, "That is the land for me." However, he probably did not mean the free constitution and government – since here the Negro children can attend the public schools, which is not possible in the former slave states in the southeastern United States – but the complete absence of the winter cold, ice, and snow.

There are plenty of excellent winter resorts, especially for patients with lung and kidney diseases. Many doctors are available.

I am quite sure that, once the Panama Canal is finished, patients from Europe will also make the refreshing ocean voyage to southern California, whereas they now have good reason to avoid the dusty and stressful land voyage across the American continent: They will be able to spend the warm season resting on the ocean, the fall on the coast, and the winter in the interior.

That afternoon, I drove through the city and its suburbs by automobile with Dr. Babcock and the Bulson family. I should mention that Dr. Babcock completed his studies in Vienna at the clinic of Fuchs, and teaches ophthalmology in Los Angeles. We visited the medical school [65], which has just established a bacteriology laboratory at great expense (20,000 dollars) and plans to start a publishing house; the rude huts from the Spanish era, the beautiful streets with huge houses, and further the avenues with electric trains that stretch for miles and are lined by pretty wooden houses and expensive mansions with beautiful gardens. However, part of the suburban area is quite disfigured by oil drilling.

A reception took place that evening at the Casa Verduga. This was once a Spanish plantation, is now an inn, and is served by an electric train that runs there (10 English miles). The specific room occupied by our group of twenty was adorned in Mexican-Indian style with blankets and tomahawks: Also the electric lighting simulated the simple lamps of a log cabin.

The food was also Spanish – peppered, the wine Californian; after dinner a Spanish brother and sister entertained us with the song "La Paloma."

The first toast by Dr. Babcock was "for our friends King William and President Roosevelt." In my response, I referred to the fact that Los Angeles was the furthest south I had been in the United States, at the same latitude as Morocco; but what a difference! Morocco is still in the Middle Ages, even in its medical practice and science [66]. In southern California there is no trace of the Middle Ages, only modern times. We exchanged many other friendly words until we parted – rather late. After returning home, another colleague drove us to the California Club, which astounded us with its combination of extreme comfort and great luxury; for Los Angeles is still just a provincial city. (Initiation 200 dollars, annual fee 60 dollars; very exclusive.)

On Saturday, July 22, I made an excursion on the Santa Fé Railroad, which is called the kite-shaped track because of its configuration. From 8:30 to 11:00 A.M. I rode through the endless fields and gardens with small stations where fruit was always being packed for shipment. I got off in Redland and saw Dr. Manges from New York, my former student and now chief at New York's beautiful Mount Sinai Hospital, along with his nephew, a medical student. We made the customary carriage ride through the fields and gardens together. It is amazing what has been done with the southern California desert with 20 years of artificial irrigation (artesian wells in the mountains, dams). You see orange groves that seem greater than the famous Spanish *huertas* that I saw in 1898; and wonderful vineyards. The fruitfulness of the land is so great that they cut the grapevines off at the ground every year. An acre here costs 1 or 2 thousand dollars, with water rights; there are owners of 250 acres and more. Millionaires have built expensive homes and created large parks, where we drove and took in the wonderful views, enjoyed the beautiful flowers, and admired the tree-like aloe plants, which I had not seen so tall since Ceylon in 1892. But you also see industrious schoolhouses and public libraries [67]. We dined very well at a simple inn, but were given nothing to drink except water that we refused. At Highlands, the next station, where we took another drive through even more wonderful fruit gardens, "prohibition" was still in effect [68]. Finally, I was able to obtain a bottle of beer for each of us by asserting as a doctor the necessity of this thirst-quenching measure.

Sunday, July 23, I rode back to San Francisco on the coastal railroad, which is cooler than the interior line, spent the night in my earlier hotel, and departed Monday evening for Denver, Colorado – a trip lasting until Thursday afternoon in blazing heat. This was certainly the most uncomfortable part of my American journey. Even stamping the round-trip ticket required for the return trip was irksome for a man accustomed to European courtesies, so that I cashed in the ticket in Denver [69] and simply bought new tickets from city to city. Even our famous Czerny wrote in his *Holiday Excursion to San Francisco*: "I was constantly amazed at the patience with which the Americans tolerate their mistreatment by the great railway companies."

I do not understand how Professor Münsterberg can advise the German traveler to bring "only a small bag with a few books for the journey": My sturdy leather handbag, which I used "around the world" and which excited the admiration of the reporters in Denver, was sufficient but was unfortunately quite difficult to store; I had to bring it to my double bed at night. Anyway, I will not mention it again, since I certainly have no wish to remake the world.

Fortunately, I withstood this trip through the deserts of Nevada and Utah [70]. In Salt Lake City, where we had a five-hour stop on Wednesday July 26, I visited not only the Mormon Temple but also their President Mr. Smith, nephew of the founder, an intelligent worthy gentleman.

Thursday the 26th at 4:00 P.M., I arrived in Denver, accompanied by Dr. Jackson and two other colleagues, who had joined me in Colorado Springs.

Once again, I was surrounded by the most thoughtful care and concern. First, we drove to a travel agent friend of Dr. Jackson, where I obtained a reasonable ticket on the best train for Chicago, including a ticket for one section of the sleeping area. Then I checked into the new Brown Palace Hotel, where I had an excellent and well-appointed room. I had just gotten out of the bath when I was interrupted by a gentleman who (falsely!) claimed he had been sent by my friend Dr. Jackson – a reporter. His questions were particularly foolish, especially related to eyeglasses, so that I had him promise not to use these words in his report. The next morning, an article appeared in the chief newspaper of Denver, with the headline in red ink "Americans are Eyeglass Fiends, Declares World-Famed Oculist." This experience convinced me not to have anything more to do with journalists.

The dinner arranged for me by my Denver colleagues, Jackson, Coover, Libby, Melville Black, and others at the Brown Palace was once again very hospitable – with real champagne but without toasts, in random collegial conversation. Sheltered on the high plains (1607 meters above sea level) in Denver, "Queen of the Plains," especially in my excellent bed, I slept much better than in the non-sleeping cars of the previous nights.

The next morning, I was picked up by Dr. Libby, a kindly, well-educated colleague who had also visited my clinic years before and who drove me in a small carriage through the city, to the Capitol, by the houses and gardens of the suburbs, to the park, where the statue of Burns has the following inscription [71]:

> A poet peasant born,
> Who more of fame's immortal dower
> Unto his country brings,
> Than all her kings.

At 11:00 A.M. I was picked up for an automobile ride through the surrounding area. We visited a lung sanitorium founded by a private individual for 120 beds, which was constructed in exemplary fashion. The patients can spend both day and night in an open veranda. The treatment regimen can be described as quite minimal for the circumstances there. All the places are occupied.

The climate in Denver is considered ideal for pulmonary patients; that of the nearby Colorado Springs is similar to Davos.

We all had lunch together at the University Club, which is nicely furnished [72].

I was earnestly queried about all the important areas of practice, especially the magnet operation. They did not hide the fact that they were "delighted" about my visit.

After this, I visited the office of Dr. Jackson and learned something new. A doctor had put up a building in a desirable area of the city, only two stories high but quite spacious, exclusively for private medical consultations, and had rented it out to a few doctors at favorable rates. This extends to private practice the benefits that we have from common or neighboring outpatient clinics.

Dr. Jackson brought me to the train and before I left put the symbol of the American Medical Association (A.M.A.) in my buttonhole [73], since I was now entitled to carry it. I had scarcely taken my place in the train when a gentleman introduced himself to me as a doctor from Chicago. He had studied in Berlin 10 years earlier and once – out of curiosity – had attended one of my lectures. Thus, I immediately had a good companion for the trip [74].

We rode through the treeless prairie. The night was fine. The cars were better than in the last train. Of course, I had a section to myself. Each section had an electric light, which (for America) was very pleasant. At night we rode through Nebraska, on Saturday July 29 through Iowa, whose endless cornfields were broken here and there by a bush or a few trees. In the evening, I reached Chicago.

Dr. Frank Allport, who of course had been informed of my arrival by telegraph, received me with his medical carriage, driven skillfully by his faithful Negro John. I was greeted and welcomed into his home like an old friend.

[p. 1191]

Chicago is without doubt one of the most remarkable cities on our planet. In my book *From New York to San Francisco* I sketched out the amazing history of the development of this city and compared the population growth to that of Berlin, "the most American city of Europe," as it is called:

> In 1840, Chicago had 4,179 inhabitants, Berlin about 400,000;
> In 1880, Chicago had 491,516 inhabitants, Berlin about 1,200,000;
> In 1905, Chicago and Berlin each have about 2 million.

Of course, it is not up to me to elaborate on the beautiful and ugly sides of Chicago – on the one hand the remarkable avenues and boulevards, the huge parks in the north and south, and the drive along the shore of Lake Michigan, on the other hand the skyscrapers, the dark streets hemmed in by the elevated train, and the slaughterhouses – since I have neither space nor time, and since the interested reader can find out about these things if he looks for them.

On Sunday morning, July 30, I drove with Dr. Allport to St. Luke's Hospital, which even the leading doctors admit is in the worst location for a hospital, although they cannot immediately change it.[25] We also drove into the very center of the giant city and I reserved a ticket and sleeping-car for the trip to Boston. In the afternoon, Dr. and Mrs. Allport and I all took a long walk through the extensive and wonderful South Park[26] and went to the Washington Club House, where Mrs. Allport had arranged a dinner where I could meet some of the leading doctors who had not been present at the ophthalmologic reception on July 3. Dr. Billings and Dr. Church, who are well known in Europe, were invited with their families, as well as the two brothers of Dr. Allport and others. We did not get home until midnight.

The next morning (July 31) I had the great pleasure of touring Chicago with Mrs. Allport: John, the worthy Colored gentleman, drove us in the carriage. We visited one of Chicago's largest banks, whose director Mr. Hubbard and his wife had traveled with us on the voyage from Bremerhaven to New York; then the largest department store on Earth (Marshall Field), and finally Dr. Allport's office. This is in a huge bank building, on the 12th floor. Three eye doctors have formed a partnership, and each has an assistant doctor. We are certainly not used to this. On the other hand, it is unfortunate that many major European cities [75] cannot overcome small-town jealousies.

Dr. Allport showed me a case of an iron splinter in the eye. Following the plan that I outlined and he adopted, he had operated successfully the next day – in the hospital, of course, not in the 12th-floor office.

Then he showed me the public Illinois Eye and Ear Hospital, which is under his direction and is very nicely equipped. I discovered that the Giant(-Magnet) was asleep, that is, without electricity. This resulted in immediate investigation and correction, so at least our visit may benefit the next case of iron splinter in the eye that requires treatment at the hospital.

Next we visited Dr. Allport's brother, a very accomplished surgeon, who has furnished his house with remarkable adornments. The entire central staircase is decorated from top to bottom with pictures of physicians. For many of them, they only knew the name under the picture; they were very pleased when I wrote down the title of the *Biographical Lexicon of Leading Physicians* by August Hirsch, and proposed that they develop a catalog for their remarkable and educational collection with the aid of this work.

After a drive through the extensive North Park [76][27] I had been invited to a dinner by Mrs. Hubbard at the private hotel where this childless couple has resided for several years. The conversation was very animated and included the Constitution of the United States and its design. It can be explained to educated Americans that we in Germany are just as free as they are in America – in many respects more free.

Tuesday, August 1, I departed from my worthy hosts and traveled by comfortable train to Boston, where I arrived on the following day, checked into the excellent Hotel Touraine and had the pleasure of spending another day with Dr. and Mrs. Holmes.

On August 3, I toured by automobile the main points of interest in Boston: Bunker Hill, where the first important battle of the Revolutionary War took place (17 July 1775), the old church, "Italian City," the memorial hall downtown. After lunch we went on foot to the beautiful State House with its opulent memorial hall [77].[28]

Then I was met by the son of my old friend and colleague Hasket Derby, Dr. George Strong Derby, who is also an ophthalmologist at the hospital, studied in Vienna and Freiburg (with Prof. Axenfeld), and is a member of the Heidelberg Ophthalmologic Society. On an interesting automobile tour, Dr. Derby showed me the beautiful parks of Boston and its suburbs, for example Brookline, which according to Baedeker is the wealthiest town on Earth. We also saw the idyllic Harvard University, surrounded by greenery, with numerous lecture halls and the residences of faculty and students [78].

Harvard University, with an undergraduate college, a law school, and philosophic graduate school, is located on the other side of the Charles River; its medical school, a beautiful still-incomplete new construction is on the Boston side, in Brookline. Right next to Harvard University is the Germanic Museum opened in 1903 with the gifts of our Emperor.[29]

Friday, August 9 at 9:00 A.M., Dr. Derby Jr. took me to the Eye Hospital. This is one of the best and largest that I saw in the U.S., and also one of the oldest, since it has been there since 1827. At the time, only the youngest doctors were active. I saw a large number of well-performed cataract cases. Dr. Quackenboss operated on two cases that I observed, with great dexterity. I myself assisted with a magnet operation – the iron splinter was visible right next to the optic disc, with a negative x-ray! Sideroscope was not available. The giant magnet pulled the splinter (which had been in the eye for 2 days) immediately into the anterior chamber; however, it heated up so quickly that it could not have been used for a longer operation [79]. The medium and small magnets were far less useful than my model.

After that, I was shown some excellent exhibits in the hospital laboratory by Dr. Verhoeff, who has also studied with us and is sufficiently known to his colleagues through publications both in English and in German.

I devoted the afternoon to visiting the famous Trinity Church, the museum [80], which is off to a respectable start, and the library.

This last (Public Library), whose façade is based on that of Ste. Geneviève de Paris and was built during 1888-1895 for 2½ million dollars, contains 836,000 volumes and is thought to be the largest public library in the world. It has a wonderful marble staircase. The historical paintings of Puvis de

Chavannes, the symbolic frescoes of Sargent, the paintings from the Grail Saga, whose long printed explanations are more eagerly and painstakingly studied by the numerous visitors than the paintings themselves, are not completely according to my taste; but that may be – just me. The mechanical equipment, which one of the librarians showed me, is quite remarkable: The tickets with the titles of the requested books are sent downstairs by a tube system, and the books are placed in baskets and returned by the same method. The library in Boston is public. I was pleased to see schoolboys and schoolgirls diligently leaning over their children's books, including some neatly dressed Negro girls; – I saw on a poster that books can be taken out for summer vacation; – I heard from the librarian that in the rare instances when a loaned book is lost, they immediately get a new copy. However, the strictly scientific department is not as abundantly supplied. At least, I looked at the subsection of books on "Ophthalmology"; these seemed rather meager.

At home, we provide for the popular readership through school, public, and municipal libraries; our distribution of these literary collections is fundamentally better and should continue to grow.

In the evening, I was taken to the University Club and dined with five colleagues in the open air on the terrace by the bank of the wide, stately Charles River. The food was good, we drank German *Steinwein*, and the conversation was animated. They asked me whatever they wanted to know. I did not hide the fact that I had omitted Boston from my first trip to America, "for hope of return," but this time had saved it for last, and did not regret doing so. It is the most European city of the United States, or perhaps the least American, and seems to me like an anomaly. Here there are historical memories, here the revolution began: The memorial in the Commons shows the Pillar of Freedom treading on the crown of the English king. Here you can see the development of art: The monument of Lincoln with the emancipated Negro slave at his feet is significant [81], the museum educational even for someone familiar with European institutions. Here I saw an ophthalmologic clinic that any European university would treasure. We did not go home until very late.

But at this point, I started getting very homesick. I gave up the plan to visit first my friend Holmes and his family on the seacoast and then his mother-in-law in the Adirondack Mountains; I traveled on August 6 to New York, stayed at the friendly home of Knapp, exchanged my return ticket for August 15 on the steamer *Kaiser Wilhelm II* for a place on the *Kaiser Wilhelm der Große* leaving August 8. I spent the afternoon at Knapp's eye clinic, and the evening with him at the famous Luna Island,[30] and the next morning departed from Hoboken and landed in Bremerhaven on the afternoon of the 15th.

The reader who has patiently followed my medical and non-medical comments, who has accompanied me through my statistical notes and meeting reports, my travel descriptions and receptions, may now rouse himself indignantly and call out, "No, you don't get off that easy! Let us see your true colors! What do you think of America? What do you think of the American universities, American medical education? Should we be exchanging professors?"

What do I think of America? Fortunately, nothing comes immediately to mind, and this is not the place to discuss that in detail. I have already given my viewpoint briefly 18 years ago [82]. I consider the developing culture beneath the stars and stripes from the viewpoint of an observer, who always holds high his own black-white-red flag. On our planet bristling with weapons, whose remotest lands have been brought so near through steam power and electricity, but whose differing people cannot in in the same way be neighbors in their hearts, it falls to us men of science to use our feeble powers to work for the unity of mankind.

In science, there are fortunately no protective tariffs and no tariff wars, but simply the free and unhindered exchange of toll-free ideas; we will not and need not be concerned about whether we are giving more than we receive [83].

Regarding American universities, it is difficult for Americans or foreigners living in America to orient themselves, and even more so for us on this side of the ocean. Also, there are no official documents corresponding to ours about "The German Universities" (Berlin 1893 and 1904) [84]. We may be directed to the excellent work written by the English statesman James Bryce, "The American Commonwealth," which is from half a generation ago – and that means a lot in the rapidly-changing life of America; or the work that was published last year by the German Hugo Münsterberg, Professor at Harvard University in Boston, which is in many ways half a generation in advance, since in addition to the current conditions it also envisions future [85] developments in lively colors.

At the time when the first English settlers came to America, the colleges [86] had become the principal teaching units in the English universities.

Therefore, the first institutions for higher learning in the New England colonies were founded on the college model. The honor of founding the first institution for higher education in the English part of America belongs to the Puritan minister John Harvard, who had studied at the Emmanuel College of Cambridge in England and at his death in 1638 left half of his fortune to establish a school in the small town of Newton (later Cambridge) near Boston. The young State of Massachusetts took the little school under its wing; later it became independent and has today become the most famous university in America.

The State of Virginia had to work for 30 years before it could establish the William and Mary College in 1693. Rev. Blair, who requested a school for preachers to save souls, was answered by Governor Seymour "Damn your souls! Make tobacco!" These were followed by Yale College in Connecticut in 1700, Princeton College in New Jersey in 1746, the University of Pennsylvania in 1749, Kings College (now Columbia College) in New York in 1754, and Rhode Island College (now Brown University) in 1764. After the Revolution there was a new impetus for founding institutions of higher learning: At Jefferson's urging, the University of Virginia was designed more on the model of the universities of the European continent.

We should not be confused by the name "university." In the West this may perhaps signify a very mediocre college corresponding to a German *secunda*.[31] In the East, a university is generally a first-rate college along with graduate schools for medicine, law, teaching, and technology. Only the actual name of the institution matters, for example Harvard College.

Prof. Münsterberg says: "The entire system of higher education can only be understood in this context, which seems self-explanatory to Americans." It seems obvious for us that only a portion of the higher education in the U.S. achieves the same level that we have throughout Germany. When he adds that "above all, there is an emphasis on the college, an unfamiliar concept in Germany; it cannot be otherwise, and under this sign America will conquer," I do not know whom it is that America will conquer. If he means the western "universities" that I just mentioned, I agree and wish them success. If he means the German universities, he is wrong. The best Americans are trying to equal our university education [87]. And even if our teaching methods are still evolving [88], nobody involved in this process is irrational enough to destroy our universities and replace them with American colleges.

Prof. Münsterberg has done a good job of describing how things have developed in America, but he consistently proceeds from the false principle that America enjoys greater freedom than Germany. We will soon cite some facts that show the opposite for the area of higher education.

The religious sects established seminaries, legal scholars united to establish law schools, physicians to establish medical schools – all without the collaboration of the national government, which over there has as little to do with higher education as it does with grammar schools. But the individual state must intervene if private efforts are insufficient – thus we come to the

"State Universities," especially in the western states of Ohio, Michigan, etc.; in addition, the state must grant the individual institutions the right to award degrees and diplomas. However, the doctoral degree generally does not require a state examination.

The college is supposed to provide a general education. Whoever has completed college is considered an educated person, regardless of chosen profession. The little prairie college is more comparable to the *tertia* and *secunda* of a German *Real-Schule*; the best correspond to the German *prima* plus perhaps three semesters in a philosophical faculty. Whoever completes college becomes a Bachelor of Arts (B.A.).

Here and there a college may have an associated graduate school, with the goal of a Doctor of Philosophy, a law school, medical school, etc.

The college is led by a Rector or President, who is chosen by the board of trustees and installed for life, usually a professor of the philosophical faculty, and who is granted almost unlimited authority [89]. The trustees serve in an honorary capacity and are chosen by the alumni.

Harvard College has 5000 students: Some of them work as hard as the specialty student; "another group, not the worst, would consider such an imposition to be an insult."

Another final word: The very large endowments available to individual American universities should not arouse our envy. Given the circumstances, Germany spends more on higher education. And not everything can be bought with money. "Can I buy Olympia?" I was asked in 1890 on the Isthmus of Corinth by a delegate of a wealthy American university; when I smiled and said no, he asked, "Can't I buy Delphi?"

As I turn from these brief and necessarily incomplete remarks about the American colleges to a consideration of their medical schools, I should mention that some individual state universities, for example that of Michigan in Ann Arbor, do have a department for medicine and surgery (and also a homeopathic college); however, most medical schools in the United States are private institutions, which have received the right to award a doctoral degree from the corresponding state.

To the credit of our American specialty colleagues, I should especially emphasize that they fight strongly against the inappropriate extension of this right to institutions that do not deserve it, and quite often declare war on their legislative bodies and threaten to exterminate their own mediocre medical schools. [90]

I have in front of me the *California State Journal of Medicine* from April 1905:

> With the deepest and most profound reverence one may well say, Thank God! The Legislature has adjourned *sine die*! Fortunately, no harm has been done so far as the relations of the physician to the public are concerned, and the standards required for eligibility to practice medicine within the state remain unchanged. . . .
> Assembly Bill No. 1164, which amended the same law in the section defining the practice of medicine in such a way as to permit any pharmacist to practice medicine or surgery, was, on the same day, refused passage by a vote of 13 to 34. The two bills representing the very acme of superlative legislative asininity, the bills creating a board of examiners of "naturopathy" (?)... died on the file. [91]

Medical education in the United States [92] has indeed made significant progress. In recent years, the requirements for entry into the medical schools as well as for graduation have risen. The examining boards for the state examinations [93] have made fundamental contributions. The number of registered medical students in the U.S. for the academic year ending 30 June 1905 was 26,147, which was a decrease of 1,995 compared to the year 1904 [94]. Of these, 24,119 were in regular medical schools, 1104 in homeopathic schools, 578 in eclectic schools, 114 in "physiomedical" schools, and 232 in unclassifiable schools. The decrease affected the latter schools, not the regular medical schools, which showed a slight increase. In the year 1905, there were 5,606 graduates. There were 1073 female medical students, that is 4.1% of the overall total [95].

Among the medical schools there are 126 regular, 18 homeopathic, 9 eclectic, 3 physiomedical, and 1 unclassifiable. In the past year, 2 homeopathic colleges merged, and 1 eclectic changed its philosophy and became a regular school. Six of the 126 regular schools do not award degrees, since they teach only the first and second years. Three colleges (2 regular and 1 homeopathic) are exclusively for women, 63 exclusively for men, and 91 coeducational. Five are exclusively for Negroes. 68 of the regular colleges, 4 homeopathic, and 1 eclectic are associated with a university or a literary college. Two colleges in Chicago only have classes in the evening [96]. There is also improvement in the duration of study. In the year before last, 56.8% of the colleges had a study period of less than 18 months, and last year this figure was only 39%; 61.8% had an academic year of 8 or 9 months.

It is of interest to consider the admission and graduation examinations of the main schools.

Every college that is a member of the American Medical Association must require for admission: a) a bachelor's degree from a recognized college or university; b) evidence of 8 years' education in a recognized secondary school; c) an examination in mathematics, English, history, languages (including Latin), and sciences: However, this examination can be replaced by an explicit testimonial. Transfer from one medical college to another is possible except for the final year, and requires a written testimonial from the dean of the first college regarding morals and effort. The candidate for the doctoral examination must give evidence of 4 years of study, each year consisting of at least 30 weeks. The entire course must include at least 4000 hours: Of this must be included [97]

	Lecture	Laboratory	Clinical Total
Histology	30	60	90
Anatomy	190	230	420
Pathology	100	140	240
Medicine	180	360	540
Surgery	180	360	540
Eye/Ear	30	30	60

They have produced a list of 63 medical schools that meet these criteria, with which a German university teacher could generally agree, if he is reconciled to the omission of Greek.

In some schools, however, instruction in the theoretical subjects (anatomy, physiology, pathology, bacteriology, pharmacology) does not seem up to the desired level [98]. On the other hand, any German reader would take pleasure in admiring the illustrations of the beautiful laboratories of the Pennsylvania University in Philadelphia that Prof. Orth [99] recently showed us in an enlightening publication.

Furthermore, we also have more clinical instruction. A student who spends the summer with us in the eye clinic has at least 60 clinical hours just for ophthalmology. Some of my young American friends, who had not even had 20 hours of eye clinic admitted to me that they saw and evaluated more clinical cases in a week with us than during their entire course at home.

The requirements of the homeopathic colleges are much fewer. For admission, they require: 1. An English essay on a given topic, at least 200 words; 2. Mathematics (fractions, decimals, quadratic and cubic roots, etc.); 3. Geography (the main facts about North America); 4. History, especially progress in art, science, and literature; 5. Latin (4 books of Caesar). By 4 is added: The examination will avoid exact dates and minor details. That is a great comfort for the examinees [100]. (In my day, if we substitute German for English and take out 4, all this would have been required for the *Unter-Secunda*.)

The eclectic schools require for admission either a diploma or an examination demonstrating a good English education, including elementary knowledge of natural history, physics, and Latin. (Here also I can only see the requirements of a *Secunda*.)

The following states and territories of the U.S. have no medical school: Arizona, Delaware, Florida, Hawaii, Idaho, Indian Territory, Montana, Nevada, New Mexico, North Dakota, Puerto Rico, Rhode Island, South Dakota, Utah, Washington, Wyoming.

They do not have collegiate fees in our sense, since the number, type, and order of the lectures, clinics, and exercises are prescribed to the students. However, the costs of instruction are published for individual medical schools. I will specify a few numbers:

Cooper Medical College, San Francisco: 4x150+80	= 680 dollars
College of Physicians and Surgeons, University of Illinois, Chicago	= 612 dollars
Johns Hopkins Medical School, J. H. University, Baltimore, Maryland	= 800 dollars
College of Physicians and Surgeons, Columbia University, New York	= 780 dollars
Medical School of Harvard University [101], Boston, Massachusetts	= 805 dollars
University of Pennsylvania Department of Medicine, Philadelphia, Pennsylvania	= 805 dollars

These fees are not high for American conditions. We should recall that for us the costs of medical instruction on average have been estimated as 2000 Mark = 500 Dollars [102].

These are the facts about medical schools that I have carefully abstracted from the official *Journal of the American Medical Association*. It is not my place to recommend improvements. At any rate, we can see that the Americans themselves are working hard to elevate and improve medical education. Finally, I will emphasize that continuing medical education is well organized and well supervised. On 4 April 1882, Prof. Roosa, an excellent eye- and ear-doctor in New York, founded the first independent Post-Graduate Medical School. This has its own hospital and journal. The course lasts for 1 year (honorarium 450 dollars); auditors are also accepted for 6 weeks. 9565 doctors have so far attended this worthy institution. (Recent American and

German publications fail to mention that Berlin is the originator of continuing education courses. The Berlin Docents' Union [103] for Vacation Courses between 1880 and 1894 has taught 16,293 doctors. This included thousands of Americans.)

"What do you conclude from your own experiences with American students?"

Well, I have taught hundreds during my 35-year career as a university teacher [104] — but these were not students; they are not the ones who come [105].

It is postgraduate doctors that want to continue their education; and these are certainly the better ones, full of curiosity, ambition, and generally in a relatively secure financial condition. They are older than our students; many of them married [106], some of them actually on their (extended) honeymoon. Their talents are no different from our German attendees, their diligence quite satisfactory, their preparation usually somewhat inferior to the German students. Thus their training takes relatively more time. Language difficulties are not a major factor. After the German lectures and in the outpatient clinic we have provided explanations in their mother tongue to anyone who wishes or needs them; our American gentlemen have learned German fairly quickly, so that they are able to examine patients after a few months, an educational opportunity they have grasped gladly and enthusiastically. My outpatient records contain hundreds of eye examinations entered by American hands. Several American doctors have spent a long time studying with me and are my friends, and have become professors at home. One of them was my assistant for three years, beloved by the patients as well as by the leader of the institute, with complete mastery of the German language (even for literary activity) and very well trained. Although as a rule I prefer not to hire foreigners [107], in a special case I am inclined not to be or seem to be exclusive.

"What do you think about an exchange of professors?" A reporter [108] asked me this question as soon as I arrived in Boston, in the lobby of the Hotel Touraine; however, I declined to give him an answer. Even here, I do not intend to answer the question in general, although I agree with the anonymous, including to me, scholars and countrymen who asserted in the German *Rundschau* [109] that a comparable status has not yet been achieved. In my specialty, none of the many professors with whom I delved into such intensive discussions about university teaching made even the mildest suggestion that this was the case; all of them recognized the advantages of German university education for young American doctors [110], and two of them wanted to send me their sons for further education. We should hesitate to offer the Americans things that they do not expect. We should hesitate to Americanize ourselves at a time when the best American scientists are trying to Germanize themselves. The friendly relations and the hospitality should remain, indeed should grow and be extended. I advise any colleague who can avoid it not to emigrate to America. I advise any colleague who can afford it to enlarge his experience by traveling to the United States. "Fewer emigrants, more visitors." It seems to me that this would be most beneficial for our fatherland.

Original Notes

1. See *Von New York nach San Francisco*, by J. Hirschberg, Leipzig 1888; *Um die Erde, eine Reisebeschreibung*, by J. Hirschberg, Leipzig 1894.
2. "The removal of foreign bodies from the eye," *Journal of the American Medical Association*, August 30, 1902. (14 pp.)
3. *The Importance of General Therapeutics in the Treatment of Ocular Diseases*, Glasgow 1905. (39 pp.)
4. Likewise on all my journeys I speak German until I see that it is not being understood. When I climbed the Great Pyramid in Egypt, I sought out a German-speaking Arab out of the crowd of guides speaking all possible languages. If I am in Switzerland or Italy and somebody asks "Do you speak English," I reply "Yes, if necessary."
5. From Berlin to Bremerhaven   408 km
   From Bremerhaven to New York   6,631 km
   From New York to Portland (Oregon)   <u>5,456 km</u>
       12,495 km

   The circumference of the Earth is 40,000 km
6. History of Ophthalmology II, 1, History of Arabic Ophthalmology, *Handbook of General Ophthalmology*. (Graefe-Saemisch), XIII, B, 243 pp. Leipzig: W. Engelmann, 1905. The special edition of this book is "Dedicated to the Ophthalmology Section of the American Medical Association in Portland, Oregon, July 1905," and I delivered the first copy there myself.
7. I would recommend this to anyone who undertakes something similar. If you write it out first in German and then translate it (or have it translated) into English, the style will not be as good. In 1877, I made this mistake with my "Historical notice concerning the doctrine of the smallest visual angle," which I published in the *Royal London Ophthalmic Hospital Reports*. But in 1879, when I was first invited to

Cork, Ireland, as guest of honor of the British Medical Association, I wrote my address "On the quantitative analysis of diplopic strabismus" directly in English and it was published in the *British Medical Journal* (1 July 1880).
8. "*Einen Vortrag halten*" in English is "to read a paper." Had I spoken in my native language, I would never have let a piece of paper separate me from my audience.
9. Whoever has not made at least one voyage to America should not dare to make this claim. But I have passed many tests. During the 65 days of ocean travel on my trip around the world, I consumed 195 main meals with a good appetite.
10. I will not describe the ship, the departure, the travelers, or life aboard ship here. Those interested in a doctor's description of these things should refer to my book *Um die Erde* [*Around the World*].
11. Even in midsummer, the Atlantic Ocean between New York and north Germany can be quite cool. A warm suit is advisable. Americans who often make this journey in the hot time of year bring a trunk with warm clothing and leave it in storage with Lloyd until they return to Bremerhaven from Italy or Switzerland.
12. What do you know? In one major American city a "former first assistant of mine" was in practice, whose name was completely unfamiliar to me.
13. *Centralblatt für Augenheilkunde*, May 1885.
14. I had also chosen this European method on my earlier journeys; it is more expensive. The American method consists of entrusting your luggage to an agent of the transportation company and personally using the ferry and streetcar; in that case, it can take several hours for your luggage to arrive.
15. Νεα ασπρορουχα and νεωτατα.
16. Actually, I had obtained a thin, black-bound, plain volume consisting only of the first 80 pages that pertained to New York.
17. C. Herzog, Imperial State Secretary found even 24 years ago that the traffic in New York was "more hasty, pushy, and energetic" than in London City at noontime. See his very readable *Reisebriefe*, I, 1884.
18. The truck drivers seem to be more considerate of the pedestrians than in dear old Berlin. Nevertheless, they tend to have more accidents than we do: First, because women and children are driving dangerous vehicles, and second, because the daring Yankees often risk their own lives by excessive speed.
19. At a reception in my honor in Tokyo in 1892, the Japanese also had a

menu showing the flag of the German Empire next to that of Japan – but the German colors were in the wrong order.

20. *Archives of Ophthalmology*, edited by H. Knapp. Volumes I-XXXIV, from 1869 to the present. Also published in a German edition with the title *Archiv für Augenheilkunde*; I edited this German edition 1879-1881 and brought it to its current form; my successor was C. Schweigger, and the current editor is Carl Hess.

    American Journal of Ophthalmology, edited by Dr. Alt, St. Louis, 1889 to the present, Volumes I-XXII.

    The Ophthalmic Record, edited by Casey Wood, Chicago, from 1891. (The first volumes were edited by Dr. Savage, Nashville, Tennessee.)

    Annals of Ophthalmology founded by Parker, Kansas City, 1891 until Volume XIII, 1903.

    Ophthalmology, edited by Wurdemann, Milwaukee, starting 1903.

    The Journal of Eye, Ear, and Throat Diseases, founded by Chisolm, 1896.

    The first American journal of ophthalmology was founded by a German, Julius Homburger, with whom I was acquainted, but it lasted only a few years. (*American Journal of Ophthalmology*, 1862-1865. Julius Homburger, Editor, New York.) I would also mention the *Transactions of the American Ophthalmologic Society*, around thirty volumes, and the reports of Eye Clinics, especially the *New York Eye and Ear Infirmary Reports* of Weeks, since 1893.

21. See also Harry Friedenwald, "The early history of ophthalmology and otology in Baltimore," *Johns Hopkins Bulletin* Aug-Sept 1897; *Progress in Ophthalmology* by Casey Wood, 1899; *Early (prior to 1860) British and American Ophthalmology*. Literature by Casey Wood, 1902.

22. I was asked to prepare the section on wound management; however, I could not take this on, because I was too busy with other work at the time.

23. The same goes for the other (French and Belgian) claims of priority. Dieffenbach performed the first strabismus operation in 1839.

24. A nice new invention are the "invisible bifocals."

25. It is remarkable that this important tool, which I myself have tried to improve, was generally absent from the ophthalmology clinics I visited this time. The eye magnets that I saw were also mostly mediocre. This is all the more surprising because electrical applications, for example illumination, are done very well in the United States. Except for street lights! These were mostly placed too low, often flickered, and were insufficiently frosted: In this area, Berlin is ahead of the American cities.

26. There is an old saying that I learned in school, whose author I cannot recall at the moment: "Empires grow by the same forces that founded them." Immigration to the United States is starting to become uncomfortable: There are more Slavs and Italians arriving instead of Germans and English. Certain guarantees may be demanded, I can understand that. But restricting immigration could be a disaster.
27. *The Sphenoidal Cavity and its Relation to the Eye.* Cincinnati 1896.
28. I can cite it from memory: "This wide world with its rivers and seas, cities and castles, hills and valleys is narrow and empty, unless there is a good friend here and there who thinks lovingly of us."
29. The room with bath rented just for the daytime was not at all expensive, 2 dollars.
30. Editor of *A Treatise on Diseases of the Eye, Nose, Throat, and Ear*, Philadelphia and New York 1903 (1233 pp.)
31. We received a printed catalog of the books, and also a complete passenger list, as is customary these days on a steamship crossing the Atlantic Ocean.
32. The text says 75%.
33. In the *Journal of the American Medical Association* issue from 2 September 1905 (XLV, Nr. 10) a report of this year's Fourth of July casualties reads "In this issue appears an annual summary of the accidents due to the idiotic methods of celebrating our national anniversary. The list, which no one can claim to be absolutely complete, is yet sufficiently appalling."
34. *Zahme Xenien*, VI.
35. See *Um die Erde*, p. 36.
36. They politely declined to be quizzed on the anatomy of the eye, since they had not yet studied it.
37. *Von New York nach San Francisco*, p. 123.
38. One building had the inscription "Katzenjammer-Palace, a great amusement." (Well!)
39. "I register" is the usual expression.
40. *Von New York nach San Francisco*, p. 128.
41. You can hardly imagine the number of business, charitable, and religious organizations, masonic brotherhoods, women's clubs, etc. who are all pleased to make use of such an opportunity.
42. See the *Journal of the American Medical Association* XLV, No. 3, 15 July 1905.
43. *Von New York nach San Francisco*, Foreword, p. vi.
44. A brief report has been published in *The Ophthalmic Record*, Chicago,

August 1905. Some of the presentations have been printed in the *Journal of the American Medical Association.*
45. Well, not quite all. In Arlt's *Klinische Darstellung der Krankheiten des Auges* from 1881 there is a chapter on rheumatic keratitis on p.123.
46. A beautiful town near Los Angeles in southern California.
47. The presenter said "x-rays," as do most English speakers. I say "Röntgen rays." Otherwise, people may forget that a German made this discovery. In Utrecht, a Londoner urged me to visit London to see his collection of "x-ray photographs." I thanked him politely, but added that we in Berlin make extensive use of this discovery by our countryman and have our own excellent collections.
48. The presenter used the term "*ex anopsia,*" which is not the appropriate term. Ανοψια means "lack of side dishes."
49. Thus it is no longer the way it was 18 years ago, when you could get a full meal and eat your fill three times a day for a dollar apiece.
50. The traveler who only meets innkeepers and transportation staff when in a foreign country can hardly get a correct impression of the population: This often leads to the negative judgments in so-called travel descriptions. It was very pleasant for me on this American journey to meet educated male and female citizens of the U.S. quite often, to address their prejudices and lose some of my own.
51. This was originally a gardening term, has been adopted in medicine ("skin graft"), but today is most often used in America to describe not the simple thievery of a pickpocket but the expropriation of governmental or corporate funds by a corrupt official. (The root of the word, by the way, is graphium, γραφειον, the metallic sharp stylus of the ancients.)
52. I have taken this figure from the education issue of the *Journal of the American Medical Association*, 19 August 1905. Baedeker gives 355,000 for 1903.
53. The same man donated to the university the famous Lick Observatory on Mount Hamilton in southern California.
54. These figures are from Baedeker.
55. It is not as large and not as varied as our Wertheim, which is fairly well known and appreciated here in San Francisco. However, in Chicago I was simply and emphatically told that their city had the largest department store on the planet.
56. See *Von New York nach San Francisco*, p. 157.
57. See *Von New York nach San Francisco*, p. 158.
58. I will mention in passing that helpfulness is one of the nicest charac-

teristics of Americans. It naturally grew out of the early experience of living in log cabins and camps.
59. They do not follow the silly example of many waiters in the fancy hotels of Lucerne or Rome, who will only speak English or French – until they run into a hard-nosed man like me who refuses to give in.
60. *Pais* = land (Spanish). *Tamal* is an Indian word.
61. In any case, none of the experienced eye doctors in the United States – and I asked many about this – had ever seen a woman perform a cataract operation, although a medical career has long been open to women.
62. *Die Amerikaner*, Berlin 1904, II, p. 88.
63. More figures taken from Baedeker.
64. Our government unfortunately does not have the money for this sort of thing.
65. The "University of Southern California College of Medicine" was founded in 1885 and has a faculty of 29 professors and 19 instructors. Clinical material is provided by the County Hospital with 200 beds, the Sisters' Hospital with 150 beds, the Children's Hospital with 20 beds, and an outpatient clinic. The student must have a high school education. There is no entrance examination. The study period is four years, each with 32 weeks. The number of students was 115 in 1904/05, with 24 graduates. In addition, a "College of Physicians and Surgeons" opened in 1903. It has 25 students for 1904/5 and graduated 13.
66. See my *History of Arabic Ophthalmology*, p. 2.
67. These were donated by Carnegie, the Steel King. However, he is not beloved any more than Rockefeller, the Oil King. People like the dollar, but start to hate anyone who has too many of them. One of Rockefeller's donations was recently returned since it was "tainted money." However, people usually accept the money.
68. I heard that this originated with some pious rich people from the northwestern states who settled here. The Californian enjoys life and is no hypocrite.
69. It is a long piece of paper in multiple parts, the "rattlesnake of the American railroads," which I keep as a memento. The Americans are remarkably patient and put up with a great deal. Whoever buys such a ticket has to sign his name and then the ticket collectors require him to repeatedly sign his name for comparison.
70. I made almost the same trip in 1887 and described it in *New York to San Francisco*, pp. 201-255.
71. It is a great failure of Baedeker not to mention such inscriptions. I had

visited the birthplace of Burns near Glasgow in 1894, driven by one of my students there, Dr. Rowan.
72. It also serves as regular living space for a colleague who lost his wife, while the office is of course in the city.
73. Almost every American wears some sort of insignia, whether from his school, his masonic order, or something similar.
74. This occasion reminded me of the international congress in Rome in 1894, when my wife and I visited the catacombs, a German monk recommended that I remove the insignia of the congress, since otherwise everyone would charge me double.
75. In my own room, I have hung next to each other the portraits of three famous eye doctors, who when alive would not have enjoyed being in the same room, even though they lived in the same city.
76. Five hours later, on a street corner that we had peacefully passed through, an automobile was stopped by the gunshots of three masked robbers, and the occupants were robbed.
77. The state seal of Massachusetts since the revolutionary era has the inscription: *Ense petit placidam sub libertate quietem*. The English politician Algernon Sidney wrote this verse in an album in Copenhagen in 1677. The well-known saying about Boston's greatest citizen, Benjamin Franklin – *Eripuit Jovi fulmen, mox sceptra tyrannis* – is from the French minister Turgot (1727-1781).
78. They have built a new football stadium, about a quarter the size of the Colosseum in Rome – apparently to hold 20,000 spectators.
79. This had been constructed by a friend of the doctor, after the Haab magnet was burned out and destroyed when somebody forgot to turn off the current. At this point, the hospital administration had not yet decided whether to get a new one.
80. There is also an "Isabella Stewart Gardner Museum," which used to be accessible at times (for an admission price of 1 dollar!). However, the lady has now decided to close her museum.
81. It is by Thomas Ball, 1877, a copy of his grouping at the Lincoln Memorial in the federal capital Washington from 1875.
82. *From New York to San Francisco*, p. vi: "The impression that America has made on me is favorable. It has an important present and, I am convinced, an even more important future."
83. But this has to be distinguished from the tariff and economic area: There Germany should and will defend its rights.
84. I did find, at least for 1882, an official report by the American Central Board of Education with some general statistics in the available litera-

ture. I do not currently have the time to look for more recent reports of this kind.
85. Volume II, p. 57: "The 'American danger' stood at the gates before we realized how rapidly American industry was increasing. Tomorrow Europe will experience the same surprise in the intellectual area." Incidentally, I can point the concerned reader to the interesting book by Hugo von Knebel-Doeberitz, *Is there an American danger for Germany?* (Berlin 1904, 88 pages.) I share the conviction of the author: "Our ship will never founder on the rocks of the American danger."
86. As is well-known, at the medieval universities there arose institutions for inexpensive and orderly communal living for teachers, and then for both teachers and students. The model was the *Collegium Sorbonicum* in Paris (1257). Oxford has colleges with nicely furnished buildings and gardens, where teachers and students live together. I had the opportunity to visit these last year. (I lived at Keble College). Each college has its Rector and a certain number of Fellows, who receive generous salaries. The Professors are chosen from among the Fellows. The tuition and boarding fees paid by the students are rather high for most colleges. – Cambridge has 17 colleges.
87. President Roosevelt holds up the status of the European continent as an example to Americans. "The American scientist, the American scholar should have the chance, at least, of winning such prizes as are open to his successful brother in Germany, England or France." (*Journal of the American Medical Association* XLV, No. 4, p. 246, 22 July 1905.)
88. As an Executive Committee member of the Berlin Union of Friends of the Humanistic *Gymnasium*, I know something about these things.
89. We cannot be pleased that recently Prof. Julius Goebel was abruptly dismissed by the President of the University of Palo Alto because of his criticism of a scientific work by President Roosevelt – very much against the wishes of Roosevelt himself. We have also sadly experienced that a diligent researcher of ancient history was dismissed by an American university president because of his Jewish religion, and are pleased that he has found employment at a German university.
90. Now the responsibility for this depressing state of affairs, to a large extent, rests with the medical profession itself, because it permits the establishment and continuance of so many medial schools that have no other reason for their existence than the purely selfish ambitions of small groups of men. *Journal of the American Medical Association* XLV, No. 4, p. 247, 22 July 1905. The seriousness and the energy of this organ of the American Medical Association deserves its reputation.

91. I have intentionally given this text in English, since it is an important piece of evidence.
92. Educational issue of the *Journal of the American Medical Association* XLV No. 8, 19 August 1905. In England (*British Medical Journal*) and in France there are also such university issues. As far as I know, we in Germany only do this in the *Hochschul-Zeitung*. Perhaps this *Medizinische Klinik* will decide to publish a university supplement at the beginning of each semester, with statistics and curricula.
93. This is a new arrangement taken from Germany and introduced in the most important states of the U.S. When I was a student, many of those who failed the state examination but had a doctorate went to the U.S., presented their diplomas, and were admitted to practice. I thought this was contrary to the honor of German medicine and not in the interest of American medicine. In 1887, when I met the Dean of the medical school where my friend Knapp worked, I asked if I could be admitted to a state medical examination; but I was not able to convince him.
94. Number of medical students in the German Empire
    Summer semester 1903   7,265
    Winter semester 1903/04   7,042
    Summer semester 1904   6,502
    Winter semester 1904/05   6,198
    Summer semester 1905   6,290
    The reason for this decrease is known.[32]
95. It can be seen that this does not come close to the situation in Bern and Zürich, where the number of female students is larger than that of the male students. – Although ophthalmology might be more comfortable for women than many other specialties, I encountered only one female eye doctor in the meeting of our section in Portland.
96. My text says "evening." The inscription that I read myself in Chicago says "night." These medical schools are for those who have to earn a living during the day, and wish to study medicine in the evening. (1.8% of medical students attend these night schools. One of those in Chicago has now closed.) The basic idea is fine, but the outcome can only be pitiful. A trade school for manual workers would not be limited to the evenings. The study of medicine requires the entire workday.
97. I have abbreviated the list.
98. *Journal of the American Medical Association* XLV, No. 4, p. 247, 22 July 1905: In ninety percent of our medical colleges the salaries offered are mere pittances, the equipment, time and opportunity of good work minimal.

99. "Ueber ärztliche Schulen und Anstalten in Nord-Amerika," *Berliner Medizinische Wochenschrift*, 1905, No. 2.
100. "Due to the strictness of entrance requirements in the medical schools of Chicago, the number of registered students in the past year has decreased significantly."
101. It is particularly striking to read in the official report of such a famous university "The laboratories and lecture rooms offer ample facilities, and the equipment is good …" But the official reports of most medical schools contain such and even more emphatic statements. Still more ringing are the announcements in the medical journals, for example X Medical School. "Buildings and equipment new. Clinical opportunities unequalled…. The recognized leader in medical education." Here an ocean separates us from America.
102. Albert Guttstadt, Medical Faculty, in *Die Deutschen Universitäten* 1904.
103. See my short report in the *Berliner Klinische Wochenschrift* 1905 Nr. 11.
104. And I have had hundreds, many hundreds of American patients. I am not only speaking about my trips to America. But I would like to respond to Dr. Münsterberg (I, 18) that he is in error when he maintains that "indeed the academic circles – he means the university teachers – are full to overflowing with prejudices against America." – We do not derive our opinions from the caustic book of Ponsonby (*The Preposterous Yankee*, London 1903). We prefer to read the kindly book *Those Delightful Americans* by Mrs. Everard Cotes (London 1903).
105. It would be even stranger to send German students to America. They would not remain for a semester.
106. In my experience, the wives never had a disturbing influence on the studies, but often an encouraging one. Sometimes, their ambition was a driving factor.
107. Those who have passed our state examination should not be regarded as foreigners from a scientific standpoint. I have found positions for them as assistants in state institutions.
108. The hotel register, in which every guest who takes a room has to enter his name, position, and home, is freely available to them or to anyone who goes into the hotel lobby.
109. XXXI, 11, p. 248, August 1905.
110. In 1903, 430 foreigners were studying medicine at German universities. Most of them were Americans. However, a much larger number of these do not officially register but are satisfied with visiting clinics, hospitals, laboratories, and vacation courses.

Biographical Source

Snyder C, "Julius Hirschberg, the neglected historian of ophthalmology," *American Journal of Ophthalmology* 1981; 91:664-676.

Publication Source

Medizinische Klinik ceased publication in 2010. Historical issues can be obtained through the Hathi Trust.

Translation Notes

1) The author hardly seems reluctant to talk about himself.
2) "*Verweile doch, du bist so schön.*" A famous quotation from *Faust* (Part I, Line 1700), in which he agrees to forfeit his soul if he ever says these words.
3) The author spells the name "Caterbau," but all other sources have "Katerbau."
4) Referring to Edward Bellamy's utopian novel *Looking Backwards* (1888).
5) Baedeker's tour guides from this time refer to the dubious sanitation in Greek hotels outside of Athens, and state that ασπρορουχα (literally "white clothing") means "linen." Thus, the Greek words in the footnote were presumably those addressed to the innkeeper, meaning "new bedsheets" and "newest."
6) The Brooklyn Bridge, completed in 1883.
7) See Pooley TR, "On the detection of the presence and location of steel and iron foreign bodies in the eye by the indication of a magnetic needle," *Archives of Ophthalmology* 1880; 8:255-271.
8) A modern discussion of heterophoria, including the issues with this terminology, is found in Kommerell G et al., "Heterophoria and fixation disparity: A review," *Strabismus* 2000; 8:127-134.
9) Sideroscopy was an extension of Pooley's magnetic needle method for localizing intraocular foreign bodies of steel or iron.
10) The Miami and Erie Canal ran from the Ohio River in Cincinnati to Lake Erie at Toledo. With the advent of railroads in the late 19th Century, it gradually fell into disuse. "Over-the-Rhine" is still a distinctive neighborhood of Cincinnati.

11) The fountain has been renovated since that time, but is still a principal feature of downtown Cincinnati.
12) The quotation is from *Wilhelm Meisters Lehrjahre*, Book 7, Chapter 5. It is actually a bit different from what Hirschberg remembered, but the same idea.
13) Now the Congress Plaza Hotel.
14) Carl Stangen was a well-known travel agent, the "German Thomas Cook."
15) Written in 1827, and discussed (in English, including the questionable geology) by Wadepuhl W, "Amerika, du hast es besser," *Germanic Review* 1932; 7:186-191. There have been many English translations of this poem, but this is my best attempt to preserve the meaning, meter, and rhyme scheme.
16) From *Faust*, Part I, Verse 2586.
17) From *Faust*, near the beginning of Part II, Verses 4695-4696.
18) *Regenbogenhautentzündung* (Rainbow membrane inflammation) is the cumbersome but colorful German word that the author uses for "iritis."
19) The extravagant City Hall collapsed in the earthquake of 1906. The Spreckels Building was damaged by fire but survived, and after several renovations is known today as the Central Tower.
20) The baths gradually lost popularity and closed. The concrete ruins can still be seen at Golden Gate Park.
21) This was probably $\Phi BK = \Phi\iota\lambda o\sigma o\phi\iota\alpha$ $B\iota ou$ $Kv\beta\varepsilon\rho\nu\eta\tau\eta\varsigma$ (Phi Beta Kappa = love of knowledge is the guide to life).
22) A Mediterranean resort on the border between France and Italy.
23) This cynical motto has also been ascribed to Louis XIV of France, and can be found on other cannons. *Ultima ratio regum* means "the final argument of kings."
24) That is, just prior to the Seven Years' War, during which Spain and Prussia were on opposite sides.
25) St. Luke's Hospital did get a new building on Michigan Avenue in 1908. It is now part of Rush University Medical Center.
26) Now Washington Park and Jackson Park.
27) Probably Lincoln Park.
28) The Latin words in the footnote mean "By the sword she seeks peace, but peace with freedom" and "He snatched the lightning from a god, and the scepter from a tyrant."
29) The St. Louis brewer Adolphus Busch donated a new building for the Germanic Museum on the Harvard campus, which opened

just after the First World War despite the unpopularity of Germans and brewers at that time. The building now houses the Minda de Gunzberg Center for European Studies.
30) Luna Park on Coney Island.
31) A student completing the *secunda* in a German *Gymnasium* still has two more years before graduating.
32) This decrease was anticipated as a result of stricter requirements for medical study introduced in 1901. See Schwalbe J, "Die neue Prüfungsordnung und die Ueberfüllung des ärztlichen Standes," *Deutsche Medizinische Wochenschrift* 1901; 27:418-419.

11
Gunnar Nyström (1905)

Erik Gunnar Nyström was born in 1877 in Stockholm, Sweden. He studied medicine at the nearby Karolinska Institute, receiving his medical license in 1902.

During the spring of 1905, at the age of 28, he traveled to the northeastern United States, and reported on his experiences later in 1905-06.

After his return, he continued surgical training and became a junior faculty member at the Karolinska. In 1915, he published his observations of the German army medical corps, emphasizing that "we can all discuss military medical work without hate or bitterness, whatever opinion we may have about this war." In 1916, he joined the faculty of the Uppsala University, becoming Professor of Surgery in 1921.

He returned at least twice to the United States. In 1930, he became an Honorary Fellow of the American Surgical Association, and in 1935 he was the Abraham Flexner Lecturer at Vanderbilt University School of Medicine.

He was appointed Emeritus Professor at Uppsala in 1942, and died in 1964.

Från en studieresa i Amerika
Allmänna Svenska Läkartidningen 1905; 2:545-553, 561-570
1906; 3:257-264, 273-278

From a study trip in America
by Gunnar Nyström

I. Medical education

During a 3-month stay in the United States of North America last spring in order to study American surgery, I naturally came into close contact with their medical education system. Since educational reform is currently under discussion here, and comparison with medical education in the great western country of the future should be of interest, I gathered information about their situation as well as time permitted. This description of medical studies in America that I will try to give the readers of *Läkartidningen* certainly does not claim to be exhaustive. In addition, that country is too large and too varied in composition, and my time was too short. What I will present is an outline of my personal impressions, information that I obtained during conversations with teachers and students, and information from catalogs, curricula, and annual reports from about twenty medical schools.

The United States is a country of contrasts, variations, and mixtures of different elements. Alaska's polar regions and semitropical Florida are included in the same vast realm, and even along the same latitude, nature changes from wild high mountains and sterile salt deserts to forested hills and plains of wonderful fertility. The same city is inhabited by Americans, English, Irish, Scandinavians, Germans, Russians, French, Italians, Greeks, Jews, Chinese, and Negroes. In New York's squalid ghetto, tens of thousands of people spend their lives in abject poverty, while nearby, at the Wall Street Stock Exchange, bankers and trust barons speculate for their millions. Such contradictions can be found in all areas, including the cultural ones.

It is impossible to specify a single level for the quality of medical education in America, any more than you could specify a single level for its elevation above sea level. Here in Sweden, there tends to be a low opinion of the doctors on the other side of the Atlantic. This is partly due to ignorance, and partly due to the fact that we meet only inferior representatives of American medicine. I well remember a Yankee doctor who visited one of our clinics a few years ago. In discussing an operation, some simple anatomical relationships became relevant. At that point, this medical doctor took a small book out of his pocket and eagerly leafed through it. It was a "vademecum," containing a summary of all medical subjects, including anatomy. I may be mistaken, but I think I remember him asking how many ribs there are in the body. An occasional medical doctor like that also comes over here to take the Swedish medical exam and amazes us with his ignorance. In Minnesota I met a Swedish-American doctor whose parents had emigrated from Sweden and who had obviously been poorly educated in America, both in medicine and other fields.[1] In the most terrible Smålandic[2] I have ever heard - he spoke it like a foreign language due to his American accent - he complained that the Swedes had such a low opinion of American doctors. In Germany, he had met an assistant from one of the Stockholm clinics, who expressed his disdain for everything called medical art across the ocean, and he felt extremely upset about it.

Such a sweeping conclusion is now unjustified. A couple of decades ago, American medical education was far from brilliant. The rapidly growing country needed a lot of doctors, and in most places a course of two to three years was then sufficient to earn an M.D. degree and obtain the right to practice. Little by little, the requirements have become stricter, as new educational institutions have been established, the supply of doctors has increased and demand has become more selective, so today there are only a few medical educational institutions that grant M.D. diplomas after less than four years of study. However, there are still few regulations on doctors in some parts of the "Wild West," and there you might have to be satisfied with any medicine man.

But the most significant thing in assessing the level of medical education in America is that during the last 5-10 years a few of the larger medical schools have had absolutely magnificent development in all areas, while most smaller schools have not kept up, except for a gradual increase in study time, and have fallen in reputation. The day will probably come when these laggards will disappear completely, as new large well-equipped institutions arise, and the leading schools are steadily expanded, while at the same time the hitherto less civilized parts of the country increase their requirements for doctors so that the small schools cannot keep up with the competition. Perhaps even in the near future it will be possible to give a more uniform assessment of America's medical education system, and it will probably be an assessment of which this future great country in the West can be justifiably proud, as it is now for most things that bear "the American stamp."

It appears that the main reason for this variable quality is that the medical schools are completely independent, without a common, central administration. A rich man decides at some point that he should do a good deed, or that his name and fortune should be remembered by posterity. He donates a certain amount for the establishment of a medical school. A Board of Trustees is appointed from among the more reputable local men and then a corporation is started, which thus assumes a completely private character, established and maintained as it is with the money of individuals, although sometimes with a contribution from the relevant state. Depending on the size of the donations, a larger or smaller school results, and depending on the equipment and teaching staff that the new institution has been able to obtain, it acquires a higher or lower reputation.

It is important to note the number of medical schools (often called medical colleges). Most states have three or more, Chicago alone has fourteen, and altogether there are currently no fewer than 160 such institutions in the United States.

From this background, I will move on to the teaching itself. The course now available at almost all schools, large or small, is for *four years*. Classes usually run from the beginning of October to the middle or end of May or the beginning of June, with a couple of weeks for Christmas holidays. At the end of each academic year, an examination is held in the subjects that were completed during the year, and after successfully completing the examination at the end of the fourth year, the student receives his doctorate in medicine, an M.D. degree, without needing to write and defend a thesis, as in our country and other European states [1]. In order to gain the right to practice, he must then pass an examination before an examination commission (The Board of Medical Examiners or simply *The State Board*) in the state where he intends to settle [2].

The length of the medical course is essentially the same in the different schools, but the quality of the teaching is much more variable. And the resulting education received by the newly graduated doctor of medicine is so different for different schools that the title itself hardly means anything unless you know that it was obtained in a reputable institution. Using this standard, we can divide the medical schools into two large groups.

The first consists of the large majority of smaller schools of low reputation. Most of these belong to the Association of American Medical Colleges, which does exercise a kind of control over teaching. The entrance requirements have until this year been a three-year high-school course or its equivalent, but have now been increased by a decision of the association (in April 1905) to a full (four-year) high-school course [3]. At several schools, admission can also be gained without a high school or equivalent educational institution after passing an examination in the following subjects: English, Latin (translation of easy prose), elementary arithmetic, algebra, and physics. The four-year medical course usually includes the same subjects that I will later mention in detail when describing the Johns Hopkins Medical School. After obtaining the M.D. degree at the smaller schools, there is usually no additional service at a hospital, but the young doctor seeks to start his practice immediately.

The second group consists of a few larger teaching institutions, where in addition to a complete high school course for entry, 2-4 years of university (liberal arts or scientific college) is expected and required, including a "medicophile" course in physics, chemistry, and biology. After completing the four-year medical course, the doctors of medicine who graduate from these schools usually continue their clinical training as interns at a hospital for one or two years. After completing their studies, the best-educated American doctors have thus worked for 7-10 years on their medical training, and they also usually further increase their experience by visiting European clinics. The studies thus approach our own in terms of duration, and I will suggest that they far exceed ours in intensity, but more on that later.

As examples of educational institutions of the latter category, I can mention Johns Hopkins in Baltimore, Rush in Chicago, Harvard in Boston, Jefferson and University in Philadelphia, and the College of Physicians and Surgeons, University and Bellevue,[3] and Cornell University Medical Colleges in New York. Due to the students' comparatively high level of education, the superiority of the teaching staff, the large clinical experience, and the excellent physical facilities, these deservedly enjoy a high reputation and can undoubtedly be placed on an equal footing with the best schools in Europe.

Nowhere was the difference between these two groups of schools so distinct as in Baltimore, and shall therefore give some impressions of the existing smaller colleges, and a more detailed description of medical education at the Johns Hopkins University.

In Baltimore, a city about the size of Copenhagen, there are no fewer than nine medical schools; of these, eight belong to the first-mentioned group and have a rather "shady reputation," as one of my friends at Johns Hopkins put it. One or the other of these schools has infamously received and graduated as Doctors of Medicine such medical men who could not be admitted to one of the better educational institutions, and one must assume that it is such institutions that turn out the not inconsiderable contingent of morally less scrupulous doctors.

Unfortunately, I was not able to personally observe the teaching itself in these colleges that produce the "cheap doctors," the doctors of lower social status. But I did make a brief tour of the city and saw the premises, and my impressions of them were consistent with the judgments about the quality of the teaching that I heard from credible people. When I entered the little Maryland Medical College[4] one afternoon during graduation time, nobody was there but a dirty old Negro dressed in rags. He served as caretaker and showed me the way around the empty building up a narrow, grimy staircase with names and drawings scrawled on the wall, and we entered a large lecture hall. Between piles of disordered chairs stood a number of large spittoons, which were sprinkled with suspicious brown spots, as was the floor around them. The whole room gave to sight and smell a more disgusting impression than a dirty third-class waiting room at a poorly managed railway station in Sweden. But on the blackboard there were some questions from the previous day's examination, which formed a strange contrast to their surroundings. They had written about the differential diagnosis between surgical shock and fat embolism, between acute appendicitis and intussusception, and eight other such excellent scientific questions about which the tobacco-chewing students had exercised their brains at the conclusion of their third and final school year.

However, the worst was the dirty little house in Ensor Street in a poor part of the town, home to an educational institution with the fine name of The Medico-Chirurgical and Theological College of Christ's Institution.[5] As the name indicates, teaching in theology and medicine is provided here. The students, numbering about 40 in the medical department, are mostly Negroes, and the annual report states that the school is "the greatest colored Medical Theological and Academic Institution in the United States." The course is four years, each year of "at least 6 months." On entering the small, cramped hall, on one side of which shelves with pharmacy goods were arranged, I was attended by a Negro and introduced to another Negro, who turned out to be the dean or superintendent of the school. I was conducted through a dirty hall, not unlike a peasant's chamber, in which a few persons were currently sitting, eating a simple dinner at a long, unpainted wooden table. Next, we entered a small room with a kind of rudimentary amphitheater, which served as a dissection *and* operating room, then passed a theological classroom about the size of a small living room and a chemist's laboratory of similar dimensions and returned to the vestibule through "The Hospital," whose few beds were occupied by some Negro patients. The hospital ward seemed to be relatively clean, but otherwise everything was pretty awful. I think it probable that this institution occupies the lowest place among all the medical colleges. In a list of medical schools in *The Journal of the American Medical Association*, it is not even mentioned, although the state of Maryland has granted it the right to create Doctors of Medicine. The very fact that Negroes can be admitted means that Americans must consider it part of the pariah caste.

One cannot formulate any conclusions about the quality of the teaching out of catalogs or curricula from such institutions, since these usually describe the school as particularly outstanding. It is quite natural to try to attract as many students as possible, especially when the school's existence is entirely or almost entirely dependent on their tuition fees [4]. And so, they describe brilliant prospects and turn a blind eye to the examinations. But one becomes suspicious of the flowery presentation of all the benefits the school has to offer, when one reads lines such as the following in the catalog of the medical-theological educational institution just described, "the great and noble institution," as it is called: "the hospital department wherein some of the most miraculous cures have been performed. The blind have been made to see, the deaf to hear, the lame to walk and leap for joy as well as some of the pronounced cases of chronic diseases have been cured; also very many surgical operations have been successfully performed ..." One gets the definite impression that the author of these lines belongs to the category of benefactors to humanity who fill the newspaper columns with illustrated advertisements for miracle cures.

I have already dwelt too long on these inconsequential institutions, but I have deemed it necessary to give some idea of the low position occupied by a large part of the medical schools, in order to fairly balance the impression of the whole, when I now proceed to a description of the teaching at the model school, which bears the name Johns Hopkins University Medical School.

In the 1870s, a university in Baltimore was established through a multi-million donation from a single man, Johns Hopkins. Medicine was not initially part of the new university, but the donor had also planned the establishment of a medical school. Physics, chemistry, and biology were therefore taught at the university as a kind of preparation for medical studies. In 1884, a professorship in pathology was established, and in 1889 the Johns Hopkins Hospital was opened. Land and buildings for this had cost over 2 million dollars. An additional sum of ½ million dollars was obtained through further donations, including from a committee of women who attached to their gift the condition that women would be allowed to participate in the education on the same terms as men. Together with available funds from the university and hospital, this enabled the university board to open the Medical Department of Johns Hopkins University in 1893. The number of students at the new medical school increased rapidly and last academic year reached 291.

Anatomy and histology are housed in one building, and physiology, physiological chemistry, and pharmacology in another, both near the hospital, to which the pathology department is attached. One of the main ideas in construction of the hospital was to facilitate clinical teaching in every way, and within the huge complex of buildings, which together occupy an area of about 5½ hectares,[6] there are large lecture halls and well-equipped laboratories, and spaces for students or doctors who want to do special work. The ample facilities, the neat interior design, and the exemplary arrangements make it a pleasure for teachers and pupils.

The medical section of the university library is housed in the hospital and is easily accessible to the students, who thus have the advantage of being able to obtain all the desired information from textbooks, encyclopedias, or journals during their clinical studies without having to leave the hospital.

The entry requirements at Johns Hopkins Medical School are an A.B. degree (Bachelor of Arts degree) from the chemical-biological department at J. H. University or its equivalent. The course for a chemical-biological A.B. degree requires 4 years after completion of high school. It includes the subjects of chemistry, physics, biology; mathematics; French, German, Latin; English literature, rhetoric, economics, history, and philosophy.

Chemistry: Labs around 5 hours a week for 1 year along with lectures. Inorganic chemistry and the basics of organic chemistry.

Physics: 1-year course with lectures 4 hours a week and laboratories 3 hours a week.

Biology: Laboratory work 9 hours a week for 1 year, including studies of several lower organisms, such as ameba, yeast, mold, bacteria, other fungi, higher plants, earthworms, lobsters; the anatomy of the frog and the development of its egg, structure and transformation of the frog larva; dissection of a mammal; chicken embryology. In addition, there are lectures.

In the subjects of chemistry, physics, and biology, the future medical man may possibly acquire slightly more knowledge than what is equivalent to our medicophile. The requirements in foreign languages and history are no greater than in the examinations of our Latin schools, in mathematics somewhat greater.

Teaching at the Johns Hopkins Medical School continues from the beginning of October until the middle of June with shorter breaks at Christmas and Easter. The academic year is considered to be nine months.

An attempt has been made to arrange the studies in a logical sequence and at the same time enable the students to concentrate their work on one or a couple of closely related subjects.

1st year, 1st trimester: Anatomy, histology.
2nd trimester: Anatomy, physiology.
3rd trimester: Physiology, physiological chemistry.

2nd year, 1st trimester: Anatomy, physiology, bacteriology.
2nd trimester: Pathology, pharmacology, toxicology.
3rd trimester: Anatomy, pathology, pharmacology.

3rd year: Clinical and outpatient work in medicine, surgery, and neurology, courses in physical diagnosis, therapy, clinical microscopy, medical and surgical anatomy, operative surgery and surgical pathology, lectures and demonstrations in obstetrics, including exercises on the mannequin, lectures in pharmacy, therapy, dietetics, hygiene, medical zoology, forensic medicine, and medical history.

4th year: The students are divided into three equal-sized groups, each group serving three months straight, successively in the medical, surgical, obstetrics and gynecology clinics and outpatient clinics. Gynecology also includes practical courses in gynecological diagnosis and gynecological pathology. In addition, 4th year lectures are given in hygiene, forensic medicine, medical zoology, and medical history.

[p. 2:561]
Some information about the specific studies in each subject may be of interest.

Anatomy. Lectures are not held. Spalteholz's Atlas[7] was usually used as a textbook, with Quain's anatomy[8] as a reference book. Due to the limited availability of material, muscles, vessels, and nerves are dissected on each specimen, and each student thus dissects through the human body only once. Dissections are at least as detailed as with us. I saw a portion of the posterior abdominal wall with the sympathic chain and the large abdominal ganglia very neatly dissected. Also, fine nerve branches and ganglia in parts of the cranial nerves were exposed. The dissection of the head and neck takes about 8-10 weeks. The students are asked to make drawings of their parts, and for this purpose they are provided with printed "outlines," i.e. contours of arms, legs, etc. The drawing is not absolutely required, but good drawings have a beneficial effect on their grade for the work.

A special course is given in neuroanatomy (brain and spinal cord) much like here.

During the second year, there is a special course in "medical anatomy," which, if I understood correctly, is intended to form a basis for the exercises in physical diagnosis [5]. There are also elective courses in topographical anatomy and surgical anatomy.

Histology. Much like with us. Sections of fresh tissue are made by the students themselves. Approximately 150 unstained sections of organs and tissues are distributed for staining and study.

Embryology. The basics are a prerequisite for entering the school (see above). An optional course is given in embryology with lectures and demonstration of preparations.

Physiology. Laboratories and lectures with demonstrations in the same style as with us; the laboratory course requires 6-9 hours of work per week for 12 weeks in the autumn of the second year, after the students have received a series of lectures on the subjects which are intended to be illustrated with the laboratories. The laboratory course was probably more detailed in some parts than with us; among other things, the students themselves do blood pressure experiments on animals, investigate the speed of the pulse wave, etc. The curves I saw were particularly nice in comparison with the crude ones that were produced in the courses at the Karolinska Institute several years ago. I would like to add that all electrical devices had visible wiring as much as possible, which is important because it spares the student from worrying about "how the current flows." The students have a freely accessible physiological library at the physiology department.

Physiological Chemistry. Laboratories: 1) Preliminary course in the examination of certain important substances, e.g. proteins. 2) Qualitative analysis of various organs and tissues, such as liver, muscles, fat, bone, blood, milk, bile, gastric juice, etc., as well as pathological fluids and calculi. 3) Enzyme action in saliva, gastric juice, and pancreatic juice. 4) Quantitative analysis of normal and pathological substances in urine, milk, gastric juice, gastric lavage, air, water, and foodstuffs. 5) Examination of feces with particular regard to processes of decay. Lectures and demonstrations. Hammarsten's *Physiological Chemistry*[9] in English translation was used as a textbook.

Toxicology, Pharmacology, and "Practical Therapy." In the first of these, a laboratory course of 6 weeks is given. It begins with toxicological experiments on anesthetized animals and then proceeds to 1) investigations on volatile poisons by distillation; 2) investigations on alkaloids and glycosides according to various methods, e.g. detection of the admixture of toxic alkaloids in food; 3) examination of metallic and non-volatile poisons; 4) examination of blood stains and spectroscopic studies of various kinds of blood pigment derivatives; 5) changes in the urine from drugs.

Pharmacology is partly studied through laboratories (animal experiments).

"Practical Therapy" is given as a course in pharmacy (prescriptions) as well as lectures on medications, their indications and dosage, hydrotherapy, diet, etc.

(Pharmaceutical chemistry is not included in the curriculum, and there are no pharmaceutical-chemical laboratories.)

Pathology. Autopsies are attended by second-, third-, and fourth-year students. Lectures and demonstrations in both general and special pathological anatomy and histology are much as with us.

Bacteriology. Practical course of about 9 hours a week for 12 weeks (preparation of nutrient substrates, principles of sterilization and disinfection, culturing, staining and study of bacteria; biological examination of air, water, and soil). Such practical skills as determining the bacterial species from an infected animal also occur. However, no examination of feces for cholera bacilli or of material from a diphtheria throat.

Medicine. Teaching occurs in the outpatient clinic, the infirmaries, and the clinical laboratories. The 2nd-year course in physical diagnosis is continued into the 3rd year, and during the fall semester diseases of the chest organs are examined in groups of 4 to 5 students. The exercises are held in the outpatient clinic and continue 4 hours a week throughout the semester; in the spring semester, physical diagnosis of the abdominal organs is performed with larger sections, 2 hours a week throughout the semester. Furthermore, there are exercises in journal writing under supervision and outpatient clinic duty in the same style as with us. Three times a week there are clinics in the medical amphitheater, following roughly the same pattern as our own. A special course is given in medical laboratory work (examination of blood, urine, stomach contents, etc.) During the summer holidays after the 3rd year, the students have the opportunity to serve as assistants at the outpatient clinic. In the 4th year, as mentioned above, the whole class is distributed among three departments. The students in each department serve 3 months at the medical clinic as "clerks," i.e. journal writers. This service corresponds very closely to that of the students in medical department of the Serafimerlasarettet,[10] and the clinics are run on the same schedule as with us, i.e. new cases are investigated, the development of previous cases is reviewed, deaths are discussed, autopsies are reviewed, and preparations from these are shown. A large laboratory is allocated exclusively to 4th year students. Each student has an assigned place here with their own microscopes, reagent storage, etc.

Surgery. Teaching occurs in the outpatient clinic, the wards, the operating rooms, and the laboratory. Principles of surgical technique have already been covered in the second year. Optional course in operative surgery (surgery exercises on live animals).

During the 4th year, the students serve 3 months in the surgical clinic as "dressers" (assistants during dressing changes), while also writing journals as in the medical department. They also observe operations and assist in them. They are allowed to perform some minor surgical procedures themselves, but only to a very small extent (they will not get the same opportunity to practice techniques of minor surgery as our medical students until much later).

Obstetrics. In the third year teaching in the anatomy and histology of the female genital organs and in obstetric pathology. Exercises with mannequins. Lectures. In the fourth year three months' service at the obstetrical clinic. Two students are on duty at each delivery, and the whole class is called in for more unusual and operative cases. The students also assist in the indigent service outside the hospital.

Gynecology. In the fourth year, service at the gynecological clinic. Teaching gynecological diagnostics on anesthetized patients, assistant duty at the outpatient clinic, one student every day. Rounds and teaching at the bedside. Observing operations 4 days a week. 2 hours a week during the period of service, a course in gynecological pathology; special emphasis is placed on the study of uterine curettings.

For work in the special departments of medicine and surgery, namely pediatrics, dermatology, urology, laryngology, rhinology, otology, and ophthalmology, the surgical and gynecological-obstetric section of the fourth-year class is divided into two subsections, each thus constituting 1/6 of the entire year class. The specialties just mentioned are reviewed by each subsection in courses of 5-6 weeks. At the end of each course is held an interview with practical tests, which constitute the final exam in the subject. Courses in neurology and ophthalmoscopy are given during the 3rd year. Teaching in orthopedic surgery is given during the 4th year in connection with surgery at the orthopedic clinic and the outpatient clinic by a professor in the subject.

Psychiatry. Lectures and demonstrations at the city hospital clinic and outpatient clinic once a week during the 4th year [6].

Instruction in *hygiene* is provided in connection with the course in pathology, bacteriology, physiology and physiological chemistry. In addition, lectures in hygiene in the 3rd and 4th years.

Medical zoology. Ten lectures on human parasites and demonstrations. Exercises in examination of meat for trichinosis.

Forensic medicine. Lectures during the 3rd and 4th year. The students themselves do not get the opportunity to testify or perform forensic autopsies [7].

Medical history. "The Historical Club" has meetings once a month during the school year, during which there are lectures about individual eras or people in the history of medicine. Students have access to these lectures, but their participation is completely voluntary. There is no structured course, nor any other teaching about medical history other than this club.

Examinations.

At the end of the first year, an examination is held in physiologic chemistry and histology; after the fall semester of the second year there is an examination in physiology including a practical exam in bacteriology; after the spring term of the same year there is an examination in anatomy and at the end of the year in bacteriology and pathology, pharmacology and toxicology. At the end of the 3rd year, an examination is held in the parts of medicine, surgery, obstetrics, and nervous diseases that have been completed. In the final spring there is an examination in medicine, surgery, and obstetrics and gynecology. Examinations are partly written, partly oral, and include practical skills. The student must pass the examinations at the end of each year to be admitted to the following year's course. Conditional promotion is allowed, but the requirements must be completed before the start of the fall semester.

Employment at the hospital.

The twelve best of the newly graduated doctors are appointed as "house officers" at the hospital clinics for a period of one year. They receive board and lodging at the hospital, but no salary. Their service can be considered as a continuation of their clinical education. Employment as a house officer is considered a great honor and selection is highly competitive. In addition to these "interns," a number of "externs" are also appointed from among the new graduates to work at the outpatient clinics, including two at the city hospital.

Tuition fees.

200 dollars per year. For the entire 4-year course, this will be a fairly substantial sum of around 3,000 *kronor*[11] in Swedish currency.

With a single glance at the curriculum of the Johns Hopkins Medical School, two of the most characteristic features of the teaching immediately stand out, the *scholastic* arrangement of the studies and the *general daily program* at clinics and institutions. The student has pretty much every hour of his day assigned to a definite task from the time he enters the anatomy room at the beginning of the first autumn semester until he leaves school as a fully trained doctor at the end of the fourth year.

Another characteristic of the studies should be highlighted at the same time, namely the *intensity* of the work. The American youth "buckle down" to a much greater degree than most of us did during our time as students, and it is absolutely necessary if they are going to make it through all their courses. I got the impression that the students at Johns Hopkins Medical School get through about as much in their four years as we did during twice that length of study. This also applies to the book learning; the American textbooks are generally just as detailed as those used here.

The intensity and interest in their studies are attributable in part to the so-called "quizzes," i.e. repetitions of reviewed parts of the subject with questioning, just as in a typical school lesson. These "discussions" are not so much about ascertaining the student's knowledge as they are about further teaching in the form of questions, reinforcing what has already been learned and increasing interest in the studies; no grades are given at these quizzes.

Studies are based on the "honor system"; it is considered the student's obligation to attend all prescribed lectures and exercises. Attendance is not taken, but a student's absence may be noticed incidentally at the above-mentioned quizzes. In such a case, he will not be formally reprimanded, and there will be no addition of service days. The penalty is considered to be the loss of teaching he incurs, and absence without a valid reason as well as any lack of enthusiasm in his studies will have a depressing effect on his final grade. However, in the last two years, and especially in the fourth year, an occasional absence is not counted so carefully.

For a large part of the students, the intensity of the work takes on the character of a real frenzy. "They run the life out of us," complained a Norwegian-American student whom I met at Rush College in Chicago.

Due to the excessive speed in the studies, the ability to retain and digest the content is of course greatly reduced, but this is compensated in some cases by the *generally excellent quality of the teaching*. The public schools of the United States are famous for their lively instruction, and even in the higher educational institutions the practical sense of the Yankee is evident. I witnessed at the Johns Hopkins clinic a demonstration of bacteriological blood examination, which was genuinely enjoyable because of the clarity and vivacity of the presentation. The entire procedure was carried out, from the washing of the patient's arm to the plating of the blood on nutrient substrate, after which the results of similar cultures from previous days were shown. And as another example, I can mention that a lecture on hip joint dislocation (at Harvard Medical School, Boston) was accompanied by dislocation and reposition exercises on cadavers, in which all the students participated in turn. I am convinced that these young students had significantly better preparation for the future practical application of what they had learned in this area than most of our new medical graduates.

The teaching also seems to produce beautiful results almost immediately. I do not think I have heard at home such coherent, neat, and concise case histories and answers to questions raised about the patient - without consulting the medical record - as the students at the Johns Hopkins clinic were generally able to give the professor on rounds.

The other major medical schools mentioned above have essentially the same plan for teaching as Johns Hopkins, although as far as I know only Harvard Medical School has such strict entrance requirements. Rush Medical College requires two years of university studies, others allow admission with only a high school education including certain subjects and a certain grade, although usually the desirability of the applicant having a university education is strongly emphasized. Teaching in chemistry and physics is given during the first year of these medical schools for those who have not previously acquired the level of knowledge in these subjects that is considered necessary for medical training. At Cornell University in New York State, the A.B. degree can be earned with three years of study in any university subjects, plus the first year studies in the medical faculty. This year is then also credited toward the continued medical studies, and the M.D. degree can be obtained with another 3 years of study. A number of other deviations from the description of the Johns Hopkins Medical School could be pointed out, for example that Rush College has no scholastic curriculum, but leaves the students free to arrange their studies according to their own wishes, that Harvard Medical School offers summer courses during June-September, covering all medical subjects, and thus provides an opportunity for organized work even outside of the regular school year, etc. But to continue the description of such differences would take me too far afield and be of no further interest.

Finally, however, I have to say a few words about a small group of medical schools, that occupy a special position because of their somewhat unscientific basis, namely the *homeopathic, eclectic*, and *osteopathic*.

Homeopathic schools with the right to graduate medical doctors are located in New York, Philadelphia, Baltimore, Chicago, and in a few other places to a total of 13. However, homeopathy itself occupies a rather modest place in the curriculum, which otherwise is quite similar to that of the other schools, with purely scientific physiology, pathology, surgery, etc. Even our usual medical therapy is taught to the students, who usually have hardly any more tendencies towards homeopathic practice when they leave school than their peers from the purely scientific teaching institutions. In addition, homeopathy in America has leaned towards the second of Hahnemann's two articles of faith. They still try to maintain the doctrine of "similia similibus,"[12] but the principle of minimal doses has been changed so that the smallest dose is given that produces a tangible effect. This is according to information from a professor of homeopathy in Chicago. One wonders how it is possible that homeopathic schools can still exist and how teaching in homeopathy and scientific medicine can be provided there at the same time, which seems to be two somewhat incompatible tendencies. The answer - which I received from a Norwegian pathologist employed at Rush College - is quite typical of America: There is probably no strong conviction about the truth and value of homeopathy, but since the money has been donated for a homeopathic educational institution, homeopathy is still included and the rest of the program is provided in accordance with the needs of the times so that it can still attract followers. Because it would be a sin against the Mammon-religion over there to sacrifice some fat donations simply because they are tied to a less tenable theory.

I do not know if this is also the situation for the eclectic schools, of which there are currently a total of 9 (with a 4-year course and the right to create medical doctors). American eclecticism in medical application, which dates its origins from the beginning of the last century, is to some extent related to homeopathy, and to some extent its opposite, but in any case, judging from essays on eclectic medicine, it has warm sympathies for Hahnemann's teachings. Its chief article of faith is "specific remedies for specific conditions." Treatment is based on the patient's own individuality and not on any classification of the diseases, "which in all probability are different in two patients, who seem to suffer from the same ailment, and also different in one and the same patient at different times." Another fundamental principle is the use only of such drugs as do not themselves produce abnormal conditions, and in accordance with this "the eclectic fathers rejected the use of antimony, arsenic, mercury, and the injudicious use of the knife." A third principle is the prescription of small, often repeated doses.

About 10,000 of the practicing physicians in the States are said to belong to the eclectic school.

Osteopathy has quite numerous supporters in the States, and even in Chicago there are one or two schools for the education of osteopathic doctors. As you know, the osteopaths proceed from the premise that many diseases are due to misalignment of some skeletal part, especially the vertebrae. You struggle to keep your mouth shut when you see their attempts to give their theories and treatment methods a scientific basis; I must quote a few pithy lines from an entertaining textbook on osteopathy (Hazzard, *Principles of Osteopathy*): "Atlas is a very important vertebra because it can press on certain nerves and affect spinal centers." H. gives an example from his own practice: "the result of displacement of the atlas was that the child could not speak; it could say 'Mamma', but everything else it tried to say was a strange sound. It could only articulate this single word. In addition, the left side was paralyzed and paretic; the child limped, the leg was short and the arm drawn up. The source of the evil actually lay entirely in the first cervical vertebra, which was displaced from its normal position, affecting the spinal cord and brain either by affecting the blood supply or by direct pressure."[13]

Such diseases are cured by manipulations, whereby the guilty bone is returned to its proper place! I do not consider it impossible that the school I mentioned in Chicago has the right to give an M.D. degree like the others, although I did not manage to get information about this. Osteopaths who have not passed the exam for the right to practice are not considered to be quacks, as long as they do not prescribe medicine but simply stick to manipulations.

Is there anything for us to learn from America's medical education system? We probably don't want to take the scholastic arrangement of the studies as a model. But on the other hand, isn't the value of the so-called academic freedom in our country overestimated? I believe that many would gladly sacrifice a good portion of this sanctified freedom in order to get on with life a little earlier, with less debt and more vitality and strength in reserve, and to get a better return on their studies. How many are there who lack the lucky natural gift of being an "exam whiz," but who are still quite capable of being competent in their future vocation? We see too many of our students procrastinating month after month in useless fooling around with exams. Academic freedom may be a very good thing, but at the same time it is a bit evil. Even if you do not want to use the maximum time to prepare for the exam, a more strictly implemented curriculum with specified times for each subject would be helpful for many and not inconvenient for the others. More practical courses, more systematic coverage of the subject in the lectures, guidance during the studies for the medical degree regarding which parts of the subject are particularly important to master for application in clinical work, and better guidance in journal writing are all to be desired. However, we hope for significant improvements in all these areas through the reforms we are now awaiting in our medical education system.

Unfortunately, it appears that this wait may be extended into an uncertain future. In our country, it not infrequently happens that an important reform proposal is suffocated when the investigating committee takes too long; it is born as a committee child, it is beaten to death by unkind criticism, or left to die in silence and oblivion by the negligence of procrastination. Our study reforms seem to be going that way. It is reasonable to be cautious with political or national economic issues that most profoundly affect the country's future. But in a matter of education, which concerns principles that are comparatively less important, but still highly significant for a more efficient use of working time, there is surely no need for such fear. A certain degree of experimentation is probably not so dangerous in this case, and mistakes can be corrected by further changes in the next few years. Anyway, it is certainly better to wait longer for an ideal reform – although it probably not be perfect since all the investigations and discussions were several years ago and there is now less general interest - than to adopt something now that will lead to a deterioration. But the proposal the examination committee is offering us is probably not so bad that it would not lead to significant improvements. The committee's work at least forms a good basis, and with some changes and additions, which were found suitable during the discussion of the proposal and of which Professor Müller's proposal for a practical year at a hospital should find active support, it should not be impossible to achieve a definitive proposal, on which all three faculties could agree, and thereby achieve a reform that most of us consider particularly needed. But that now requires some effort and a little more American enterprise.

[p. 3:257]
II. This and that from American hospitals (written in the fall of 1905)

A Swede disembarking in New York or Boston immediately gets the vivid impression of restlessly pulsating life, and soon experiences the Americans' intensity of work, their desire and ability to maximize efficiency; but to these impressions soon comes another, perhaps the more dominant: the wealth and colossal natural resources for the production of more wealth! It is not only their enterprising nature and hard work that allow the Americans to celebrate one triumph after another in the material struggle of the nations. This new country, united into a huge unit with almost inexhaustible resources, is fundamentally able to give its population significantly better conditions for victory in the struggle for existence than overpopulated and exhausted Europe, divided as it is into a multitude of states, some of which are overcultivated, or lax and indulgent, or politically, socially, and morally "on the downhill slope." The United States is currently populated by about 80 million people, but the Americans estimate that well over 200 million can be accommodated within the country's borders. Most old American families are rich, and according to our concepts, at least the Germanic immigrants usually become wealthy after several years of residence in the country. However, what especially determines the character of American wealth is of course the massive accumulation of dollars in private hands, and its concentration at certain places in the American land into volcanoes of money, which not only shake the financial world, but also erupt to spread the wealth across the country in the form of donations to science and art, education, health care, etc. And its millionaires, Carnegie, Morgan, Rockefeller, Astor, Gould, Lenox, Vanderbilt, and others, are the ones that the United States has to thank for many of its universities, schools, libraries, etc. A couple of examples are sufficient to give an idea of American donations – Chicago's new university has come about mainly through donations of Mr. John D. Rockefeller, amounting to about 40 million *kronor*, and according to one of the university's teachers, Mr. R. still makes contributions each year sufficient to cover a small annual shortfall of about 1½ million *kronor*. When the Harvard Medical School a few years ago became too crowded, it was decided to build a new one; Messrs. Morgan, Rockefeller, and some other millionaires were called and immediately gave about 10 million *kronor* (verbal information), and now a group of huge white marble palaces is arising in the southern part of Boston, whose magnificently equipped laboratories, study rooms, and lecture halls will soon open for the non-clinical departments of Harvard Medical School. And finally, I need only mention how Johns Hopkins in Baltimore, having first established a university through donation of several million dollars, also appropriated over 2 million dollars for construction of a clinical hospital. When a great fire in Baltimore in 1904 destroyed a lot of real estate, from which the hospital had income and through which a loss of several hundred thousand dollars arose, a letter immediately arrived from the sympathetic J. D. Rockefeller, in which he offered to donate a half million dollars to cover the shortfall.

Wealth and the liberality of private individuals for non-profit purposes constitute two indispensable conditions for the economic support of a large number of public institutions in America, and I have begun by seeking to give a concept of them in order to establish some important premises, before I now proceed to briefly describe the finances, administration, working arrangements, etc. of American clinics.

Of course, it is mainly the large new hospitals or those modernized according to the latest patterns that have been the subject of my study, and I will try to describe one or the other of these, which, especially in comparison with our own conditions, may be of some interest, thereby taking as a basis my impressions from Johns Hopkins Hospital in Baltimore, Pennsylvania Hospital and University Hospital in Philadelphia, Boston City Hospital and Massachusetts General Hospital in Boston, Roosevelt, St. Luke's, Presbyterian, and Mount Sinai Hospitals in New York,[14] and others. Some details may not fit all the mentioned hospitals, but they can all be considered to belong to the most modern type of "American Hospital."

It is largely *English* role models, that have left their mark on American institutions. A Swede, who is accustomed to being taken care of in all possible conditions of life by the state and municipality as if by a guardian, is at first surprised when he sees how in England and America the state leaves as much as possible to the initiative of the individual members of society. The Americans have no national railways, no national telegraph or national telephone; all of these are provided by private companies. In fact, politics has shown such a pernicious influence on the administration of state institutions that public services are left in private hands with the risk of having them monopolized by trusts or autocratic individuals rather than putting the same "job" into the hands of "politicians." This concession of public companies to the initiative of individual members of society applies above all in the field of health care.

The small federal army, about 70,000 men including in the colonies, as well as their new, splendid navy, naturally have their own state-maintained medical care; the individual states, or rather their county subdivisions, take responsibility for mental health care, and some of the largest cities have municipal hospitals (e.g., Bellevue Hospital in New York, City Hospital in Boston). *But otherwise, health care is of a private nature.*

As far as the large modern private hospitals are concerned, they have been created either by one or a couple of millionaires or a millionaire family paying for all or most of the enterprise (e.g., Johns Hopkins Hospital in Baltimore and Roosevelt Hospital in New York); or else - and this is a more common situation - it is a special religious community, which through some of its wealthiest members starts the hospital, which is then maintained by "voluntary subscriptions," charitable contributions from the public. For example, the Presbyterian Hospital in New York was built by the church community of the same name, and the magnificent new *Swedish* hospital in Chicago, the Augustana Hospital,[15] was founded by the Swedish Lutheran Church in Illinois. To a large extent, the influence of public contributions is guaranteed year after year. The new and magnificent Jewish hospital, Mount

Sinai in New York, thus has 6,000 "donors" who each give 10-100 dollars a year.

The need for voluntary subscriptions is regularly announced to the public; one hospital thus emphasizes that for next year so and so many thousand dollars are needed to furnish the new pavilion donated by millionaire X, which for the time being must remain empty due to lack of funds, another announces its need for a pathology laboratory, a third simply says that an additional 500,000 dollars is needed in order to continue with the health care at the same level as last year, etc. Free health care is also usually provided on a very large scale – thus in 1904 no less than 75% of the patients were cared for in free beds at Mount Sinai Hospital – which of course further increases the demands one must make on the public generosity. However, the money keeps coming in, even though more than a few coins are needed to fill the holes. The total annual shortfall of the hospitals in New York the last year (1904) amounted to a sum of more than 1 million *kronor*. But that is how they can maintain an extremely lavish scale for the construction and operation of hospitals in America today. A few numbers and a comparison with the conditions at home should be of interest. I thereby transfer to *kronor* the sums in dollars that I found in some of the excellent reports of the American hospitals. The nominal value of the dollar is 3.75 *kronor*, but its real value is currently only 2-3 *kronor*, and varies for different goods. I calculate its value in the following at only 2 *kronor*, whereby I should not be guilty of overestimation. Using this basis of calculation, the most important financial items for the year 1904 were as follows (with the larger numbers rounded off):

Presbyterian Hospital, New York
    Average number of patients per day 196, of which 9% in individual rooms.
    Total cost per year 400,000 *kronor*.
    Cost for each patient per day: for a private room about 7 *kronor*, for a general ward about 5 *kronor*.

St. Luke's Hospital, New York
    Average number of patients per day 209, of which 10% in individual rooms.
    Total cost per year 375,000 *kronor*.
    Cost for each patient per day: for a private room about 6 *kronor* for a general ward about 4 *kronor*.

Mount Sinai Hospital, New York
   Number of beds 480.
   Construction cost 5½ million *kronor*.
   Average patients per day (1904) 220. [8]
   Total cost of operation (1904) 400,000 *kronor*.
   Cost per patient per day 5 *kronor*.

Boston City Hospital (municipal hospital)
   The hospital itself [9].
   Average number of patients per day 425.
   Cost per patient per day 4 *kronor*.
   Total cost of operation per year 650,000 *kronor*.

Johns Hopkins Hospital
   Number of beds about 350.
   Construction cost > 4 million *kronor*.
   Average number of patients per day 276.
   Total cost of operation per year 450,000 *kronor*.
   Cost per patient per day on average 4.50 *kronor*.

Academic Hospital, Uppsala
   Number of beds 298.
   Construction cost (original building construction and equipment + new buildings and improvements 1902-1904) 900,000 *kronor*.
   Average number of patients per day 235, of which about 7% in individual rooms.
   Total cost of operation per year 184,000 *kronor*.
   Cost per patient per day 2.15 *kronor*.

Serafimerlasarettet
   Average number of patients per day 346, of which about 3% in individual rooms.
   Total cost of operation per year 385,000 *kronor*.
   Cost per patient per day about 3 *kronor*.

As can be seen from above, the daily cost per patient in the American hospitals is significantly higher than in the Swedish ones. From two of the former, there is specified information for individual rooms and wards, and the daily cost for ward care amounts to 5 and 4 *kronor*, respectively, compared to 3 and 2.15 *kronor* for the Swedish hospitals on average for both wards and private rooms. The percentage of patients in individual rooms and the costs for these are specifically stated in the annual reports of the three American hospitals, but as far as I could tell, the medical care in private rooms was not of such an extent that it could significantly increase the average cost per day and patient, which for these three hospitals amounted to 5, 4, and 4.50 *kronor* respectively. The hospitals' facility costs are also significant, 11-12,000 *kronor* per bed for Mount Sinai and Johns Hopkins Hospital, and all these figures agree well with the impression of richly lavish, in some cases luxurious, equipment that one gets when visiting the American hospitals.

When you enter through the doors of the free-standing St. Luke's Hospital on a hill beside New York's beautiful Central Park and find yourself in the huge, beautiful marble hall, where uniformed attendants stand ready to give information or show you the way to the various departments, you feel like you have entered the castle of a prince. As a rule, a lot of marble is used in the halls, staircases, and corridors of American hospitals and, especially in the operating rooms, this contributes greatly to the impression of cleanliness, light, and order that is encountered everywhere. The hospital's *administration department* is usually located in a special building, which forms the center of the hospital's architecture and occupies the large main entrance. In front of this are the business and financial office and – of course – in the most easily accessible and most eye-catching place in the large hall inside the gate "the bureau of inquiries," the information agency. Such a thing is considered indispensable in America for every major public institution. There are secretaries here throughout the day, who manage the hospital's ongoing operations and provide the visitor with the desired information, inform them of available places, conditions for admission, give instructions on which ward this and that patient is being cared for, where Dr. X or Y is currently located, etc. This is also where the hospital's *telephone exchange* is located, which is connected to all the wards and operating rooms, the office of the executive director, the head doctor, and the housekeepers, the nursing home, and other important locations. The bureau of inquiries is thus a kind of nerve center, which greatly facilitates and simplifies communication within the hospital.

The *wards* are usually arranged according to our usual pattern, with 10-20 patients in each ward. The space is well managed, and you do not have the unpleasant sight of overcrowded halls.

The children are cared for in special rooms, which are furnished and equipped in a way that appeals to the little ones, with storage for toys, etc.

The surgery department is always separate; it usually consists of several operating rooms, preparation (wash) rooms for the patients, anesthesia rooms, sterilization and dressing rooms, toilets and bathrooms for the surgeons; in addition, there is a sufficient number of *special rooms for postoperative patients,* a facility of great humanitarian importance, which does not generally seem to gain sufficient consideration in the case of new and renovating hospitals in our country. It often happens that postoperative patients and other sick people disturb a whole lot of others in the same ward, perhaps for several nights in a row, by crying, loud talking when upset, vomiting, etc., and it should be a reasonable demand that such patients, as well as the dying, should be isolated.

Each major hospital has its own *pathology department.* As is well known, Americans favor a consistent division of labor, whereby the greatest possible time saving is achieved, and accordingly one finds that the pathology department not only takes care of the autopsies and the bacteriological and histological-pathological examinations, but also all the clinical laboratories, urinalysis, gastric juice, blood, sputum, fecal examinations, etc. Since the pathology department is immediately available within the hospital itself and is equipped with sufficient personnel to immediately handle even difficult analyses, the significant advantage is achieved that laboratory studies that may contribute to the diagnosis or inform the therapy reach the clinical doctors in the shortest possible time. This displacement of the laboratory work does restrict the activity of the clinical assistants, but on the other hand, the few assistants in our surgical clinics have plenty to do with work in hospitals and operating rooms, indeed are often overworked due to lack of time, and sometimes postpone or completely abandon laboratory work that might be important for practical assessment of a case or for scientific studies.

The *nurses* have their residence in a separate building or a large separate part of the hospital. In addition to the sleeping rooms - in general, each nurse or student has her own room - there are bathrooms and toilets, one or more lounges with newspapers and periodicals, a library, piano, rooms for teaching, etc. Overall, the nurses are treated much better than in our country, which admittedly in many places does not mean much. At Johns Hopkins and Boston City Hospital, the *"nurses' home"* has its own large, magnificent building; but the record for expensive accommodation for nurses must be held by the Presbyterian Hospital in New York (average 209 patients), whose nurses and students reside in the recently built Florence Nightingale Hall at a cost of nearly 1 million *kronor*. The money was simply donated by a member of the hospital management when the space for nurses within the hospital became too crowded.

So far, I have not mentioned anything about the hospital's *relationship to medical education*, but I want to say a few words about it in passing. Most of the large hospitals in the medical teaching centers I visited in New York, Boston, Baltimore, Philadelphia, and Chicago are clinical hospitals. Often a medical school makes agreements with several of the hospitals for clinical teaching of their students, and the clinicians participate in rounds, write journals, and perform operations just as we do. Usually, the largest operating room is built as an amphitheater for educational purposes, but many of the clinical hospitals are otherwise not specifically set up for teaching. This is so far occurred only with a few; the model for these is the *Johns Hopkins Hospital in Baltimore* (350 beds, approximately 150 clinicians), which was created in conjunction with the medical school of the same name, and which was planned from the beginning with the purpose of benefiting teaching to the greatest possible extent. A special clinical building has recently been erected there, placed at the corner between the two huge perpendicular wings of the hospital. Among other things, the *clinical building* houses the *surgery department* with three operating rooms, one of which is constructed as an amphitheater, sterilization room, anesthetic room, changing room, examination room, and room for postoperative patients; also the *radiology department* and regular *photography studio*, a splendidly equipped department of *surgical pathology* located in close proximity to the operating rooms, where the preparations from the operations are examined and demonstrated for the staff [10], *lecture halls* with adjacent smaller *examination rooms* and *waiting rooms* for patients, special rooms for examination of people who have previously been cared for at the hospital, regarding the final result of the operation or other treatment, rooms for *special studies*, and a couple rooms for *record storage and cataloging*, etc. Space has been provided far beyond the current need, and several rooms are reserved for temporary or future purposes. Right next to the clinical building are the *outpatient clinics*, and the ground floor of the former contains operating rooms, anesthesia, sterilization rooms, and "recovery rooms" for postoperative patients, but exclusively for the needs of the outpatient clinics. In addition, there are a number of smaller *rooms for accident patients* that need to be admitted to the hospital, and you thereby avoid disturbing a large number of other patients, as in many of our hospitals, when a patient who arrived during the night is wheeled into the hall.

The outpatient clinics have their own entrance, separate from the large main entrance, which is thereby freed from the crowds of outpatients and gives the visitors a more pleasant impression than would otherwise be the case.

The general tendency within American institutions to run as expediently and efficiently as possible is shown by the facilities at the *new outpatient clinic at the Massachusetts General Hospital in Boston.*

The building consists of a 4-story L-shaped building with the main entrance at the angle and the various departments distributed in both directions from it. You first enter a large waiting hall. The patient goes to a table, where a doctor asks a few questions to find out which department the patient should be sent to, and stamps the name of the department (surgical, throat, skin, etc.) on a cardboard form in regular book format, which is given to the patient. On this form, a female "clerk" at an adjacent table now fills in the patient's name, age, address, etc. The rest of the form is reserved for the medical history and other notes by the doctor. Now the patient goes with his form to the "central office" in the same hall and leaves the form there and instead receives a piece of paper with a sequential number. While the patients are taken to their respective departments, they are registered in the central office according to the information on the forms, which are then sent out in small electric conveyors to their destinations on the various floors and automatically emptied into a basket in some central place. The doctors enter the medical histories, notes on treatment, etc. on the forms and leave them unorganized on their desks when they leave their work, after which all the forms left out by any employee in the entire outpatient clinic are gathered back into the administrative heart of the outpatient clinic, the central office. Here they are catalogued by name and by disease into one of the sanctified card-catalog-systems so beloved by Americans. All the different outpatient clinic departments are in telephone contact with the central office, and if the patient visits the outpatient clinic again, whether it is the same department as before or another one, the relevant doctor has only to request his medical history by phone, which is sent up to him within a few seconds from the central office. Doctors never engage in such menial and time-wasting tasks as "booking" or arranging and keeping track of medical records; to allow a doctor, whose time and energy are fully needed for health care, to deal with purely mechanical administrative tasks, such as registration of patients, would be considered an unreasonable waste of energy.

The new outpatient clinic gives a first-class impression throughout. Each department has its own laboratory. At the surgical outpatient clinic there are, among other things, rooms for postoperative patients, separate changing rooms for clean and dirty cases; the medical department has special rooms for examining the heart and lungs, equipped with soft rubber mats to make percussion and auscultation as undisturbed as possible. The changing rooms are supervised by a special person, and clothing is hung in insulated compartments, which are ventilated by a stream of fresh air. Each department has one or two lecture halls; the hall of the medical department, which is built in amphitheater form, has the practical arrangement of a wide corridor in front of each row of benches to allow demonstrated patients to pass "close by." The nose-throat department has teaching rooms with practically arranged examination places, equipped with tripod lamps, tables for instruments, a large spittoon by the patient's chair, etc. But it would take me too long to continue with the details; as a conclusion from my outpatient clinic description, would only mention that in America nowadays more and more importance is placed on isolation and special care of *tuberculosis in the outpatient clinics*. At Johns Hopkins, a large sum of money was donated in 1903 for the establishment of a tuberculosis clinic. A nurse is also employed at this hospital, who is especially assigned to visit the tuberculosis outpatients in their own homes and to help teach them to the best of her ability. Similar arrangements have been made in other major hospitals.

Some of the larger hospitals have their own *automobile ambulances*.

[p. 3: 273]

I will continue with a few words about the *staff* of American hospitals and again choose the Johns Hopkins Hospital as the basis for my description.

However, it should first be mentioned that the hospital's *management*, the Board of Trustees, generally do not have medical members but consist of businessmen. Moreover, the composition of hospital boards varies so significantly for different hospitals that I refrain from giving any kind of general description and only briefly outline conditions at the Johns Hopkins Hospital. Here, the board consists here of about 12 members, very respected businessmen, who appoint a president and a vice president from among themselves, as well as various committees for the administration of the hospital. At their side, as an advisory authority, stands a *medical board*, composed of the hospital's department heads and a *superintendent* or managing director.

At the larger hospitals, the latter is usually a reputable physician who does not belong to the hospital's medical staff; he is the intermediary between the management and the hospital staff.

Compared to our conditions, one characteristic of the American hospitals is their very large *staff*, which is considered necessary for the operation of the hospital and its clinical teaching. If you include doctors, nurses, financial staff, and everyone else having to do with the actual operation of the hospital, their number usually reaches or exceeds the number of patients. For Johns Hopkins, I don't have exact numbers, but there the ratio was calculated to be 1:1.

St. Luke's Hospital ...	209 patients,	275 staff
Mt. Sinai Hospital now ...	220 patients,	263 staff
anticipated at full operation ...	480 patients,	570 staff

For comparison with Swedish conditions, I only have figures from the Academic Hospital available. There the relationship is: patients 235, staff 107, thus approximately 2:1.

The nursing system is generally organized according to the English pattern. Almost every major American hospital has its own nursing school, the *training school for nurses*, and the clinical work is carried out for the most part by the *students*. The few graduate nurses permanently employed at the hospital serve as supervisors for the students. For example, St. Luke's Hospital with just over 200 patients has one operating room nurse, one night nurse, one outpatient clinic nurse, one private room nurse, and two ward nurses, for a total of 6 fully-qualified nurses. The total required number of nurses is otherwise composed of students. And at Johns Hopkins Hospital, the nursing corps directly participating in nursing work consists of 8 head nurses and 93 students. But then the students also get a thorough education. The course is usually *2-3 years*; a good scholastic foundation is required for admission (St. Luke's Hospital requires a high-school diploma [11] or equivalent), so in general it is only *educated girls who are recruited into the corps* at the more reputable hospitals. The nursing education at Johns Hopkins Hospital, which can probably be considered typical of the modern American nursing school, consists of a 3-year course. For the *first half year*, there is no clinical work. The student must go through home economics training within the hospital, learn to cook food for diets and compose diet menus, to keep household utensils in good condition, to cook, make beds, and clean (in the nurses' home), laundry, etc. She also receives lessons in hygiene, including the most important health care regulations, anatomy, physiology, pharmacology, and some theoretical teaching about health care. During this time, the student is called a *probationer*; her suitability for the calling is evaluated, and if she is found unsuitable in one respect or another, she is dismissed, usually after only a short time. At the end of the probationary period, i.e. after half year, an oral and written *exam* is held in the subjects covered; those who pass this continue as *juniors* for the *rest of the first year*; the second year is called the *intermediate* and the third year the *senior year*. During these 2½ years, the students work in the hospitals and operating rooms as day and night nurses; the working day in health care is 8 hours, and in addition, lessons are held every day for 1-2 hours by the headmistress of the nursing school or her assistant or by a doctor. The nurses become quite well educated in America. What can you say about the following lessons: The changes in the surrounding atmosphere through respiration, harmful organic and inorganic substances in water, mechanics of the human body, quantitative analysis of urea and albumin, diseases of the adrenal glands? But on the whole, the teaching focuses on those things that are specifically interesting or practically useful for a nurse. During the junior year the student receives lectures in hygiene, bacteriology, general medicine, diseases of the digestive system, orthopedics, infectious diseases, during the middle year lectures and exercises in urinalysis, lessons in medicine, surgery, gynecology, instruction in massage, and during the senior year teaching in obstetrics, pediatrics, nervous and mental diseases, skin diseases, eye, ear, throat and nose diseases. *Oral and written exams* with practical tests are held at the end of every year; and after successfully passing the exam at the end of the 3rd year, the student receives her diploma as a "graduate nurse." She can then seek employment as a head nurse. The students receive no salary; they get room and board, and the hospital also provides them with a uniform (after the probationary period), linen, and textbooks. A head nurse earns 30-50 dollars a month, and the headmistress of the nursing school (a former head nurse) earns 1500 dollars a year (St. Luke's), which may serve to give an idea of the wage conditions of American nurses.

As far as *the medical staff* is concerned, it has been increased in the same grand style as the staff elsewhere. The Johns Hopkins surgical department has approximately 120 beds, and for this there are: 1 chief and professor of surgery, 4 associate professors – 1 in general surgery, 1 in neurosurgery, 1 in urology, 1 in surgical pathology[16] – plus 2 instructors (assistant doctors, who do some of the teaching), one specialist in orthopedic surgery and a doctor at the hospital's orthopedic department, 3 assistants, and 4 "interns" (newly graduated doctors), for a total of 14 people. Two of the mentioned associate professors and the orthopedist are also employed at the surgical outpatient departments, but otherwise these are managed by 8 special doctors. Ear and eye disorders are assigned to a joint special department.

A comparison between the American and our Swedish clinics is not fully possible because at the former the number of clinicians, who within a certain time complete their duties and receive a degree in surgery, is greater than at any of our clinics and requires more teachers. But this much is clear, that in our country people have a significantly different perception of the required number of doctors and teaching staff at a surgical clinic. For example, at the Academic Hospital surgery department in Uppsala, with a number of patients approximately equivalent to that at Johns Hopkins, 1 senior physician and professor of surgery, 1 assistant teacher in surgery, and 3 junior physicians are considered sufficient for the medical care and teaching. And of these, only 4 are clinically active, whereas at Johns Hopkins all the 14 doctors participate.

Such an abundant clinic staff would be completely unthinkable for our small circumstances; and one could imagine that in this, as in many other areas, the Americans are using an unnecessarily large standard. However, from a purely financial point of view, this is not actually true. The surgeon-in-chief receives a large salary, but the assistant doctors get quite modest fees – and the associate professors, who most closely correspond to our docents, have to be content with name and reputation, while the interns get housing and board, but no salary. (This according to oral information, which I hope I have not misunderstood).

One would also be inclined to believe that the 14 surgeons at Johns Hopkins stepped on each other's feet or had too little to do; but this is by no means the case. The work is systematic and well distributed, and everyone works intensively in their own areas. In particular, *teaching* is well provided for. The clinics are held by the chief surgeon and two of the associates alternately, so that one lectures and one operates, the professors of surgical pathology and urology each give a special course in their subject, the orthopedist has rounds with lectures and interviews in his department, and the neurosurgeon gives a special course in surgical technique (operations on live animals). Because of this division of labor, every one of these teachers has plenty of time to prepare their teaching and to develop it in the best possible way.

There is something else, for which the modern American clinics largely owe their abundant staff, and that is the patterned *order* which usually characterizes these institutions. Consider how the personnel records are checked, completed, organized, and stored at Johns Hopkins Hospital! The doctors very often make long additions and explanatory remarks in the journals, using for this purpose the most readable style one could ask for, namely that of the typewriter; once a week, all the assistant doctors in the various departments gather for a joint medical record conference, where the patients' medical records issued during the week are reviewed, corrected and completed, so that they become fully reliable for possible scientific studies. A special records secretary then takes charge of them and arranges them according to the card-catalogue-system with names and numbers in one series of cards, illness and treatment in the other. If I want to bring out all the cases of the last five years with incarcerated hernia with intestinal resection, I only need to pull out one drawer of cards and on the letter H, look for the word "hernia" and then in the next row of cards select the subsection "resection" and write down the numbers on the cards standing here in order to have what I need within a couple of minutes. I can do it myself, but it is even faster to ask the secretary to pull the records.

And I can't help thinking with pleasure in this context about the surgical-pathological laboratory. Preparations of special interest in teaching are collected in special accounts; the material is never stored in a pile for eventual processing en masse, but is managed immediately; careful descriptions and explanatory remarks are written down with typewriters, photographers and draftsmen are put to work, and so the whole thing is collected bit by bit into an ever-growing academic handbook locally manufactured with illustrations.

With pride, Dr. B, the head of the department, showed me a beautiful little book on skin sarcoma, which was currently being revised.

It is probably precisely in the area *of scientific production* that the modern American clinic has the greatest advantages from its rich staff of doctors. Where even one of these has plenty of time left over from clinical work to devote to scientific work, and as he also - at least in the higher grades - focuses his energies both in the practical and the theoretical field of work to a definite specialty of his special science, he has prerequisites to become, although limited in scope, a master in his field. My highly valued friend, the young associate professor of neurological surgery at Johns Hopkins, had previously as an assistant devoted himself to general surgery and there made several good contributions; however, he became increasingly interested in the still underdeveloped field of neurosurgery and was made an associate professor in this subject; now he has completely put away thoughts of laparotomies and herniorrhaphies and thrown all his energy and interest into the new subject, and so you do not need to wonder "will it be enough?" Johns Hopkins Hospital publishes journals, *Reports of the Johns Hopkins Hospital* for larger works and *Bulletin of the Johns Hopkins Hospital* for shorter essays, both of them known and appreciated throughout the world. And the hospital does not shy away from financial sacrifices in order to support the scientific work in every possible way, for example through the employment of secretaries, draftsmen, and photographers for this purpose; works from J.H.H. often contain fine illustrations and thereby become particularly appealing and useful. The annual report for 1903-1904 gives a good idea of the intensity of the scientific work at the clinic; the members of the hospital staff at that time had published 149 major and minor works during that year! In addition, it should be noted a thesis is not required for the M.D. degree in America, which thereby differs favorably from Germany, where small, often worthless doctoral theses pad the medical literature, already cluttered with the mass products of a chronic writing itch.

In connection with this description of an exemplary American clinic, I cannot help but think of our own clinics. A comparison would certainly be interesting in many respects, but I just want to touch in passing on some deficits in our surgical clinics. Here, above all, the lack of assistants makes itself felt. Fully occupied, often rushed and greatly overworked, in at least at one of our clinics usually working 10-12 hours at the operating table and in hospital rooms, the assistant doctors have neither time nor energy left for other work. Those on duty are allowed to do whatever they want without the guidance of the assistant doctor, which should be an important contribution to teaching, the medical records are left unorganized and unchecked due to lack of time, patients seeking admission have to wait hours to be examined, some have to wait for surgery for a week or more unnecessarily, simply because the doctors are overwhelmed with work, and during all this there is no respite for studying books and journals for further research on the subject; the professor does not get the help he needs from his assistant doctors in scientific processing of the clinical material and even less, of course, do these have time left for independent work. And there is plenty of good material. I do not think I am exaggerating if I say that our clinical material could produce twice as much as it does now. However, we can hope that a remedy for these severe shortcomings can be found, if the new proposal is approved to introduce a certain period of compulsory assistantship at hospitals into Swedish medical education. The clinics' assistant staffs would then be able to obtain the required increase without financial difficulties, and the junior doctors would also have time for academic studies and scientific work.

In America one may be quite sure that, as soon as private institutions, such as the hospitals, are concerned, the most important positions will be found filled with the ablest men it is generally possible to obtain. The hospital board calls for the medical positions whom it deems most suitable, regardless of age and paper merits, and no appeal is made against its selection. The 'merit gap' between applicants, which we have to deal with but find repellent, is relatively unknown there, since I believe there is no application process for the medical positions.

Finally, I cannot fail to mention a few words about the amiable and friendly treatment, which especially at Johns Hopkins Hospital, visiting colleagues enjoyed. The pleasant impression of my time at this institution was also increased by the relaxed and cheerful, fine and gentlemanly social tone that prevailed there. The students have a good university education as a basis for the medical studies, and this certainly contributed to the university spirit in its best sense, which marked the J.H. medical school and clinics.

Add to that an unusual freshness and vigor in the work. "We are all boys here," the famous surgeon Kelly said, when he introduced me to his clinic, and he described in these words one of the great qualities of Americans. You do not see professorial loftiness over there; the *Geheimrat*[17] of Berlin would seem completely out of place in America. But then the Americans are also a sports-loving people – even clinical professors participate there in athletic exercises – and sport certainly has its essential share in the origin of their healthy and brisk demeanor.

In the foregoing, I have in some places touched on conditions within our hospital system in connection with the depiction of the American system. I would not want to make any kind of comparative valuation; the conditions here and those on the other side of the Atlantic are so different that such an evaluation would be pointless. The economic conditions are already largely not comparable. Considering that America with impunity engages in the most reckless waste, let us here in Sweden try to get by with our very limited resources and make the best of it, and the ratio between what is achieved in really good health care and the costs incurred is probably quite satisfactory here in our country.

However, in this as in other areas, it is important not to fall behind in development; in particular, this should especially be considered when building and renovating hospitals – more than has happened in some places – and in the teaching and scientific work in our clinics. In these areas, I believe that the American institutions, although founded on a different basis than ours, will be able to give us quite a few good suggestions.

Original Notes

1. In some quarters, efforts are being made to have the course increased further. For example Rush Medical College in Chicago has just decided to introduce a voluntary fifth year.
2. These examinations, which constitute the only public control over medical training, are very easy, but the combined number of those passed in all the states during the year 1904 was only 19% of the total number of examinees. Those who fail can try their luck at a future examination or in another state, where they are not as particular. New York State is considered to have the strictest requirements.
3. High school or secondary school teaching could be compared most closely with the upper secondary school in our general education, and a complete 4-year course should generally impart the amount of

knowledge considered necessary for the matriculation exam. But such a comparison is greatly hampered by the fact that an American "high school student" has far more freedom than ours to choose subjects that are considered suitable or required as a basis for his future vocation, and the high school could thus be described as a lower university. For example, a young man receiving his high school diploma may not have studied more history or language than our fourth or fifth classmen, while he is at least as well versed in physics and chemistry as our *realstudenter* and knows enough Latin to match our sixth lower class.

4. In the smaller colleges this usually amounts to 50-75 dollars, to which in some cases extra laboratory charges are added.
5. I specifically asked whether this course included anatomical aspects of vaginal and rectal examinations, but the answer was that it did not.
6. An M.D. without special training in psychiatry is not considered competent to render an opinion about mental status, etc. Psychiatric matters are left entirely to the decision of specialists (private or hospital doctors).
7. Forensic medicine is an unfortunate aspect of the American medical system. To fully understand this, one needs to understand the fundamental corruption of political life and public administration in the States. Forensic matters are managed according to the old English pattern by non-medically trained persons, so-called coroners, who are elected by the people at the same time as they elect the governor etc., and this election is based on purely political considerations. The coroner is a sort of intermediary between medicine and law. Forensic autopsies are assigned by the coroner to a doctor hired by his office as the "coroner's physician" and paid by the state (salary of 2500 dollars in Illinois). The coroner's physician does not need to have special training as a forensic doctor or pathological anatomist, but in complicated cases, pathologists are called in for an expert opinion. Furthermore, doctors or medical students do not have access to coroner's autopsies. A coroner's physician devotes himself exclusively to his work for the coroner, as he has practically no time for any other work.

In Massachusetts and possibly some other states, the institution of coroner has been abolished and replaced by a system of medical examiners, with a certain number assigned to each county in proportion to the population. These doctors stand in much the same relationship to the police authorities as our doctors in forensic cases; they do not have any special training for their position as a coroner.

There is widespread dissatisfaction with the institution of coroners.

This office is considered to be completely superfluous, and it is perpetuated only through the influence of "politicians," who find the position of coroner to be a lucrative position to reward party members with no real qualification. It is likely that the coroner system will be abolished and the entire system of forensic medicine reorganized when there is less corruption and more order in the politics and administration of the States.

8. Mount Sinai Hospital, the great new Jewish hospital, was completed in 1904. The small average number of patients in relation to the number of beds is due to the fact that the hospital could only gradually be put into full use during the course of the year. The operating cost at "full operation" is estimated at 600,000 *kronor* per year.

9. Boston City Hospital also includes an epidemic hospital, a convalescent home, etc., totaling over 900 beds.

10. Surgical pathology is split off as a separate department from the general pathology department, which is located in another part of the hospital. Having access to a pathology laboratory in close proximity to the operating room is considered to be of great importance in some cases, for example tumors about whose benign or malignant nature one is uncertain. I particularly remember an operation for a lip tumor of questionable malignancy at another American clinic. The excised tumor was submitted to the pathologist, and while the wound was sutured, frozen microtome sections were made which were stained and examined, and in three minutes the diagnosis of cancer was made, which led the operator to also remove the regional glands of the neck. I was also able to see one of the stained sections, which was a really beautiful preparation of squamous cell cancer.

11. See above essay in *Läkartidningen* No. 35, 1905 [Part I].

Biographical Sources

Vem är det: Svensk biografisk handbok 1963. Accessed through https://sv.wikipedia.org.

Nyström G. *Där stridens sår läkas*. Stockholm, 1915.

Nyström G. Experiences with the Trendelenburg operation for pulmonary embolism. *Annals of Surgery* 1930; 92:498-532.

Nyström G, Blalock A. Contributions to the technic of pulmonary embolectomy. *Journal of Thoracic Surgery* 1935; 5:169-188.

Publication Source

Allmänna Svenska Läkartidningen [General Swedish Medical News] is today simply called *Läkartidningen*. Historical issues have been digitized by Google Books.

Translation Notes

1) The author visited Minnesota, and Andrea Majocchi (Volume 2, Chapter 17) says that "Nistron di Upsala" visited the Mayo brothers in Rochester, but there is no mention in this report of such a visit. William Mayo's description of his visit to Sweden several years later (*Journal-Lancet* 1914; 34:351-456,475-480) suggests that he first met Nyström there.
2) Småland is a region of southern Sweden that was the original home of many American immigrants. It has a distinctive regional dialect.
3) The medical schools of New York University and Bellevue Hospital had merged in 1898 to form the University and Bellevue Hospital Medical College. This is now part of the NYU Grossman School of Medicine.
4) Closed after the Flexner Report.
5) Closed after the Flexner Report. See Tkacic C., "Where the healing happened: Dilapidated East Baltimore church was a place of medicine, faith," *Baltimore Sun*, 1 March 2018.
6) About 13½ acres.
7) See Williams DJ, "The history of Werner Spalteholz's *Handatlas der Anatomie des Menschen*," *Journal of Audiovisual Media in Medicine* 1999; 22:164-170. Max Brödel got his start as an illustrator working with Spalteholz.
8) Jones Quain (1796-1865) was an Irish anatomist, whose *Elements of Anatomy* was a standard for many years.
9) Olof Hammarsten (1841-1932) was a Swedish biochemist, whose textbook was a standard for many years.
10) The Serafimerlasarettet was a major hospital in Stockholm until it closed in 1980.
11) The *krone* (plural *kronor*) was and still is the monetary unit of Sweden. As stated later in this article, the official exchange rate in 1904 was 3.75 *kronor* to the dollar.
12) *Similia similibus curentur* (let like be cured by like), the doctrine that

medications should produce similar symptoms as the disease.
13) Hazzard C, *Principles of Osteopathy*, 3rd Edition, Detroit, 1899. The anecdote about the child with a subluxation of the atlas is on Page 19.
14) The Roosevelt Hospital, founded by a distant cousin of the presidents with that name, is now the Mount Sinai West Hospital. St. Luke's Hospital became the Mount Sinai Morningside Hospital. The Presbyterian Hospital is now part of the New York – Presbyterian Hospital system.
15) Augustana Hospital was later called the Lutheran General Hospital, and closed in 1989. The name Augustana refers to the Augsburg Confession (*Confessio Augustana*), the fundamental document of the Lutheran Church.
16) The Associate Professors were J. M. T. Finney (general surgery), Harvey Cushing (neurosurgery), Hugh H. Young (urology), and Joseph Bloodgood (surgical pathology). The author seems reluctant to give their names, although he does later refer to "Dr. B."
17) "*Geheimrat*" was a title bestowed by the emperor on deserving subjects. The British equivalent is "Privy Councillor," and even this sounds rather silly to Americans.

12

Edvin Helling (1906-1907)

Edvin August Helling was born in 1873 in Gothenburg (Göteborg). He studied at Uppsala University, receiving his medical license in 1903, and then occupied junior surgical positions at the Sahlgrenska Hospital in Gothenburg.

In 1906-1907, at the age of 33, he traveled to Great Britain and the United States on a Hwasser Fellowship, and his experiences in America are described in the following pages.

After returning to Sweden, he also studied in Munich and Vienna, and continued his surgical training in Gothenburg at the Sahlgrenska and Children's Hospitals.

He spent some time at a military hospital in Austria during the First World War and made another visit to the United States in 1922. However, he primarily devoted himself to general medical and surgical practice in central Sweden, mostly in the small city of Mora. His dedication and good humor were still recalled in local histories many years later. He retired in 1938 and died in 1951.

Några anteckningar från en studieresa i Förenta Staterna
Upsala Läkareförenings Förhandlingar 1907-1908; 13:169-204

Some notes from a study trip in the United States
by Edvin Helling

It was not without very great expectations that I, as a Hwasser Fellow, embarked in September 1906 on a trip to the United States to study American surgery as it is practiced at the larger clinics in the eastern and northern states under the direction of men such as Halsted, Kelly, Young, Cushing, Keen, Deaver, Murphy, Ochsner, the Mayo brothers, Munro, Richardson, etc. I have to say that these expectations were not only met but also in many cases exceeded.

It became quite clear that the best American surgery is in no way inferior to the best European surgery.

Only the most superficial observer would fail to be impressed that this is a surgical community whose practitioners received their basic education according to the German model, on which basis they have constructed a healing profession that can completely measure up to that of their teachers, and could be largely considered a development of the same. The German influence is noticeable everywhere: Most clinical chiefs have spent several years at German hospitals, partly as first assistants; a number of management positions are held by Germans, usually former first assistants at one of the larger German clinics, and "last but not least" one finds everywhere a thorough and detailed knowledge of not only the German but also the English, French, and Italian surgical literatures and of everything important that has taken place in the larger European clinics, especially the German ones. It is precisely in this way that I think American surgery has an advantage over European surgery; if it is not compensated by a similar knowledge of American surgical conditions here in Europe, the "center of gravity" in the field of surgery will shift from the Old World to the New, perhaps sooner than expected.

An equally brief and apt characterization of all the American surgery I have had the opportunity to see was given by an old doctor far from the "Wild West." After seeing a day's operations at the Mayo clinic, now a place of pilgrimage for all American surgeons and also a good many European surgeons, he said "this surgery is really just simple common sense."

Dr. Gunnar Nyström has recently described American hospital conditions in general, as well as the medical teaching at both the best and some mediocre schools (and there are many of these). Since my experiences in these respects agree completely with his, I shall confine myself to a brief account of some observations of more special surgical interest, which I had occasion to make at the Johns Hopkins Hospital in Baltimore; the Pennsylvania, Jefferson, and German Hospitals[1] in Philadelphia; the Mayo clinic in Rochester; the Hotel Dieu, Augustana, and Mercy Hospitals[2] in Chicago; the Swedish Hospitals[3] in St. Paul and Minneapolis; the Massachusetts General, Carney, and City Hospitals in Boston; the Mount Sinai and Presbyterian Hospitals in New York; and during the Society of Clinical Surgery meeting in Philadelphia.

The clinical experience at each of these institutions was extremely large, with the exception of the smaller Swedish Hospitals in St. Paul and Minneapolis, since all of the others except the Mayo clinic are located in large cities; the operative statistics in their annual reports are colossal. The number of laparotomies alone amounted to 2,750 at the Mayo clinic (two surgeons) in 1906, at the Swedish Augustana Hospital in Chicago the same year 882, etc. Many assistants are available to the chief physicians (for example, in the Department of Surgery at the Johns Hopkins Hospital, with 130 beds, there are no fewer than 16) and the work is distributed to the smallest detail.

The experience here was also usually richer than that which I had been able to obtain in the European clinics that I had visited; this was not only because of the extreme accuracy with which diagnosis, prognosis, operation, indications, surgical technique, and postoperative treatment are reviewed for each particular case, but perhaps to an even greater degree that anyone in the audience is permitted to raise objections, ask questions, or request further information during both the lectures and the operations, all of which are addressed or answered by the surgeon as far as possible, without the operation being apparently affected adversely in any way. Most American surgeons also spontaneously impart a lot of both diagnostic and purely technical advice during the course of their operations, which is extremely valuable information usually drawn from their extensive personal experiences.

Model institutions in this respect are the Johns Hopkins Hospital and the Murphy and Mayo clinics. At the latter, a special discussion club has been formed by the visiting doctors, where every afternoon the cases shown during the morning are carefully reviewed by representatives appointed by the club each day and presented for further discussion; usually one of the clinic's assistants is also present to provide additional information.

This method of presentation puts great demands on the operator's endurance as well as his technical skill, and it was astounding how Murphy or the Mayo brothers could each perform 6-7 major operations between 8 A.M. and 2 P.M. while continuously lecturing with their faces covered by a thick mask.

Asepsis at the clinics I visited largely met the highest standards. Dry asepsis seems to predominate. All drying is done with sterile gauze, and flushing of a wound or a serous cavity is rarely seen.

Operators as well as assistants and nurses were always wearing sterile gowns or aprons and wearing rubber gloves, as well as sterile caps and a face mask or at least a sterile gauze placed over the nose and mouth and tied at the neck. The gloves generally extended well up the forearm and over the sleeves of the surgical gown. One clinic director in New York commented somewhat disparagingly during a lecture about the kind of asepsis sometimes seen where surgeons had gloved hands, but rather hairy arms sticking out of elbow-length gowns.

The gloves were sterilized either by heating in dry air or by boiling or by storage in sublimate[4] or formalin. Hand disinfection and the disinfection of the surgical field differed little from our methods. Sublimate and alcohol were used as antiseptics for washing both hands and surgical fields, and sometimes potassium permanganate, oxalic acid, creolin, or the so-called Harrington's solution (a mixture of strong hydrochloric acid, sublimate, alcohol, and water).[5]

The day before the operation, the patient was given a bath if possible and placed in a clean bed, with or without an antiseptic dressing for laparotomies, and in most cases this was the only cleansing that took place until the final washing immediately before the operation, which was usually started after the induction of anesthesia.

The instruments used during the operation are usually dry.

Catgut was used almost exclusively as suture and ligature material, for skin sutures silkworm gut or silver wire. Buried nonabsorbable intestinal sutures were almost always made with celluloid linen. Silk was generally used very little. Sutures through the skin were systematically avoided in many places and the skin edges were united by a subcutaneous suture of catgut or silver wire, which could later be removed without difficulty after healing to be used again. This method produced almost imperceptible scars and the antiseptic properties of silver were thought to play a significant role in healing.

Catgut was sterilized in several ways, sometimes with hot dry air, but usually one or another kind of iodine catgut was prepared according to the method of Moschcowitz (potassium iodine and alcohol) or according to the so-called paraffin method, in which raw catgut was dried in hot air (140° C. for 3 hours), placed in liquid paraffin for 12 hours, slowly heated in this (150° C. for 2 hours), and then stored in a solution of 2% phenol in paraffin or in tincture of iodine. This method produced a suture and ligature material that was at the same time extremely strong as well as flexible and absolutely sterile. Also, several kinds of chromic catgut were widely used.

Anesthesia

The anesthetic used in all the northern states was almost exclusively ether, in those of the southern states, which have a more or less tropical climate, exclusively chloroform. On repeated inquiries as to the cause of this apparently strange relationship, I never succeeded in obtaining any other answer than that ether is not suitable for narcotic purposes in the tropics. The ether was always given by the drip method (only in one place did I see a modification of the Clover mask[6] used) and on a normal open chloroform mask, around which a towel or gauze compress was usually folded several times, in order to reduce the access of air. The patient's face is often coated with a thin layer of Vaseline or lanolin and the eyes are in many cases covered with small pieces of rubber tape. This naturally made it impossible to test the corneal reflexes, which did not seem to be necessary since the administration of the anesthetic is never entrusted to someone who is not fully competent [1]. Once in a while, the ether was combined with chloroform and somewhat more often with nitrous oxide.

The ether was almost always dripped from the original metal containers, through a small strip of gauze inserted between the neck of the bottle and the stopper.

In most places, the patient received 10-20 milligrams of morphine subcutaneously a half hour before the start of anesthesia. Gastric lavage was occasionally done before the anesthesia, but this was more commonly done immediately after the operation and before the patient had even woken up; in other places oxygen inhalations were given instead, and both procedures were said to significantly reduce the discomfort after a longer anesthesia.

For special indications, oxygen was often given throughout the anesthesia along with the ether through a tube leading directly from the storage cylinder, attached to a hook-shaped bent feeding tube, which was placed under the mask and hung in one corner of the patient's mouth. I saw several examples of the Roth-Draeger anesthetic apparatus, but never saw it used. The anesthetists on duty generally seemed to be unusually skilled, at least compared to our far from ideal conditions in many places, and during the several hundred operations I witnessed, I never observed anything that could be called an "anesthetic complication."

The conditions in this respect at the Mayo clinic were particularly ideal. In all major operations, the anesthetist was a lady who had devoted herself exclusively to this for more than 10 years and who during that time had administered over 15,000 pure ether anesthetics according to the drip method without a single death.[7] It was surprising to see, with the help of the smallest possible amounts of ether, how she could talk the patients to sleep, as it were, including big, strong men. As a not insignificant contributing factor, she particularly emphasized the importance of almost complete silence around a patient who is being put to sleep. He should hear nothing but the anesthetist's voice. She said that under such conditions she could put a patient under anesthesia with half the amount of ether that would be needed in a room where the patient is distracted at every moment by talking, clattering instruments, scales, etc.

This is of course a fact known to every surgeon, but it seems to me that the offenses against this simple and yet so important rule are so numerous that it should be pointed out again.

Regarding local anesthesia or the spinal anesthesia developed by Bier, it is surprising that these methods are rarely used, especially since the American literature has many valuable papers especially in the former area (Cushing's works on local anesthesia in hernia operations, etc.)[8] The reason for this may be found in the patients themselves, who almost always refuse to undergo an operation without general anesthesia and are generally far from being as compliant as they should be. The American physician, and especially the younger surgeon, must take into account the wishes and whims of the patient and his relatives, to a degree which we would often consider almost ridiculous, even when these extend into the purely medical area. During my entire stay in America, I only saw one operation (for ingrown toenail) performed under local anesthesia.

Regarding general surgical technique and instrumentation, there is probably not much to record.

With one exception, I never saw anyone fall for the temptation to "operate against the clock."

All operations were performed with extreme, sometimes almost agonizing meticulousness, thereby sometimes dragging on unnecessarily long and increasing the duration of anesthesia.

The most prominent surgeons operate with amazing speed, despite the fact that most of them simultaneously hold an instructive lecture on the case in question and do not appear the least bit rushed, but this is not surprising in view of their enormous experience. Many of them perform over 1,000 laparotomies annually in addition to a host of other operations. At the Mayo clinic, a gastroenterostomy never took more than 40 minutes, a gastrectomy not more than an hour, an enucleation or extirpation of a goiter even in very severe cases not over 20 minutes; perineal prostatectomies were often done in less than 10 minutes, evulsion of the infraorbital, lingual, and mandibular nerves in less than a quarter hour, etc., all without any appearance of inaccuracy.

When a doctor refers a patient to a colleague for surgery, the Americans consider it his duty to attend the operation if possible. This practice is particularly appropriate and would be well worth following here at home to a far greater extent than is now the case.

This would provide a significantly increased experience, especially in the pathological anatomy of the abdominal organs and in the indications for the special operative treatments of intraperitoneal diseases. Furthermore, this desirable practice could certainly prove to be an effective means of preventing or ironing out any misunderstandings that might arise between the referring physician and his operating colleague.

Regarding general postoperative care, it was particularly noteworthy that patients were kept in bed for a relatively short time, in most places.

Simple laparotomy cases (appendectomies, gastroenterostomies, most gynecological cases) were not kept in bed for more than 8-9 days, since the abdominal wall was closed primarily. After perineal prostatectomies, patients at the Johns Hopkins Hospital were usually mobilized on the third postoperative day, after extirpation of the Gasserian ganglion likewise on the third day. The most complicated surgical cases on the biliary tract were kept in bed until all or most of the drains were removed, thus about 12 or at most 14 days.

In general, the principle was that patients should not remain in bed after an operation without reason simply to "gain strength," a concept which the vast majority completely reject.

On the contrary, they believe that patients who were not debilitated before the operation will regain strength much more quickly by being discharged early than by the opposite.

The risk of postoperative thrombosis is also thought to be significantly reduced.

Such a way of thinking is starting to make itself felt here in Europe as well, which can be seen from a recently published report from the Landau clinic in Berlin.

After these general remarks, I will try to give a brief account of the most important observations in special surgical areas that I have had the opportunity to make at the above-mentioned hospitals and clinics.

Brain and nerve surgery has representatives in men like Harvey Cushing, Frazier, and Murphy, who are well known and highly esteemed all over the world. The first in particular is now the most respected specialist in this field in his home country.

He proposes that most "decompressive" operations should be performed in cases of inoperable brain tumors, serous meningitis, etc. by removing pieces of the skull below the temporal muscle on both sides after bluntly splitting the muscle in the direction of its fibers. This avoids hernias, which are otherwise often very troublesome in such cases.[9] A particularly ingenious way of achieving permanent drainage of the subdural space is that used by Charles Mayo. After turning a normal skin-periosteum-bone flap with the base downwards, a similar flap incision is made in the dura. The base of the reflected bone piece is cut along its entire width to a height of about 1 cm., after which the dural flap is folded down and brought through the gap created in the bone out under the temporal muscle outside the periosteum and thus is in contact with the lymphatic system of the face and neck. The skin-periosteum-bone flap is then replaced. I saw several cases of traumatic epilepsy operated on in this way, where nothing was found but edema in the arachnoid and pia, and according to Mayo, out of a whole series of similar cases, many were completely cured and the vast majority significantly improved, provided that the operation was not undertaken too late. In case of emergency, bilateral surgery has been undertaken. In cases of serous meningitis and ependymitis, Mayo said he had used a similar approach with the difference that he split the dural flap from the tip down to the base, bringing one part out under the temporal muscle, then folding the other into a string and inserting it through the frontal lobe into the lateral ventricle, after which the craniotomy was closed. Both he and Cushing and several others have pointed out the importance of early operative treatment of serous meningitis and the extremely favorable results which can be expected from this.[10]

As elsewhere, in recent years also in America extensive studies have been devoted to investigations into the possibility of reasonably effective drainage of the cerebrospinal intradural space and have recently successfully operated on several cases of acute permanent leptomeningitis. In these cases, Murphy does not hesitate to open the dural sac in the sacral region (the lower end of the dural sac is at the middle of 3rd sacral vertebra) and flush the entire spinal dural sac after trepanation in the occipital region just behind the foramen magnum. He also has demonstrated the possibility of draining the ventricular system of the brain through a similar opening in the skull and, if the foramen of Magendie is occluded, to open it through a small V-shaped incision in the velum. In an extensive[11] and otherwise very instructive essay on the surgery of the nervous system in general, he recommends a similar procedure in some cases of tuberculous meningitis. (See the April 1907 issue of "Surgery, Gynecology and Obstetrics.")

In this context, Cushing's method for surgery of spina bifida should be mentioned.[12] To prevent the occurrence of secondary hydrocephalus, after opening the sac, one of the vertebral bodies lying in front of it is pierced with a fine trephine, and through this a fine silver cannula constructed for the purpose is inserted into the peritoneal cavity. Through a laparotomy incision, it is verified that the cannula will not press on any vessel or other structure. The laparotomy incision is closed, and the sac is treated in the usual way, leaving behind the small silver tube. In this way, the subdural space is drained as intended.

The oldest of the patients thus treated, a girl of 8 years, died of scarlet fever during my time in Baltimore - but up until a couple of weeks before her death she had been perfectly healthy.

Of all the remarkable cases in this field which I had occasion to see, two were shown at the Society of Clinical Surgery meeting in Philadelphia:

One case was a 14-year-old boy, who at the age of 7 months had fallen into a coal fire and had the entire upper part of his head badly burned. Necrosis and sequestration of most of both parietal and both frontal bones, a total area of 17x11 cm. Gradual onset of epilepsy and mental dullness due to pressure from the scar mass on the scalp formed by remnants of skin and dura.

In December 1904, Keen performed a subcutaneous circular craniotomy to relieve the pressure, requiring 2 sessions and 8 incisions, and creating a 7 mm.-wide defect around the entire head to mobilize the entire overlying part of the skull. Two years later, noticeable improvement, with fewer seizures and less lethargy. (The case published in *Annals of Surgery*, May 1907).

The second case, likewise demonstrated at the above-mentioned meeting and of great theoretical as well as practical interest, was a woman about 25 years old, who 2½ years earlier had the spinal cord completely severed in the lower dorsal region by two revolver shots with consequent paralysis of the entire lower part of the body. The ends of the cord had been united by means of catgut sutures shortly after the trauma, with the result that the bladder and rectal paralysis quickly disappeared. During the demonstration, the patient was able to walk with the help of support rails for the legs and two canes. The sensitivity disorders had almost completely disappeared.[13]

Trigeminal neuralgia and its treatment received special attention in several places. The greatest interest was attached to the extirpations of the Gasserian ganglion, as performed by Cushing, of which I had the opportunity to see six – the most recent in a series of 48 with only 2 deaths.[14]

His surgical method differs somewhat from the usual ones of Krause (the so-called high or temporal method), Rose-Andrews (pterygomaxillary) or Doyen, in that access to the ganglion is obtained through a small arcuate incision immediately above the zygoma in the hairline, blunt parting of the temporal muscle, permanent resection of the zygomatic arch, and trepanation of the middle cranial fossa near its base. After this, pieces of the outer side wall and the bottom of the fossa are rongeured away, thereby creating a defect which often did not need to be larger than a 2-*krona* coin[15] and which extended inward to only 1 to 2 cm. from the ganglion. With blunt dissectors and spatulas, the dura was lifted extremely carefully, and precisely at this point the advantage of the "low" trepanation was apparent, in that the tension on the dura and its vessels could thereby be made much less than would be necessary if approaching the ganglion through a higher incision. The ganglion itself was dissected free with blunt instruments. One of these was inserted behind it, and by a prying motion the central root was severed. In many cases, as suggested by Frazier, it was sufficient simply to fold the ganglion forward and allow the dura to sink in between the ganglion and the central stump, since complete extirpation was often associated with great difficulties and profuse bleeding. In none of the cases operated on in this way had any recurrence been observed. In some cases, the entire operation could be performed in about 35 minutes, but in others, even with an operator as experienced as Cushing, it could take more than 2 hours. The wound was closed primarily in all the cases I observed, and the patient was already out of bed by the third postoperative day.

In milder or earlier cases, where such a major intervention as the one mentioned above is not considered indicated, Charles Mayo has used a method of evulsion of nerve branches combined with sealing or closure of the bony canals through which they had exited.[16] For the supraorbital notch this was accomplished by means of a periosteal flap taken from the forehead, which was folded downwards and inserted into the opening; the infraorbital and mental foramina were closed with small silver screws; in some cases, the lower jaw was trepanned near the angulus, the nerve was evulsed, and the canal was sealed with silver amalgam or lead. In all cases, Mayo evulses the lingual nerve, whether or not it is symptomatic. Several cases of this kind with no recurrence over 10 years were shown at the Mayo clinic. Some surgeons were mostly using the old osmium injections, and others, especially Kiliani in New York, had replaced them with alcohol injections, Schloesser's method.

I saw only one plastic facial operation, performed by Prof. Finney in Baltimore. The case involved a complete defect due to syphilis of the nasal bones, cartilage, and septum, but with the skin intact. A new "Nasengerüst"[17] was formed out of one of the little fingers, incised along the dorsal side and in the middle joint bent almost at right angles and ankylosed, which was brought up under the loosened skin. The two outermost joints thus formed the bridge of the nose and the proximal one a kind of septum. Plaster cast was applied for 2 to 3 weeks, after which the finger was disarticulated and the proximal phalanx was folded into the nasal cavity. A case operated on in the same way two years earlier was shown and the result was surprisingly good. The patient stated that he could now enter a streetcar without having to feel stared at. Cases of cleft palate were generally operated on very early, preferably before the children were 6 months old, at which time both maxillas were fractured with an instrument like a lion's claw. Then a strong needle reinforced with silk, silkworm gut or silver was pushed through both bones, which were brought close to each other and held in position by 2 to 3 such sutures tied in the oral cavity. These were only removed after 14 days, when they usually had cut through (I never saw any plates used to prevent this). The suturing of the soft parts, except for the lips, was often postponed for some time but was generally done before the child began to talk.

Otology in America is almost always connected with ophthalmology, so I was not in a position to devote much attention to this area. After radical surgery for chronic, persistent otitis media, the wound is primarily closed in the vast majority of cases, which is probably the method used by most people here at home, too. The opening of the ear canal was large enough to allow visualization of almost the entire operating field. The entire postoperative treatment was then managed from within the ear canal, usually such that the holes were tamponed firmly to reduce granulation formation as much as possible, usually with four pieces of iodoform gauze, one in the middle ear and one in the atticus (both pressed hard against the bone), as well as one in the upper and one in the lower part of the defect in the mastoid process. The tamponade is changed after the 4th day, then daily during the first 4 weeks, and then can be replaced with a powder or another treatment, as long as the granulation formation is kept within appropriate limits and not allowed to hinder the proliferation of epithelium.

During the last few years, research on the tonsils and their diseases has been zealously conducted at many centers in the "States," and related questions were always on the program at every major medical meeting. Several times I heard this organ referred to in clinical lectures as the point of entry for almost all imaginable diseases, and the great importance of the rational treatment of tonsillitis is carefully emphasized.

At the Mayo clinic, serial sections were made with bacterial stains on all removed tonsils, and, among other things, tubercle bacilli were demonstrated in no less than 16% of cases, where the patient otherwise showed no signs of tuberculosis. Similarly, mass examinations of school children recently conducted in Chicago showed that tubercle bacilli could be detected in the extirpated tonsils in no less than 22-28% of cases with tonsillar hypertrophy without other signs of tuberculosis. In connection with this, they also strongly emphasize the need to completely extirpate these organs and not be satisfied with simply cutting off a larger or smaller part of them. At the Mayo clinic, the tonsils were first cut off and then the remnants were scraped away, after which the last bits were removed by blotting the wound bed with a coarse compress. The operation was always performed under anesthesia and with the head dependent. Since a complete removal of the tonsils can only be achieved this way in children, extirpation of the tonsils by circumcision was done in older people, with subsequent blunt ablation. A method for performing this operation under local anesthesia is described by Worthington in the *Journal of the American Medical Association*, 25 May 1907.

In cases of lip cancer, both the submental and submaxillary spaces were always cleared out first.

The thyroid and parathyroid glands seemed to be of particular interest to surgeons and physiologists. The Mayo clinic had a particularly large amount of material to offer in this area. In 1906, they had 73 simple goiters and 57 cases of toxic goiter.[18] Special interest was devoted to the operated cases of toxic goiter and the exceptionally good results that Charles Mayo managed to achieve. This disease he calls hyperthyroidism, and the quickest and surest remedy, according to him, is the removal of greater or lesser parts of thyroid tissue. He emphasizes that this operation must not be considered harmless, but he also demonstrated that the mortality rate can be minimized by operator experience, a careful selection of cases, and appropriate pretreatment. Four of his first 16 cases died, two of the next 30, and two of the following 62.

Far-advanced cases were not operated on, or were experimentally subjected to preliminary treatment, often lasting several months, consisting of X-ray irradiation and refracted doses of quinine and atropine in combination with bed rest.

The operations were always performed under anesthesia, several times in my presence, despite a pulse rate of 170-180. Patients with an irregular pulse were not operated on. Mayo did not think he had lost a single one of these patients because of the anesthetic. But, as mentioned earlier, the anesthesia management was in unusually safe hands. The patient lay during the operation with the upper body elevated and an extra pillow under the neck. The incision used was always the curved Kocher incision; the muscles were divided transversely along a line located a little higher than the incision in the skin and fascia.

Usually, one thyroid lobe and isthmus were extirpated, and particular emphasis was placed on the fact that the dissection took place in the subcapsular plane to avoid as far as possible injuring the parathyroid glands. In the few cases where tetany was observed after such operations, the parathyroids had been excised on one side. This finding after the removal of these organs or damage to their vessels – they each have only a single artery – is consistent with the tetany that occurs in experimental animals subjected to this procedure, as MacCallum and others have demonstrated. The wound was always drained after rinsing with "Harrington's solution" (see above), through whose irritating and "serum-attracting" effect the wound cavity flushes itself, as it were. Not counting the deaths, Mayo estimates that 50% of his cases have had rapid improvement and complete recovery. Among the remainder, symptoms have gradually returned in half over the course of several months, and in the rest, despite appreciable improvement, temporary relapses of tachycardia and tremors have occurred.

It was surprising to see how quickly the symptoms disappeared in many of the very responsive cases; in a couple of these, the patients could hardly be recognized 10 days after the operation, because their exophthalmos had regressed so much.

A couple of cases of mild recurrence were operated on by extirpation of the lower part of the remaining lobe, and Mayo said that in none of his 6 or 7 reoperated cases had he observed any further recurrence of the old symptoms. Möbius' serum[19] had been used here as in several other places, but without any obvious success. The preliminary X-ray treatment was said to increase the connective tissue around the gland and thus facilitate its dissection. All deaths (9 out of 100 cases, of which, as previously mentioned: 4 were among the first 16) had occurred within 24 hours after the operation.

At the above-mentioned surgical meeting in Philadelphia, among other things, a lot of interesting cases in the field of thoracic surgery were shown. For example, one of the city's hospitals situated between the Italian and Negro neighborhoods recently had no fewer than three cases of sutured stab wounds to the heart, and three cases of huge aortic aneurysms which protruded above the sternum and the clavicle like tumors larger than a child's head. One of these was operated on in such a way that, through a fine cannula, no less than 14 feet of gold wire was introduced into the aneurysm, after which the cannula was withdrawn, a procedure which scarcely occupied 10 minutes, and during which the patient only lost a few drops of blood. A similar patient was presented who had been operated upon about 2 years before following the same method, with an external mass slightly smaller than the one just mentioned; now no trace of the mass could be seen except for some faint pulsations above the manubrium. The patient could even support himself through light work.

Pleural empyema was treated in most places according to standard methods. An exception to this was made by Murphy, who in quite a few cases used an approach which is not yet published, as far as I know. The principle was repeated aspirations or evacuations of the materal by means of a trocar, with subsequent injections into the pleural cavity of smaller amounts of a 2% formalin-glycerin solution. After one or two aspirations, usually 3 to 4 days apart, the exudate had in most cases already changed character, becoming less thick, odorless, and hemorrhagic. In this way, the initially persistent exudate was quickly transformed into an almost serous one. According to this method I saw him treat not only milder metapneumonic exudates, but also in a couple of cases pure streptococcal exudates, all of which recovered within the short space of about 3 weeks. The amounts of formalin-glycerin used varied between 10 and 20 cc. each time. There is no doubt that the method has advantages in many cases over rib resections, which is confirmed by eight cases successfully treated using this method since my return to the Sahlgrenska Hospital in Gothenburg, which I hope to publish later.

A similar procedure was also used with apparent success by Murphy in several cases of septic arthritis and other infections. Here, not only the strong bactericidal effect of formalin must be important, but perhaps to an even greater degree its ability to bring about a strong influx of lymph to the treated part. A few cc. of a weak formalin solution instilled into the healthy peritoneal cavity of a rabbit usually brings about an increase of more than 100 cc. in the amount of free fluid.

Breast cancer was treated operatively everywhere according to the Halsted method, and Halsted himself always dissects out the supraclavicular fossa with or without temporary resection of the clavicle. The sternal portion of the pectoralis major and the entire pectoralis minor are always removed, and an especially meticulous dissection is performed to remove the fascia and connective tissue of the remaining muscles. The dressing includes elevating the upper arm at a right angle to the chest for 4 days. The patient is then allowed to move the arm under competent supervision.

For many reasons, the greatest interest is attached to abdominal surgery, and this is probably the area in which American surgery has achieved its greatest success. The large American clinics can present here a truly outstanding clinical experience. The Mayo clinic stands out with its approximately 2,500 (2,750 in 1906) laparotomies with a mortality of only 2.07%, although this is at least partly due to the relatively rare occurrence of acute cases there. When Kehr published his first thousand laparotomies for gallstones, the Mayo brothers were already well into their second thousand, and at the time of my visit there were almost up to 3,000. The number of patients with appendicitis undergoing operation annually is between 800 and 900, operations on the bile ducts amount to 300-400 (385 in 1906), on the stomach and duodenum to over 200, etc. It is not unusual to see 8 to 10 major laparotomies there in one morning. In addition, the records for each individual case are very detailed and both the diagnosis and indications for surgery are carried out with extreme accuracy and care, and a lot of practical hints and advice are given during the operation itself. I think I can say that it is hardly possible to surpass the teaching about abdominal surgery that is provided at this hospital in a small town far out on the prairie in Minnesota. At the Swedish hospital[20] in Chicago (chief surgeon A. Ochsner), more major abdominal operations are performed annually than at many large hospitals altogether (882 in the year 1906). Operators such as Murphy, Deaver, Kelly, Meyer, etc. have surgical statistics, in which the number of laparotomies annually amounts to over 1,000. All these places, with the possible exception of the Ochsner clinic, provide extremely instructive and comprehensive teaching.

Undoubtedly, the most interesting subject in this area was the treatment of generalized purulent peritonitis. Murphy has developed a method of treatment which has quickly gained acceptance in almost all the larger hospitals, and has reportedly lowered the mortality rate for both localized and generalized purulent processes in the abdomen most significantly.

His views coincide most closely with those that appear in the following 6 points, constituting a summary of a presentation by Wathen on this subject, held before the American Medical Association in June of this year.

1. Operate as soon as the surgical diagnosis has been established. Before surgery, perform a gastric lavage, if there is no perforation of this organ or the duodenum, and remove possibly accumulated feces

from the rectum.
2. If possible, operate quickly ("get in quick – but get out quicker" – Murphy) and concentrate on treating the source of infection; be careful to prevent unnecessary trauma to the peritoneum, which reduces its resistance to the infection.
3. Expose and handle the intestines as little as possible. Never tear adhesions. Avoid irrigating and also drying except in the immediate vicinity of the primary source of infection. Always drain the true pelvis through a suprapubic or vaginal incision and, if necessary, insert a somewhat larger drain in and around the primary focus. Place the patient in bed with the upper body raised or in a sitting position ("Fowler's position").
4. Give the patient copious amounts of physiological saline solution, preferably according to the continuous Murphy method. In appropriate cases, stimulate leukocyte formation by subcutaneous injections, or in limited infections intraperitoneal infusion, using warm horse serum or another similar agent.
5. Avoid both laxatives and opium immediately after surgery. Do not give enemas or bowel irrigations during the first 24 hours after surgery. Nothing facilitates the spread of infectious agents in the abdomen as much as intestinal peristalsis.
6. Enterotomy is rarely indicated and then only in occasional neglected cases with severe intestinal paresis. Enterostomy is contraindicated.

I saw many cases treated, mainly following these principles, with apparently very good results. The era of large incisions and widespread intestinal tamponade seems to be past.

For example, peritonitis from a ruptured appendix was treated with a McBurney incision (transverse or oblique incision with blunt division of the musculature in the direction of its fibers) in the iliac fossa just large enough for the removal of appendix. After this, a smaller midline suprapubic incision was made. "Through these two openings, as much of the exudate was removed that could be aspirated without too much agitation" of the nearest intestinal loops. A crude, slit rubber tube, filled with sterile or iodoform gauze, was passed behind the symphysis to the bottom of the true pelvis, and a tampon, usually not large, was inserted into the iliac fossa to the primary focus. This tampon usually consisted of a finer gauze-filled rubber tube, which was sometimes brought down to the pelvic floor, as well as a few (3-4) iodoform gauze strips, always wrapped in a rubber sheet. (Rubber was indeed a very popular drain material everywhere, and small folded pieces of it were widely used for draining wounds on the neck after lymphoma and goiter extirpations, draining the axilla after surgery for breast cancer, etc.) Occasionally, an incision was also made over the left iliac fossa.

Immediately after the operation, the patient was placed in bed in the so-called Fowler's position, that is with the upper body raised to between 45° and 60° and sometimes up to a 90° angle to the horizontal plane. This is usually achieved by raising the head end of the bed or by means of backrests placed in the bed. Sometimes, the patient was placed prone, tied down, and actually suspended in this position. The intention here was to divert as much of the exudate from the most absorbent part of the peritoneum at the diaphragm and to try to collect it in the least absorbent true pelvis, in order to remove as much as possible from there by drainage. The improved statistics obtained by most operators in recent years is unanimously attributed to the reduced manipulation of the contents of the peritoneal cavity. Great importance is also placed on the administration of fairly large amounts of saline solution during the first 24 hours after surgery. This was always done through the rectum and usually according to the so-called continuous method specified by Murphy.

Through a small Nelaton catheter no larger than No. 12, physiologic saline solution was introduced into the rectal ampulla very gently (drop by drop!) from a container placed at the foot of the bed approximately at the height of the patient's elbows. The intent of this arrangement is to supply the liquid approximately as quickly as it is resorbed and thus prevent distention of the rectum and the flexures. In this way, from 250 cc. to half a liter or more of liquid can be given to the patient per hour without any discomfort, and the flatus can pass easily around the small tube. When pausing the procedure to avoid irritation of the rectal and anal mucosa, the container can be disconnected.

According to Murphy, this addition of large amounts of liquid accomplishes:

1. A reversal of the current in the lymphatic vessels of the peritoneum, so that the peritoneum changes from being an absorbing surface to being a secreting surface. The sitting position together with the movements of the diaphragm contribute to the descent of debris towards the pelvis and its removal from there by drainage. However, this rather bold hypothesis, supported mainly by the significantly increased secretion from the wounds that follows the treatment in question, has encountered quite a lot of resistance.
2. The abundant supply of liquid is an extremely good heart and kidney

stimulant and increases the diuresis significantly, thus eliminating the toxic products that have already entered the circulation. In fact, the amount of urine per day can often more than quadruple in this way and at least for the first 48 hours after the operation it satisfies the patient's need for nutrition.

During this time, nothing is done to increase intestinal peristalsis, rather the opposite. In a few places, opium was even given in small doses by the anal route during the first two days, and no solid or liquid food was given by mouth.

When directly asked if the treatment method described above did not in some cases lead to an increased number of secondary abscess formations, Murphy replied that some insignificant increase in their number possibly took place, but that they always appeared in the true pelvis and were relatively easy to drain, and that the newer method of treatment would still be preferable. At the Mount Sinai Hospital in New York, the analysis of 2,000 cases compiled by Moschcowitz led to the conclusion that the mortality rate in operated cases of acute appendicitis with peritonitis has decreased from 25-30% to around 3% with this treatment method.

Drawing any conclusions from statistical material obtained from various sources regarding the best method of treatment for so-called diffuse peritonitis (= septic general peritonitis) is almost impossible, and I believe that one of the main reasons for this is the great confusion in America as well as here at home concerning the terminology in this field. For example, one operator might find a perforated appendix and generalized peritonitis in the right iliac fossa and call this diffuse peritonitis; another uses the same term, if he ascertains the presence of an exudate in the greater part of the peritoneal cavity below the transverse colon regardless of the nature of this exudate; a third uses the same term only for an exudate of the extent just mentioned which is clearly purulent, but without regard to whether it has a different character in the immediate surroundings of the source of infection and somewhat further from it.

In many of these cases, the more remote exudate is sterile and usually due to loose adhesions separating it from the more virulent process, a difference which may easily escape observation.

Several surgeons (e.g. Moynihan) exclude all cases of peritonitis after acute gastric and duodenal perforations from the category of "general septic peritonitis," since the exudate in most of these cases has been found to be sterile or only slightly virulent.

Especially in English and American statistics, one often finds cases described as "generalized peritonitis," which at first were treated expectantly and which then, when the process has progressed to "resolution into abscess," as the difficult to understand term goes, only need a simple incision to drain the completely contained abscess. Such cases can hardly be explained in any other way than that one or more local infections provoked a "reactive peritoneal cavity," which in turn causes a greater or lesser part of the remaining peritoneal cavity to fill with a serous, sero-purulent, or frankly purulent exudate, which is often demonstrable by physical signs but is sterile or at least not virulent. As long as the primary focus is contained and the adhesions gain in strength, the *raison d'être* for the diffuse exudate ceases, it is resorbed, and the primary focus appears more and more clearly as a discrete abscess, sometimes accompanied by one or more others, depending on whether some portion of the free exudate has had time to become infected. To include such cases under the heading of "diffuse peritonitis" and thus advocate expectant treatment of general peritonitis is incorrect. The above should sufficiently illustrate the difficulties encountered when trying to draw conclusions from the statistics of different surgeons regarding the treatment of "diffuse peritonitis." It will only be possible when a uniform terminology in this area has been established.

On the other hand, if a surgeon with access to a large amount of his own material, comparing similar cases, considers himself to have achieved better results with a certain method of treatment than with another, then his opinion must be given importance. For example, knowing the terminology that Murphy uses, this is why I must consider the above-described method of treatment well worth *testing*.

In regard to surgical diseases of the stomach, duodenum, and biliary tract, the opinions and methods of treatment asserted at the Mayo clinic may be considered to represent, for the most part, the general view in these fields among surgeons of the United States.

Gastric and duodenal ulcers

An experience amounting (1 June 1906) to over 600 cases operated on and carefully investigated has given W. Mayo reason for the following conclusions:

Acute ulcers should generally not be treated operatively. Acute bleeding may be an indication for surgery. In that case, the bleeding site should be sought out and sutured from the inside, but also the serous surface should preferably be covered by means of a few musculo-peritoneal mattress sutures.

Chronic bleeding can sometimes be counteracted by gastrojejunostomy, especially if the ulcer is located in the pylorus or duodenum, otherwise it should be excised if possible.

The frequency of chronic duodenal ulcers is greater than previously thought. Out of 100 cases of ulcers operated on during the last 2 years, no less than 47 were located in the duodenum or had originated there, while 44 were in the stomach. In 9 cases, ulcers were found in both the stomach and duodenum.

Many ulcers observed during surgery are thought to be in the stomach, when in fact they are in the duodenum. The reason for this is a shallow contracture which often occurs at the distal edge of the ulceration and which may be interpreted as the boundary between the pylorus and the duodenum, a mistake which is easily corrected by noting the distribution of vessels to these two parts.

Chronic ulcers are conveniently divided from a surgical point of view into mucosal and indurated, the latter constituting 85% of the entire number. The frequency of non-indurated wounds has been significantly exaggerated in the past.

A chronic duodenal ulcer can occasionally spread to the pylorus, but a gastric ulcer almost never extends into the duodenum. Gastric ulcers were multiple in 15% of all cases, while duodenal ulcers were multiple 5 times in 135 cases (3.7%).

Gastric ulcer is as common in women as in men. Duodenal ulcer is more common in men than in women.

Gastrojejunostomy is the operation "par excellence" in patients with indurated ulcers of the pylorus and duodenum when they constitute an obstruction to the emptying of the stomach, and in these cases is a pure drainage operation.

If there is no obstruction to the passage of food through the pylorus or duodenum, it will continue to pass this way even if a gastrojejunostomy opening is created, which has been conclusively proven both experimentally and clinically [2].

For a simple mucosal ulceration, where the gastric outlet obstruction is due to muscle spasm but nonsurgical therapy has been unsuccessful, good results from gastroenterostomy are less certain, and in these cases it can usually be advantageously replaced by a gastroduodenostomy using the method of Finney.

Gastrojejunostomy is contraindicated in all cases of ptosis or dilatation of the stomach, if there are no obvious retention symptoms, depending on whether a mechanical obstruction in the pylorus can be demonstrated. A cold gastric ulcer that is not causing obstruction should simply be excised. Gastrojejunostomy in these cases is of questionable benefit.

An "hourglass stomach" should be treated with some form of gastrogastrostomy or better yet resection. A gastrojejunostomy to the proximal part in most cases does not prevent a large part of the contents from passing into the distal part, where it usually stagnates due to its lack of motility.

Most duodenal ulcers are an indication for gastrojejunostomy. Occasionally, a resection or excision can give better results.

The form of gastroenterostomy which is now used almost exclusively in the United States is that of Mayo and Paterson,[21] who describe a posterior gastrojejunostomy with a short anti-peristaltic loop and no adjunctive entero-enteric anastomosis.

The opening in the stomach is placed on its posterior surface on the greater curvature vertically below the cardia, runs obliquely from the top right down to the left and reaches a short distance forward onto the front wall of the stomach. This is precisely where the stomach wall and the duodenojejunal flexure normally lie almost immediately next to each other and therefore the opening in the jejunum is placed somewhere in its first 7 centimeters, counted from the duodenojejunal flexure. If the anastomosis is made in this place, the efferent loop leads almost straight down and slightly to the left, thus preventing stenosis of the opening. This loop, because it is so close to the duodenum, almost always has an alkaline content, so that a marginal ulcer is unlikely to develop.

Reversing the top the jejunal loop before the anastomosis was performed was not considered to be a guarantee against a vicious circle or secondary stenosis of the opening, rather the opposite. The Murphy button is never used in posterior gastroenterostomy. Anterior gastroenterostomy is only done in cases of inoperable cancer, or when a posterior one is not possible.

Anterior gastroenterostomies were often done with the button or McGraw's elastic ligature. Ochsner used a newer method of rapidly creating an enteroanastomosis, developed by the Swede Werelius. After the first seromuscular suture was placed, a long needle reinforced with a piece of fine but strong fishing line was threaded into the lumen of one viscus and out through the same wall at a distance from the insertion site, which corresponded to the length of the future opening; in the corresponding place on the other side of the primary suture, the needle was then inserted into the lumen of the second viscus and brought out at a point opposite the first insertion opening on the other side of the primary suture. In this way, the two ends of the fishing line protruded through each of its fine openings, one on each side of the first suture. After this, a second row of sutures was placed, and the inserted thread loop was tightened with the exception of the adjacent free ends. By then using this as a wire saw, the enclosed parts of the visceral walls were cut through in a few seconds. The small opening through which the wire loop was pulled out was closed, and another row of reinforcing sutures was placed. One would expect that there would be a great risk of postoperative bleeding from such an operation, but none of the many operations of this kind performed on animals and the few on humans were said to have had this result.

The principle of Finney's above-mentioned gastroduodenostomy consists of mobilizing the pylorus and adjacent parts of the duodenum and stomach and attaching them to each other with a seromuscular suture. Close to this, an incision is made in the duodenum, which goes up through the pylorus and then onto the stomach and a short distance down the greater curvature such that the entire incision takes the shape of an inverted U. The two sides of the incision are then joined as a regular enteroanastomosis. This operation has almost entirely supplanted all the old forms of pyloroplasty.

Numerous cases of gastric cancer were treated at the Mayo clinic by means of resection, but palliative operations were performed very rarely in cases of cancer that could not be operated on radically, since the life expectancy after such interventions both according to European and American statistics has been shown not to exceed 6 months on average.

As a radical operation, they generally used the Billroth II gastrectomy (gastroenterostomy with a short non-reversed loop) or sometimes Kocher's method.

The edges of the wound on the gastric pouch were united by what seemed to me for this purpose as well as for intestinal sutures in general a particularly practical method, the so-called Connell suture, slightly modified by Charles Mayo (described in *Surgery, Gynecology and Obstetrics*, April 1907). This suture is usually performed with a straight needle, starting approximately ¾ cm. from the free edge and going through all the layers. The needle is passed from the peritoneal surface through the mucosa into the lumen and then from the mucosa out through the peritoneum on the same side; from here the thread is passed over to the other side, the needle is inserted from the peritoneal surface through the mucosa and from this out through the peritoneum on the same side, etc. The gap between the stitches in sewing the gastric wall is barely 6 mm.

When tightened, the wound edges fold in spontaneously, and mucosal folds do not protrude. Instead of Lembert's continuous sutures, the so-called Cushing suture[22] is always used, which is performed in such a way that a straight needle is passed through a piece of the serosa parallel to the incision line, is then passed over the same, a similar stitch is taken on this side, etc.; thus, the suture line lies perpendicular to the incision line instead of diagonally across it as with the Lembert suture.

During gastric resections, the entire lesser curvature was always removed on the grounds that its lymphatic vessels, in contrast to those from the greater curvature, run in the gastric wall itself and only to a lesser extent pass through the lesser omentum.

Of the cases treated by radical surgery, 10% had died as a result of surgery, but of the remainder 25% had survived for at least 3 years. Among the cases of stomach cancer referred to the clinic, no more than 10 to 12% were operable (palpable tumor was not by itself considered a contraindication, nor even cachexia with 30% hemoglobin [compared to normal][23]).

In 50% of the operated cases, ulcer symptoms could be detected in the history, and in 54% they could be demonstrated on anatomic pathology after the operation.

Of course, the importance of an early diagnosis was strongly emphasized, and much valuable advice and instructions in this regard was given, all culminating in the emphasis on the only safe means currently available to us for an early diagnosis, and thus to a more satisfactory treatment of stomach cancer – exploratory laparotomy performed early and even on mere suspicion.

Regarding surgery of the biliary tract, the Mayo clinic with its colossal experience was also the most influential, and nowhere did I find opinions or procedures contrary to those that were practiced there.

Cholecystectomy is currently not at all regarded as a normal operation for gallstones, despite the fact that this was the case in many places just a short time ago. The indications for cholecystectomy were gangrene, chronic infection with contraction or malignant degeneration of the gallbladder, and obliteration of the cystic duct. Occasionally an acutely inflamed gallbladder was extirpated, if it was absolutely certain that the infection was strictly confined to the gallbladder.

If there is the slightest suspicion of infection in the bile ducts, or if the patient has ever had jaundice during the course of his illness, or if there is any pathological change in the pancreas, then cholecystectomy is contraindicated. As a technically important point, they often emphasized the ease with which possible cystic duct stones can be pushed into the gallbladder before it has been opened, or its contents aspirated, something which can otherwise be difficult. At the Mayo clinic, 50% of biliary tract operations consisted of cholecystostomies, 25% were cholecystectomies, and the remaining 25% were cholecystostomies with drainage of the bile ducts, cholecystoduodenostomies, etc.

In cases with very strong adhesions around and contraction of the gallbladder, the mucosa was often excised without disrupting the adhesions, or it was destroyed with thermocautery.

Cystic or hepatic duct drainage is often achieved by means of a tube inserted through the cystic duct with the inner end of the tube cut off in the shape of a fish tail and inserted in such a way that the possibility of drainage existed both through the common bile duct, as well as through the tube.

Any necessary drainage was always done with "cigarette drains" or thin rubber sheets, and in many cases the gallbladder is attached to the parietal peritoneum with one or two catgut sutures.

Cholecystenterostomies were made if possible in the form of a cholecystoduodenostomy and very often with a Murphy button.

The abdominal incision was usually pararectal, and if necessary was extended upwards and medially along the costal margin.

All drains around the gallbladder were removed on about the 8th day, in severe cases after 10-12 days, and the patient was allowed to leave the bed immediately afterwards. Regarding the often difficult differential diagnosis between stomach diseases, cholelithiasis, and appendicitis, a lot of valuable information has been provided in an article "Gastric ulcer and cancer" (*Boston Medical and Surgical Journal*, August 1906) by one of the Mayo clinic's many "internal medicine" specialists.

The above-mentioned Connell suture was used for all possible intestinal closures and anastomoses, and it was considered particularly suitable for "end-to-end" connections of intestinal loops; in these cases, it was often made in the form of a series of interrupted sutures with all the knots, even the last one, lying inside the lumen of the intestine and without any additional reinforcing suture line. In none of the cases I saw treated in this way did any inconvenience appear from this method. When using the button, however, even Murphy himself used a series of reinforcing sutures, always as interrupted sutures, which for this purpose were considered much safer than a continuous suture; the latter was considered by most to be absolutely contraindicated for this purpose, because of the danger of the button not coming off in time and a consequent gangrene and leak at the anastomosis that would be substantially increased by such a suture placement.

In cases of ileocecal intussusception, where resection is not required, it was considered possible to prevent recurrence by rotating the most distal loop of ileum for an extent of 10-20 cm., wrapping one half around its longitudinal axis as if rolling it into the mesentery, and fixing it in this position.

In operations for appendicitis, the appendiceal stump was treated in many different ways, usually with invagination with or without previous cauterization or clamping with a crushing clamp; in one place without invagination but only ligation and cauterization. In a few places, surgery was performed in non-emergency cases according to the Edebohls method with invagination of the entire appendix into the cecum after ligating the mesoappendix, but most surgeons advised against doing this. In one of the Philadelphia hospitals, within a short time, four patients had to undergo another operation because of "fecal impactions" that formed around this invaginated residual appendix. Very often a healthy appendix was removed in the course of laparotomies for other ailments, and in every laparotomy, it was inspected and the stomach and bile ducts were palpated.

The abdominal incision for appendicitis surgery was in most cases the McBurney or the Lennander incision through the rectus sheath, the latter very often used in acute cases with drainage.

Hernia operations were largely performed according to the same principles and methods as are used here at home. The suture material was generally catgut, sometimes silver thread, and more rarely silkworm gut or silk. As far as possible, aponeuroses were overlapped, especially in the case of inguinal hernias, but the same principle was also applied when closing other abdominal incisions.

Inguinal hernias were mostly operated using the methods of Bassini or Halsted. (The latter method differs little in principle from the method of Schultén). The suggestion of Halsted a few years ago to excise the veins of the spermatic cord has been abandoned even at Johns Hopkins Hospital. In almost all the Chicago hospitals, the Andrews method of suturing was used in hernia operations, according to which the lower border of the internal oblique and transversus muscles, often in conjunction with the upper edge of the external oblique aponeurosis, is attached to the inguinal ligament in front or behind the cord with mattress sutures passed through the ligament and tied on the outside of it, after which the lower edge of the divided external oblique aponeurosis was attached to the outside of the upper portion. Many also placed great emphasis on the placement of one or two deep sutures laterally to the cord.

Femoral hernias were operated on radically in a number of different ways, most of them not deviating from the operation of Fabricius. The Mayo brothers, who have tried most of them on their large group of patients, have reverted to simply amputating the hernia sac and believe they get at least as good results in this way as with any other method. Moschcowitz (Mount Sinai Hospital, New York) makes an incision above the inguinal ligament through the external oblique aponeurosis, descends extraperitoneally behind the inguinal ligament, retracts the hernial sac, amputates it, and constricts the femoral canal with sutures from the inside laid through the inguinal ligament and Cooper's ligament.

Umbilical hernias were generally operated upon according to Mayo's extremely simple method. The hernia sac with adjacent skin and fat is freely dissected through a transverse curved incision. The sac is opened, and the contents reduced, dividing omental adhesions as needed. The sac is not closed or sutured separately. The of aponeuroses and recti forming the hernia defect are exposed. A strongly curved needle reinforced with a strong linen thread is passed from the outside inward through all the tissue layers behind the superficial fascia and peritoneum approximately 6 cm above the upper edge of the opening. The needle is pulled down and out through the hernia opening. The lower border is punctured approximately ½ cm from its edge with a strong mattress stitch through the peritoneum and all extraneous muscular and aponeurotic layers, the needle is brought back into the peritoneal cavity and brought out again approximately 1 cm to the side of the first insertion. To the sides of this first median suture, other similar ones are placed using thick chromic catgut. During the tying, the entire lower border, together with the peritoneum, will be pulled up under the upper border, which is then fixed in its future position with an additional series of sutures. The entire operation thus consists in the lower border of the hernial ring being pulled up behind the upper one with mattress sutures, passing through the peritoneum, posterior rectus sheath, musculature, and anterior rectus sheath.

In particular, it was often emphasized that this method of overlapping the layers from top to bottom was greatly preferable to overlapping from side to side, especially in surgery of obese patients with large hernias. Overlapping is done from top to bottom is usually surprisingly easy, but when it is done from side to side there is usually great tension in the tissues generally requiring "relaxing" incisions. During the years 1894-1905, William Mayo operated on 88 cases; 75 were subsequently examined, and among these there was only one recurrence.

The method is described in the *Annals of Surgery*, January 1899 and August 1901, as well as in the *Journal of the American Medical Association*, June 1907.

Postoperative abdominal hernias, especially those arising after appendicitis operations, are often operated on using the same method.

It was often emphasized during laparotomies in the lower midline, when one rectus muscle had been exposed before suturing, that it was important to expose the other as well, suture the muscles together, and then carefully suture the aponeuroses in front of them. Failure to do this was considered in many cases to result in a tear, and predispose to the appearance of a hernia.

Of the many methods of functional kidney diagnostics, most were in use everywhere. However, cryoscopy[24] seemed to be the least popular, and at Johns Hopkins Hospital, for example, they thought they could get by without it in most cases.

Tuberculin injections are widely used for the diagnosis of renal tuberculosis. For testing of urine from each kidney they always used ureteral catheterization, never the segregator.

At Kelly's clinic, his method was used for cystoscopy and ureteral catheterization, and it was astonishing to see how quickly and safely a bilateral ureteral catheterization could be performed there.

In cases of suspected kidney or ureteral stones, where X-rays could not provide full certainty, a small piece of wax was attached to the end of a ureteral sound, which was then inserted up to the suspected kidney. After removal, the piece of wax was examined with a loupe, whereby possibly scratches or indentations could clearly indicate the presence of stone. In almost all clinics, the patient was lying prone during kidney operations. I did not see the lateral position used anywhere.

Renal tuberculosis was always treated by nephrectomy, and an affected ureter was usually completely extirpated. If it appeared healthy, 20-25 drops of pure carbolic acid were injected into it. For ureterectomy, the Mayo brothers made a very small McBurney incision immediately above the inguinal ligament, dissected extraperitoneally down to the ureter, lifted it up into the wound together with part of the bladder, possibly resected a piece of this, and then pulled out the severed ureter through the lumbar wound. They never removed just a piece of the ureter. It was either completely extirpated or left intact.

The crushing of stones was in most places an abandoned method, and it was not without some surprise that, at a lecture given in Bigelow's own operating room, I heard his successor Richardson strongly warn against this method of operation, which he considered highly risky in untrained hands and which, even when performed by the most experienced surgeons, is not without its dangers.

The management of prostatic hypertrophy has occupied American surgeons in recent years, and several methods of prostatectomy and the indications for this operation have been the subject of extensive discussion. The indication for this operation was considered by most to occur when the patient would otherwise be consigned to a "catheter life," as long as his general condition did not constitute a definite contraindication.

Both perineal and suprapubic methods were in use. The perineal ones and especially the one described by Young were, however, the ones used preferentially. One method, which I believe was described by Goodfellow, utilizes a single median incision through which one index finger is inserted into the prostatic urethra, and a small curved knife is used to cut lengthwise through each lateral lobe from the inside, after which these are shelled out from the inside with the finger; this method is much used by Charles Mayo, and the whole operation was often performed this way in 5 to 10 minutes. The importance of accurately determining the size of the lobes cystoscopically prior to prostatectomy was strongly emphasized, and Young has devised an excellent method for this purpose, which allows the examination to be performed with an ordinary cystoscope (*Johns Hopkins Hospital Bulletin*, Nov. 1904).

The final results of these operations are presented in a whole series of statistics, which in no way confirm the claims of Rovsing and others that these would be far from brilliant, and one can hardly escape the suspicion that the sharpest critics of these operations belong to those who have rarely or perhaps never performed such operations.

In the gynecological field, there were rich opportunities for study, especially at the Kelly clinic with its large and fully utilized patient experience.

I think the speed and safety with which the largest gynecological procedures were performed there can hardly be surpassed anywhere. This particularly applied to cases of widespread, chronic inflammation of the adnexa with the formation of dense adhesions. In these cases, the uterus was first amputated after being divided lengthwise, following which the adnexa, so to speak, were released from below from surrounding adhesions and without the nearby firmly adherent intestinal loops being manipulated or otherwise disturbed to any significant degree.

Cervical cancer was operated on in most cases using the method of Wertheim, in some cases by myself, during the time when I was a specially invited guest of the clinic.

Among the operations for malposition of the uterus, the ventrofixation was universally condemned, but ligament-shortening operations were often used. It seemed to me that in many of these cases the unusually definite indications elsewhere left something to be desired.

The operation was usually performed in such a way that after a short laparotomy incision in the midline each rectus sheath was opened, a curved forceps was passed behind the rectus aponeurosis and in front of the muscle out through the superficial inguinal ring into the inguinal canal, the ligament was pushed through from the peritoneum as far into the canal as possible, grasped with the forceps, pulled back the same way, sutured to the similarly pulled forward ligament from the other side in front of the rectus, and attached to both the muscle and the rectus sheath in the midline. (Method described by Charles Mayo in *Surgery, Gynecology and Obstetrics*, February 1906).

With regard to the surgery of the extremities, the main interest was related to the mobilization of ankylotic joints by resection and the insertion of pedicled soft-tissue flaps between the ends of the bones, following a method developed by Murphy.

A lot of beautiful pictures of such successful mobilizations were shown in many places, although there were also less successful ones.

At the above-mentioned surgical meeting, some cases of subacute diaphyseal osteomyelitis were shown, treated with complete subperiosteal extirpation of the diaphysis, after which the periosteum was sewn together around a drainage tube inserted as a frame, achieving an almost ideal reconstruction of the bone.

At Mount Sinai Hospital, iodoform packings were made in such a way that the Mosetig-Moorhof mass[25] was pressed into the bone cavity only after it had almost solidified, whereby part of the otherwise often difficult hemostastic measures could be avoided.

In cases suitable for this, varicose veins in the leg not too tortuous or intimately connected to the skin were operated on by Charles Mayo by ligating the saphenous vein at the fossa ovalis, after which the entire vein was dissected out subcutaneously with an instrument designed for this purpose down to an area just below the knee, from where it was extracted through a centimeter-long incision and cut off. The remaining part down to the foot was then treated in the same way, thus the whole saphenous vein was removed through three small incisions. I did not observe any significant postoperative bleeding in any case.

Superficial wounds for which rapid epithelialization was desired were always treated open, and this was especially the case with burns. For the treatment of widespread burns, several places had a special heated room, in which the patients were laid completely naked on a table, where they had to spend most of the healing time without any sort of bandage. Only if the secretions became too active were the secretion-covered surfaces carefully dried, and crusts with underlying material removed several times a day and sprinkled with some nonspecific powder.

In pedicled skin flaps, a number of shallow, parallel incisions were often made on the epithelial side, and these could then be stretched to a surprising degree without risk of necrosis.

Covering skin defects after operations for breast cancer with pedicled regional flaps was considered by most and especially by Halsted as absolutely wrong. All such defects were covered with Thiersch grafts.

Finally, I cannot fail to mention with gratitude the extremely cordial and accommodating reception that I received everywhere, both from clinic directors and from other individuals. Anyone who wants to study a medical discipline on the other side of the ocean and who shows that he has really come to learn something immediately becomes part of the extremely good and, in the best sense, democratic relationship between teachers and students that exists in most medical teaching institutions. For a Swede, there also the almost unlimited goodwill and hospitality shown to him by his American compatriots, which can contribute to making such a study trip, regardless of the purely professional benefit, also in other respects the most educational and pleasant trip imaginable.

Original Notes

1. In America, an "anesthesia complication" which could be proven to be caused by a incompetence on the part of the anesthetist, would entail a very significant liability for damages from the surgeon.
2. Kelling, *Archiv für klinische Chirurgie*, Vol. LXX, p. 289. Berg, *Annals of Surgery*, May 1907; *Annals of Surgery*, November 1905.

Biographical Sources

Vem är det: Svensk biografisk handbok, 1957. Accessed through https://sv.wikipedia.org.
Olssen DK, *Berättelser från Sollerön: Den mörka hösten (Spanska sjukan)*, 1978. Accessed at sollero-hembygd.se.
Sandström B, *Emma Zorn*, Stockholm: Norstedts, 2014.

Publication Source

Upsala Läkareförenings Förhandlingar [Uppsala Medical Society Transactions] was also called *Acta Societatis Medicorum Upsalensis* and is today published in English as the *Upsala Journal of Medical Sciences*. Whether in Swedish, Latin, or English, the journal has used the ancient spelling Upsala rather than Uppsala.

Translation Notes

1) The German Hospital in Philadelphia was renamed the Lankenau Hospital in 1917 and is today the Lankenau Medical Center.
2) St. Bernard's Hotel Dieu opened in 1905, and was renamed St. Bernard Hospital in 1962. Augustana Hospital was later called the Lutheran General Hospital, and closed in 1989. The name Augustana refers to the Augsburg Confession (*Confessio Augustana*), the fundamental document of the Lutheran Church. Mercy Hospital just closed in 2021.
3) The Swedish hospital in St. Paul was called the Bethesda Hospital, which became a long-term care facility in 1989 and transferred its services to St. Joseph's Hospital in 2021. The Swedish Hospital in Minneapolis merged with St. Barnabas Hospital in 1970 to become the Metropolitan Medical Center, which then closed in 1991.
4) Mercuric chloride, no longer used.
5) See Harrington C, "Some studies in asepsis," *Annals of Surgery* 1904; 40:475-485.
6) A description and depiction of the Clover mask is given in Romero-Ávila P, Márquez-Espinós C, Cabrera-Afonso JR, "Historical development of the anesthetic machine: from Morton to the integration of the mechanical ventilator," *Brazilian Journal of Anesthesiology* 2021; 71:148-161.
7) Alice Magaw, "A review of over fourteen thousand surgical anesthesias," *Surgery, Gynecology & Obstetrics* 1906; 3:795-799.
8) Cushing H, "The employment of local anaesthesia in the radical cure of certain cases of hernia, with a note upon the nervous anatomy of the inguinal region," *Annals of Surgery* 1900; 31:1-34.
9) Cushing H, "The establishment of cerebral hernia as a decompressive measure for inaccessible brain tumors; with the description of intermuscular methods of making the bone defect in temporal and occipital regions," *Surgery, Gynecology and Obstetrics* 1905; 1:297-314.
10) Serous meningitis was and is a poorly-understood disease later called pseudotumor cerebri and today called idiopathic intracranial hypertension, still treated with decompressive procedures.
11) 115 pages long!
12) See Chesler DA, Pendleton C, Ahn ES, Quinones-Hinojosa A, "Harvey Cushing's early management of hydrocephalus," *Clinical Neurology and Neurosurgery* 2013; 115:699-701.

13) This rather unbelievable case had also been described by J. B. Murphy in the *Transactions of the American Surgical Association* 1906; 24:513-585, in a review of spinal cord surgery slightly less extensive than the one cited above. The original report is Stewart FT, Harte RH, "A case of severed spinal cord in which myelorrhaphy was followed by partial return of function," *Philadelphia Medical Journal* 1902; 9:1016-1020.

14) See Adams H, *et al.*, "Harvey Cushing's case series of trigeminal neuralgia at the Johns Hopkins Hospital: a surgeon's quest to advance the treatment of the 'suicide disease'," *Acta Neurochir* (Wien) 2011; 153:1043-1050.

15) A Swedish two-kronor coin at that time had a diameter of 31mm.

16) See Mayo CM, "Peripheral versus intracranial operations for tic-douloureux," *Surgery, Gynecology and Obstetrics* 1906; 3:731-733.

17) A scaffold or framework for the reconstructed nose (German).

18) Like others on the European continent, the author calls toxic goiter "Basedow's disease"; in English-speaking countries it has often been called "Graves' disease."

19) Möbius PJ, "Ueber das Antithyreoidin," *Münchener Medizinische Wochenschrift* 1903; 50:149-150.

20) The Augustana Hospital.

21) Paterson HJ, *Gastric Surgery, being the Hunterian Lectures delivered before the Royal College of Surgeons of England*, London: Ballière, Tindall and Cox, 1906.

22) Not Harvey Cushing, but Hayward W. Cushing of Boston, who first described a running suture for bowel anastomosis while Harvey was still a freshman at Yale. He eventually wrote it up for publication in the *Boston Medical and Surgical Journal* 1899; 141:57-59.

23) The standard measure of hemoglobin at that time. See Dacosta JC, *Clinical Hematology*, Philadelphia, P. Blakiston's Son & Co., 1905

24) A method to estimate specific gravity by freezing point depression. See "Cryoscopy of the urine," *Journal of the American Medical Association* 1901; 36:1254-1255

25) A form of bone wax. See Das JM, "Bone wax in neurosurgery: A review," *World Neurosurgery* 2018; 116:72-76.

www.ingramcontent.com/pod-product-compliance
Lightning Source LLC
Chambersburg PA
CBHW050326010526
44119CB00030B/428/J